Essentials in Clinical Pharmacokinetics

- Concepts, Dose Optimization, and Biologics

First Edition

Guohua An, MD, PhD
College of Pharmacy,
University of Iowa
Iowa City, IA, USA

Fiona-Ann Publishing

Name: Guohua An, author
Title: Essentials in Clinical Pharmacokinetics - Concepts, Dose Optimization, and Biologics/ Guohua An
Description: First edition
Identifier: ISBN: 978-1-964623-00-9 (paperback)

University Disclaimer: Any views, opinions, data, documentation and other information presented in this book are solely those of the author and do not represent those of the University of Iowa.

I would like to dedicate this book to all my past, current, and future PharmD students at the College of Pharmacy, University of Iowa.

ABOUT THE AUTHOR

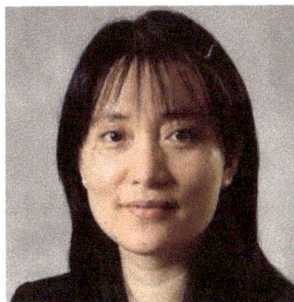

Guohua An, MD, PhD, currently is an Associate Professor in the Department of Pharmaceutical Sciences and Experimental Therapeutics, College of Pharmacy at the University of Iowa. She holds MD from Taishan Medical College (China), MS in Clinical Pharmacology from Fudan University (China), and PhD in Pharmaceutical Sciences from SUNY, University at Buffalo (USA). Prior to joining academia, she worked for two and half years at Abbott (currently known as AbbVie), where she gained extensive hands-on experience in clinical drug development, pharmacokinetics (PK)/pharmacodynamics (PD) modeling and simulation. Her research interests include mechanism-based PK/PD modeling of small-molecule compounds and protein drugs; model-informed drug development (MIDD); model-informed clinical care (MICC); population pharmacokinetic modeling of drugs in special populations; and quantitative systems pharmacology (QSP). Dr. An has been in the PK/PD field for 18 years and has published 94 peer-reviewed articles. Dr. An is an editor of Journal of Pharmaceutical Sciences, and she serves as an editorial board member of Journal of Clinical Pharmacology, The AAPS Journal, and Journal of Pharmacokinetics and Pharmacodynamics. Courses she teaches include "Pharmacokinetics and Dose Optimization" (PharmD course; 2-credit; sole instructor), "Advanced Pharmacokinetics and Pharmacodynamics" (graduate course; 3-credit; sole instructor), and "Concepts in Preclinical Drug Development" (graduate course; 1-credit; sole instructor).

CONTENTS

PREFACE

I have been teaching the PharmD course "Pharmacokinetics and Dose Optimization" every spring semester since 2016. The class size ranges from 80 to 108 students. This is neither a simple course to teach nor an easy topic to learn because this clinically relevant course is math driven. Over the years, I put a lot of effort in developing the content, adjusting the pace, and coming up with outside examples to explain those hard-to-understand terms. After I taught this course for several rounds, I developed a strong desire to write a single author pharmacokinetics (PK) textbook. I started to write this book in late January 2024. Many late nights. Many weekends. This was not a trivial task, and I am glad that I made it. I tried my best to make it easy to follow. This book was written in an unconventional way, with the goal of being engaging and informative. In this book, I provided many case examples, magazine interviews, interesting real-world stories, etc. I hope you find this book useful.

How This Book Is Organized

This introductory level PK textbook has three parts:

- Part I covers fundamental concepts, including fundamental principles and basic PK calculations (Chapter 1), absorption (Chapter 2), distribution (Chapter 3), and elimination (i.e., metabolism + excretion, Chapter 4). To better comprehend the knowledge, these four chapters should be read sequentially. Part I lays the foundation of the study topic and should be read prior to Part II and Part III.

- Part II introduces the utilization of compartment models for dose optimization under different dosing routes, such as single IV bolus (Chapter 5), multiple IV bolus (Chapter 6), IV infusion (Chapter 7), and oral administration (Chapter 8). Part II also covers PK characterization and dose optimization for drugs with biexponential decline (Chapter 9), and drugs with nonlinear pharmacokinetics (Chapter 10). In addition, Part II also touch upon drug PK in special populations (Chapter 11), including children, the elderly, people with obesity, patients with renal disease, as well as pregnant Women. Same as Part I, all case examples used in Part II focus on small-molecule drugs.

- Part III serves as a "primer" on PK and clinical pharmacology of biologic medicines, especially antibodies (Chapter 13), antibody-drug conjugates (Chapter 14), oligonucleotide products (Chapter 15), and Chimeric antigen receptor (CAR) T-cell therapy (Chapter 16). Within Chapter 15, two modalities are discussed in detail: antisense oligonucleotides (ASOs) and small-interfering RNAs (siRNAs). Prior to discussing these individual drug modalities, a basic introduction to biologics is provided in Chapter 12.

Highlights of This Book

There are two valuable aspects of my book:

- This book not only covers small-molecule drugs but also introduces biotherapeutic products, including monoclonal antibodies, antibody-drug conjugates, ASOs, siRNAs, and CAR-T cell therapy. Most of the existing PK textbooks focus on small-molecule drugs only. I consider Part III of my book a big advantage compared to other PK textbooks.
- As noted earlier, I included various case examples, magazine interviews, and interesting real-world stories in this book. Basically, I wrote this book in an unconventional way. My goal was to make this book simple, fun, practical, and easy to follow. Whether this goal is achieved or not, I leave it to readers to evaluate.

Who This Book Was Written For

This is an introductory level PK textbook. It could be a useful reference book for the following readers:

- PharmD students.
- Graduate students with a major in pharmaceutical sciences, medicinal chemistry, biomedical engineering, or toxicology, etc.
- Medical students who want to learn essentials in clinical PK.
- Undergraduate students with a major in Pharmacy.
- Healthcare professionals who work in close proximity with the patients.
- Pharmaceutical researchers who work in the pharmaceutical industry, including formulation scientists, clinical pharmacologists, scientists in drug discovery team or preclinical PK group.
- Pharmaceutical researchers who are experts of small-molecules but have limited knowledge on large-molecule drugs.

In addition, this book is ideal for a 3-credit hour basic PK course. So, it could be used as a useful reference book for any teacher who teaches this type of PK course.

Acknowledgments

Before I joined the current institute, I worked at the University of Florida for a short period of time as an Assistant Professor. Besides conducting research, I also gave lectures in a Dose Optimization course to PharmD students. Dr. Guenther Hochhaus generously shared all his slides with me so that I didn't have to start from scratch. After I moved to the University of Iowa, I continued using his slides as the base for my PharmD PK course. I would say that the first 9 chapters were built upon the slides that Guenther shared with me. THANK YOU. I am very grateful for this.

When I wrote this book, three of my graduate students, Xuanzhen (Mandy) Yuan, Joshua Reeder, and Peizhi (Paige) Li provided huge help. Xuanzhen is very good at writing, and she performed proofreading of this book, all 16 chapters; that is a lot of work. For the figures in this book, most of them were generated by Josh and

Peizhi using Biorender and Sigmaplot. Xuanzhen, Josh, Peizhi – THANK YOU all for your help. Special thanks to Dr. Fiorenza Lanzini, who performed nice and timely proofreading of Part I and Part III of this book.

Also I would like to thank all PharmD students I taught so far. All the questions you asked during the class helped me identify and address those potentially confusing or hard to understand concepts. All the anonymous feedback I received over the years, regardless of positive or negative, has been extremely helpful. This book is dedicated to all my past, current, and future PharmD students at the College of Pharmacy, University of Iowa.

Finally, I would like to thank my husband Shumin Liu and my daughter Fiona Ann Liu for their love and support. Everyday with you two is a blessing. I am so lucky to have you in my life.

Additional Notes

I hope readers will find this book useful and provide comments, good or bad, so that I can continue improving this book. In addition, this is my first single author book but will not be the last one. I plan to write another textbook "Advanced Pharmacokinetics and Pharmacodynamics" next year based on a graduate course that I have been teaching over the years. So, if you are interested in my future book(s), please follow or connect me at LinkedIn (https://www.linkedin.com/in/guohua-an-4b389525/), which is the main platform I use for posting, including book announcement.

x

PART I

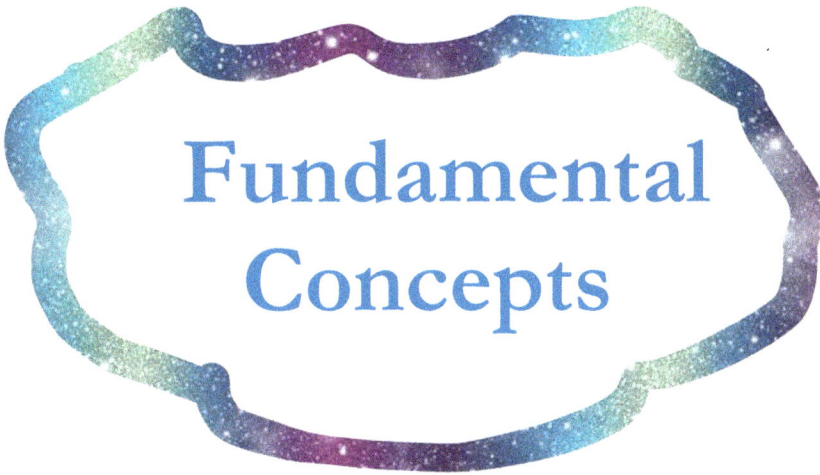

Fundamental Concepts

Chapter 1.

Fundamental Principles and
Basic Pharmacokinetics Considerations

Learning Objectives

After reading this chapter, the reader shall be able to:

1. Define pharmacokinetics and pharmacodynamics; understand why studying pharmacokinetics is important.

2. Get familiar with compartment models.

3. Understand zero-order and first-order kinetics.

4. Define elimination rate constant, half-life, volume of distribution, and clearance.

5. Use equations to calculate k_e, $t_{1/2}$, V_d, and CL, and have a fundamental understanding of the relationship among these parameters.

6. Understand the importance of pharmacokinetics in drug development and clinical practice.

7. Define therapeutic drug monitoring.

8. Predict drug concentration over time using mathematical equations.

Pharmacokinetics has a rich history, with the earliest studies can be traced back to the 1920s. The word *pharmacokinetics* comes from the Greek words "*pharmakon*", meaning "drug", and "*kinetikos*", meaning "moving". Therefore, pharmacokinetics is the mathematical expression of the movement of drugs into, through, and out of the body. As the start of the clinically relevant and math-driven learning journey, this chapter aims to introduce fundamental concepts and basic considerations in pharmacokinetics.

1.1 What Happens After a Drug is Administered?

Pharmacokinetics can be viewed as "what the body does to the drug". The fate of a drug can be broken down into the following different processes:

- For a drug that is given through an extravascular route (i.e. not directly introduced into the blood stream), such as oral, subcutaneous (S.C.), intramuscular (I.M.), intradermal (I.D.) administrations, it needs to be absorbed first before reaching systemic circulation. This process is known as **absorption**. Drugs administered via intravenous (I.V.) route bypass the absorption phase.

- After entering systemic circulation, the drug does not just stay in blood. It will travel with blood and be transferred throughout the body, including various tissues. This process is known as **distribution**.

- In parallel with the distribution process, our body comes up with a few strategies to get rid of drug molecules to ensure that these "foreigners" will not stay in the body forever. One common strategy is to use drug metabolizing enzymes to structurally modify the drug to a different molecule (known as metabolite) which usually is more polar (i.e., water soluble) and consequently can be eliminated more easily. This process is known as **metabolism**. The chief organ operating the process of drug metabolism is the liver. Another common strategy is to directly remove the drug from the body in its intact form. This process is known as **excretion**. The main organ that handles drug excretion is the kidney.

In summary, pharmacokinetics studies the time course of drug absorption, distribution, metabolism, and excretion (**ADME**). Pharmacokinetics profiles, as illustrated in Figure 1-1, typically present drug concentration on the Y-axis and time on the X-axis. The commonly used units of concentration include ng/mL (or µg/L) and µg/mL (or mg/L), and the unit of time is hours.

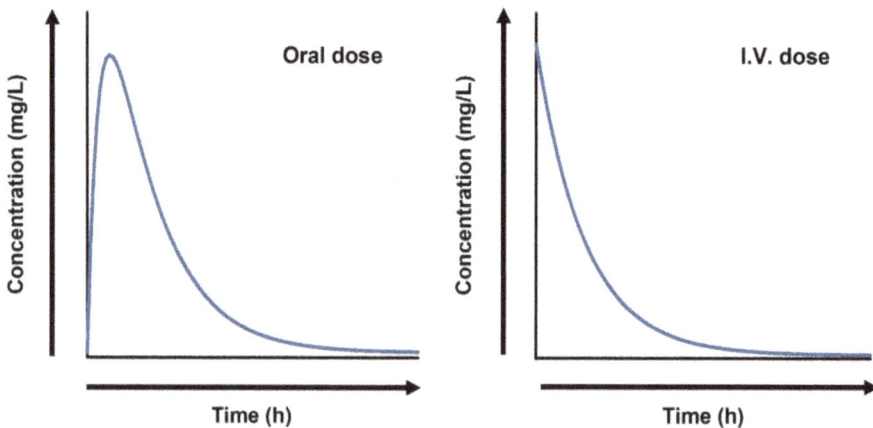

Figure 1-1. The time course of drug concentrations following a single oral dose (left) or single I.V. dose (right). In this figure, linear scale is used for both X- and Y-axis.

Over the years, I noticed, from time to time, that some wrong terms were used for ADME in some research papers and even in my own graduate students' research manuscript drafts. One misuse is the **E** part, where *excretion* is mistakenly replaced with *elimination*. This is certainly inappropriate as **elimination** is the sum of the processes of removing a drug from the body. Therefore, elimination includes both metabolism and excretion (i.e., **Elimination = Metabolism + Excretion**). Another misuse is the **D** part, where *distribution* is inappropriately replaced with *disposition*. **Disposition** is defined as all the kinetic processes that occur to a drug after its systemic absorption; in other words, disposition encompasses both distribution and elimination (i.e., **Disposition = Distribution + Metabolism + Excretion**).

The drug does not have a journey through the body just for fun. It carries a mission – binding to its pharmacological targets to elicit desirable effects to treat whatever condition it is indicated for (i.e., *efficacy*). The targets could be proteins, such as receptors, enzymes, ion channels, transporters, or genetic material, such as DNA. The effect of a drug is not always desirable, it can be harmful sometimes; this is known as *adverse effect*, which can be *on-target* (i.e., exaggerated effects at the target of interest), or *off-target* (i.e., unwanted responses due to modulation of other targets). Both efficacy and adverse effects are the response of our body to the drug. The study of drug effects is known as *pharmacodynamics,* a word originated from the Greek words "*pharmakon*" meaning "drug", and "*dynamikós*" meaning "power".

In contrast to pharmacokinetics, which describes "what the body does to the drug", pharmacodynamics can be viewed as "what the drug does to the body". After learning these definitions, you may immediately realize that pharmacodynamics is more important than pharmacokinetics, because we care more about the fate of our body than the fate of the drug. A natural question arises – why do we study pharmacokinetics if what matters is pharmacodynamics? This question is addressed in the next section.

1.2 Why Do We Study Pharmacokinetics?

Pharmacodynamics refers to the intensity and time course of the drug effects, including both desired and adverse effects. While we all agree that pharmacodynamics is important, evaluating it directly can be challenging as the intensity and time course of the drug effects are often difficult or inconvenient to measure. This is especially true if the response of the body to the drug is binary. For example, for anticonvulsant medications, it is difficult to directly measure the drug effect, and it is certainly too risky and too late to optimize dose regimen till seizure relapse. Similarly, for immunosuppressive agents, the doctor cannot just give an empirical dose regimen and wait till organ transplant rejection occurs to adjust the doses. There are similar situations for many other types of drugs, such as antibiotics, cardiovascular drugs, drugs with severe adverse effects, drugs with narrow therapeutic window, etc.

Of course, there are always exceptions. For example, for antidiabetic and antihypertension drugs, their effects can be easily evaluated by measuring blood glucose and blood pressure. But for many other drugs, it remains true that the intensity and time course of the drug effects, desired or unwanted, are often difficult or inconvenient to measure. Therefore, there is a gap between dose and pharmacodynamics. This explains why studying pharmacokinetics is important – pharmacokinetics bridges the gap between dose and pharmacodynamics, and it can be used to guide dosing regimen selection.

Pharmacokinetics is easy to measure and is known to be tied closely to pharmacodynamics. As shown in Figure 1-2, a drug's effect is often related to drug concentrations at the site of action with a sigmoidal relationship. This relationship can be easily explained by target binding and target occupancy principles: at very low drug concentrations, there are not many drug molecules bound to the target, and accordingly there is very little drug effect. With the increase in drug concentrations, the drug effect increases as more drug molecules interact with the target. The drug concentration at which 50% of the maximum effect is achieved is known as EC_{50}. Once all target binding sites are occupied, the maximum effect is reached. Beyond this point, further increases in concentration will not correspondingly enhance drug effect, which is why we see a plateau in the curve.

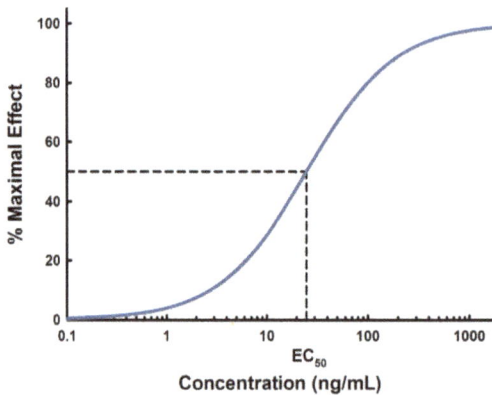

Figure 1-2. Relationship of drug concentration at the site of action to drug effect.

It should be noted that the drug concentration shown in Figure 1-2 is the concentration at the site of action. In most cases, pharmacological targets are expressed in tissues. Consequently, directly measuring drug concentrations at the site of action becomes impractical in humans, as collecting tissue samples is usually unrealistic. Fortunately, there is often a linear relationship between drug concentrations in tissues, including the site of action, and drug concentrations in blood, the latter is easily accessible.

For the blood samples collected, there are three matrix choices for drug measurement - plasma, serum, and whole blood:

- *Plasma* is the fluid portion of blood, and it contains soluble proteins that often bind drugs. When whole blood is centrifuged after adding an anticoagulant, blood cells are precipitated, and the supernatant fluid is plasma.
- *Serum* is also the fluid portion of blood. The difference between serum and plasma is that serum does not contain fibrinogen, a soluble protein that forms the blood clot. When whole blood is centrifuged after the blood has been clotted, the supernatant fluid is serum.
- *Whole blood* contains both the fluid portion and the cells.

Most drug concentrations are measured using plasma. Although drug concentrations in serum and plasma are virtually identical, plasma is preferred because it is easier to prepare and does not have the risk of hemolysis as seen in serum during the blood clotting process. Compared to plasma and serum, whole blood is the least used in clinical practice because whole blood samples are harder to assay. However, for drugs that are extensively taken up by red blood cells (e.g. antimalarial drugs), whole blood concentrations would be more relevant and should be considered.

Considering the importance of pharmacokinetics, it is tempting to find a way to quantitatively characterize pharmacokinetic profiles to facilitate data extrapolation and drug concentration prediction after drug administration. One way of accomplishing this task is utilizing compartmental models, as described in the next section.

1.3 Compartment Models

The handling of a drug by the body is complicated due to the involvement of several intertwined processes and the complexities of human anatomy and physiology. To predict a drug's behavior in the body, simplifications of physiological processes and drug kinetics are needed. One way is to use *compartment models*, which simplify the fate of a drug in the body by dividing the whole body into one or more compartments. The simplest of such models is the *one-compartment model*, where all organs and tissues are considered as a single and uniform compartment and the drug distributes instantaneously to all body areas once it enters the body (Figure 1-3, left). One-compartment model is the most frequently used model in clinical practice and is extensively discussed in this book.

One-compartment model assumes immediate distribution. This assumption works well for many drugs, but not for all. For some drugs, after entering systemic circulation, they rapidly arrive at highly perfused organs (e.g. heart, lung, liver, kidneys), then reach poorly perfused organs (e.g. fat, skin, bone) at a slower rate. This distribution pattern can be captured by a *two-compartment model*, where all organs and tissues are divided into two compartments: a *central compartment* which represents plasma and highly perfused organs, and a *peripheral compartment* which represents poorly perfused organs (Figure 1-3, right). In clinical practice, two-compartment model has been applied to some drugs, such as vancomycin and digoxin, and is covered in detail in Chapter 9.

In addition to one- and two-compartment models, there are more complicated compartment models, such as multicompartment models with ≥ 3 compartments as well as the whole-body physiologically based pharmacokinetic (PBPK) model, in which each organ represents a compartment and links to each other by organ blood flow. These complicated models are rarely used in clinical practice and are beyond the scope of this book.

When building a model, visual representation is helpful. In model diagrams, a compartment is often represented by a circle or a rectangle, and the rate of drug transfer is represented by straight arrows. Arrows pointing into/out of the box indicate that the drug is entering/leaving the compartment. Figure 1-3 shows a schematic representation illustrating both a one-compartment model and a two-compartment model.

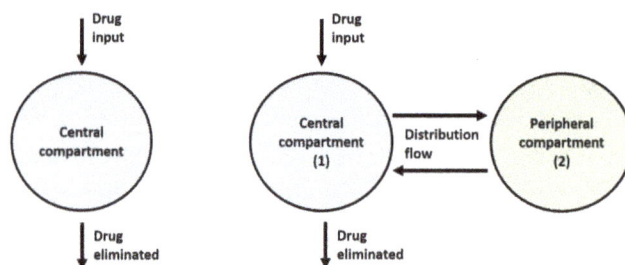

Figure 1-3. Schematic representation of a one-compartment model (left) and a two-compartment model (right).

Regarding the rate of drug transfer, as represented by the straight arrows in the model diagram, there could be different patterns, such as zero-order and first-order processes. It is important to understand these concepts, recognize their difference, and be familiar with the distinctive pharmacokinetics profiles associated with zero-order and first-order kinetics. This is the topic of the next section.

1.4 Zero-Order and First-Order Kinetics

First, let's start with an outside example. Imagine there are two undergraduate students, Tom and Jerry, both are freshman and excited to live on campus. They both received $2,000 pocket money, which is a one-time deal, from their parents on the first day of school. Tom and Jerry have different ways of spending money. Table 1-1 shows the monthly records of their remaining balances.

Tom spent $200 every month till all the money was used up in month 10. How much Tom spent each month was not dependent on the balance he had in that specific month. He always spent the same $ amount every month. Tom's bank record is a *zero-order process*.

Jerry spent different amounts of money every month. How much Jerry spent each month was directly proportional to the balance he had in that specific month. He spent more when he had a higher remaining balance and spent less when he had less money left in his bank account. Although the amount of money Jerry spent every month differs, the fraction of money he spent remains constant. Jerry's bank record is a *first-order process*.

In pharmacokinetics world, some drugs behave like Tom and others like Jerry. If we replace "Tom/Jerry" with "drugs" and "$2000 pocket money" with "single I.V. bolus dose", we will have a good blueprint for what the pharmacokinetics profiles look like under zero-order and first-order kinetics.

Table 1-1. Tom and Jerry's monthly balance of their pocket money.

Month	Tom	$amount spent	Fraction of $amount spent per month	Jerry	$amount spent	Fraction of $amount spent per month
0	$2,000			$2,000		
1	$1,800	$200	0.10	$1,000	$100	0.5
2	$1,600	$200	0.11	$500	$500	0.5
3	$1,400	$200	0.13	$250	$250	0.5
4	$1,200	$200	0.14	$125	$125	0.5
5	$1,000	$200	0.17	$63	$63	0.5
6	$800	$200	0.20	$31	$31	0.5
7	$600	$200	0.25	$16	$16	0.5
8	$400	$200	0.33	$8	$8	0.5
9	$200	$200	0.50	$4	$4	0.5
10	$0	$200	1.00	$2	$2	0.5
11	$0	$200		$1	$1	0.5
12	$0	$200		$0.5	$0.5	0.5

Next, let's dive in to learn the mathematical equations that can be used to describe each type of process.

1.4.1 Zero-order kinetics

Let's use the simplest example – a one-compartment model following a single I.V. bolus dose of a drug. For drugs that are eliminated under zero-order kinetics (i.e. drugs behave like Tom), the decrease in drug concentration during each fixed time period is a constant value. The change of drug concentration in the body per given time is expressed as below:

$$\frac{dC}{dt} = -k_e \qquad\qquad [1\text{-}1]$$

where C represents the concentration; k_e represents the elimination rate constant, which is always a positive value. A negative sign is put in front of k_e since the concentration is dropping due to drug elimination.

Equation 1-1 can be easily solved to obtain the following explicit equation:

$$C = C_0 - k_e \times t \qquad\qquad [1\text{-}2]$$

where C_0 represents the initial concentration.

Figure 1-4 shows an example dataset and the time course of plasma drug concentrations after an I.V. bolus dose, assuming a one-compartment model with zero-order elimination. As it is shown, for drugs following zero-order elimination, the decline of drug concentration is a straight line.

Time (h)	Conc. (ng/mL)
0	100
1	90
2	80
3	70
4	60
5	50
6	40
7	30
8	20
9	10
10	0

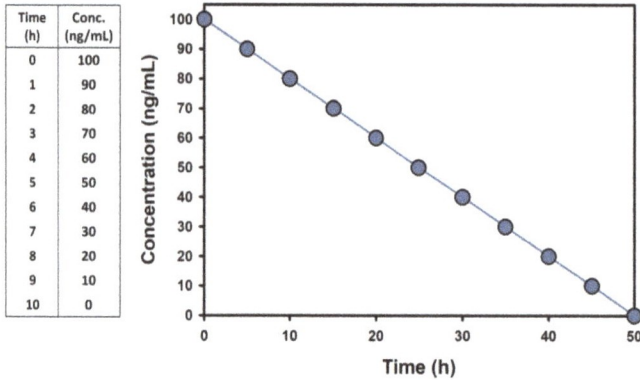

Figure 1-4. Example dataset (left) and the time course of plasma drug concentrations after an I.V. bolus dose (right), assuming a one-compartment model with zero-order elimination.

In the real world, very few drugs are eliminated by a zero-order process when the doses are within the therapeutic dose range. Some drugs, such as phenytoin, may display zero-order elimination when high doses are given. Zero-order elimination happens when the body's ability to clear a drug has reached its maximum capacity (e.g. all drug metabolizing enzymes are being used). Once this capacity is reached, the amount of drug being eliminated per given time will remain constant, regardless of how high the concentrations/doses are. For most drugs, the recommended dose range is well below the body's maximum elimination capacity. Therefore, very few drugs behave like Tom. However, when a drug is given at a dose high enough to exceed the body's ability to clear it, theoretically any drug could display zero-order kinetics. There is a saying "All drugs are poisons, it is just a matter of dose". Here we could make a similar statement "All drugs could have zero-order elimination, it is just a matter of dose".

1.4.2 First-order kinetics

Like in the previous section, let's use the simplest example – a one-compartment model following a single I.V. bolus dose of a drug. For drugs that are eliminated under first-order kinetics (i.e., drugs behave like Jerry), the decrease in drug concentration during each fixed time period changes and is directly proportional to the concentration. The change of drug concentration in the body per given time is expressed as below:

$$\frac{dC}{dt} = -k_e \times C \qquad\qquad [1\text{-}3]$$

where C represents the concentration; k_e represents the elimination rate constant, which is always a positive value. A negative sign is put in front of k_e since the concentration is decreasing over time.

Equation 1-3 can be solved to obtain the following explicit equation:

$$C = C_0 \cdot e^{-k_e \cdot t}$$ [1-4]

where C_0 represents the initial concentration.

Figure 1-5 shows an example dataset and the time course of plasma drug concentrations after an I.V. bolus dose, assuming a one-compartment model with first-order elimination. As it is shown, for drugs following first-order elimination, the decline in drug concentration is a curve instead of a straight line.

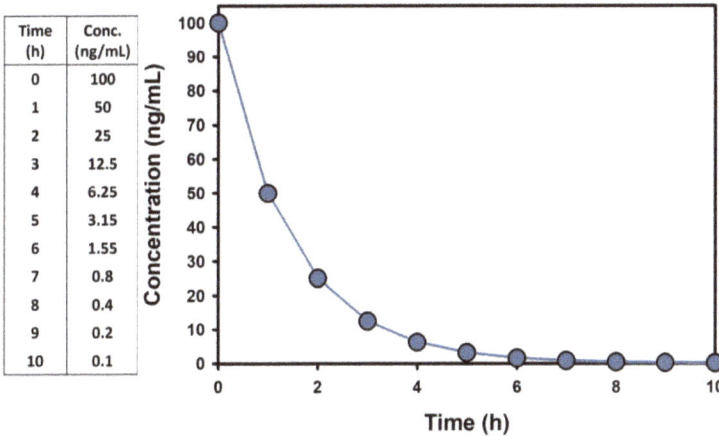

Time (h)	Conc. (ng/mL)
0	100
1	50
2	25
3	12.5
4	6.25
5	3.15
6	1.55
7	0.8
8	0.4
9	0.2
10	0.1

Figure 1-5. Example dataset (left) and the time course of plasma drug concentrations after an I.V. bolus dose, assuming a one-compartment model with first-order elimination.

Most drugs are cleared in the body by a first-order process. *In the rest of this book, unless specified, the pharmacokinetic parameters, equations, problem sets, and case studies covered are all based on drugs with first-order elimination*. The scenario of a one-compartment model with first-order elimination, and an I.V. bolus dose not only is the simplest situation from the mathematical standpoint, but also is frequently applied in clinical practice. This means that Equation 1-4 is very useful since it can be used to predict drug concentration at any time after an I.V. bolus dose once we know the values of the parameters, such as the elimination rate constant k_e. The definition and calculation of several key pharmacokinetic parameters, including k_e, are provided in the next section.

1.5 Key Pharmacokinetic Parameters

1.5.1. Elimination rate constant (k_e)

The elimination rate constant k_e determines how fast the drug concentration declines in the plasma over time. One way to calculate k_e is based on observed concentration data points. However, as shown in Equation 1-4, $C = C_0 \cdot e^{-k_e \cdot t}$, k_e

sits on the shoulder of the exponential function and cannot be calculated directly from a curve. To calculate k_e, we need to use a logarithm transformation to convert a curve to a straight line so that k_e can be pulled to the ground. Following are a few basic principles of logarithm transformation:

- logarithms turn multiplication into addition.
  For example, $\ln(a \times b) = \ln(a) + \ln(b)$
- the e and natural log will cancel out when put together.
  For example, $\ln(e^{-b}) = -b$

Based on the above principles, the logarithm transformation of Equation 1-4 is expressed as:

$$\ln C = \ln C_0 - k_e \cdot t \qquad\qquad [1\text{-}5]$$

This is an equation of straight line since it has the form of Y=a + bX, with Y being the natural log transformed concentrations (i.e., lnC) and X being time. Accordingly, k_e can be obtained by calculating the slope of the straight line using the following formula:

$$k_e = -\text{slope} = -\frac{\Delta C}{\Delta t} = -\frac{\ln C_2 - \ln C_1}{t_2 - t_1} \qquad\qquad [1\text{-}6]$$

Where k_e, represented by the negative slope, can be calculated with as few as two data points. The unit of k_e is time^{-1}, typically hr^{-1}. The larger the k_e value, the steeper the slope, the faster the drug cleared out of the body. On the other hand, the smaller the k_e value, the shallower the slope, and the slower the drug concentration decreases over time.

As shown in Figure 1-6, the original concentration-time curve (upper left) turns into a straight line when lnC versus time is plotted (upper right). However, in the real world, lnC vs time plot is not commonly used as the natural log transformed value of each concentration needs to be calculated first, which is inconvenient. A common way to overcome this issue is to plot the actual concentrations on a log scale. The Y-axis is a base-10 log scale, with equal distance between 0.01 to 0.1, 0.1 to 1, 1 to 10, and so forth. In other words, the logarithm transformation has been taken care of by the Y-axis. Therefore, a straight line can be obtained when the actual concentrations are plotted on a log scale (Figure 1-6, lower left). This is known as a semi-logarithmic plot since the Y-axis (for concentration) is on a log scale and the X-axis (for time) is on a linear scale.

For semi-log concentration-time plot, it should be noted that the slope of the straight line is not $-k_e$. A conversion factor of 2.303 needs to be used to account for the difference between log base 10 and natural log. The relevant equations are provided in Figure 1-6.

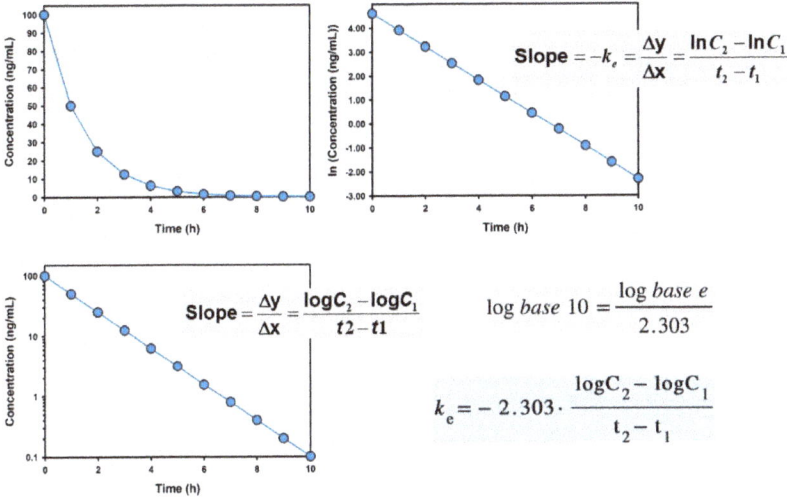

Figure 1-6. Time course of concentrations on a linear scale (upper left), natural log transformed concentrations (lnC) on a linear scale (upper right), and concentrations on a log scale (lower left).

1.5.2. Half-life ($t_{1/2}$)

Half-life ($t_{1/2}$) is the time needed for the plasma concentration of a drug to decrease by one-half. For a drug with first-order elimination, its half-life remains unchanged regardless of the drug concentration in the body; in other words, half-life is a concentration-independent parameter. Sometimes the half-life can be obtained by visual examination of the dataset. For example, if we look at Jerry's monthly balance (Table 1-1), each month Jerry spent half of the money he had at the beginning of that month. For Jerry's case, the half-life is one month.

Elimination rate constant and half-life tie closely to each other as both indicate how quickly the drug is eliminated out of the body. Their relationship can be described by the following calculations:

At time 0, $C = C_0 \cdot e^{-k_e \cdot 0} \rightarrow C = C_0$

After one half-life, the concentration drops to half of C_0:

$$\frac{1}{2}C_0 = C_0 \cdot e^{-k_e \cdot t_{1/2}} \quad \rightarrow \quad \frac{1}{2} = e^{-k_e \cdot t_{1/2}} \quad \rightarrow \quad \ln\frac{1}{2} = -k_e \cdot t_{1/2}$$

Based on the above calculation steps, we obtain the following equations:

$$t_{1/2} = \frac{0.693}{k_e} \qquad\qquad\qquad [1\text{-}7]$$

$$k_e = \frac{0.693}{t_{1/2}} \qquad\qquad\qquad [1\text{-}8]$$

Therefore, half-life and elimination rate constant are "buddies" - once one parameter is determined, the other one can be promptly calculated. While both parameters indicate how fast the drug is cleared from the plasma, half-life is a more often quoted parameter. This is likely because $t_{1/2}$ has a unit of time which is easier to understand than k_e, whose unit is time^{-1}. In addition, the name "half-life" is more intuitive. In drug package inserts, the half-life of a drug is often provided rather than the elimination rate constant.

1.5.3. Volume of distribution (V_d)

Volume of distribution (V_d) is a fundamental pharmacokinetics parameter, and it reflects the extent of drug distribution into extravascular fluids and tissues. A large volume of distribution indicates that the drug is extensively distributed into tissues, while a small volume of distribution suggests that more drug molecules are present in plasma. V_d is the "apparent" volume of the body if a drug is present throughout the body at the same concentration as it is in plasma:

$$\text{Volume of distribution} = \frac{Amount\ of\ drug\ in\ the\ body}{plasma\ concentration}$$

For drugs given via I.V. bolus dose, the initial plasma concentration is C_0, and the amount of drug in the body at time 0 equals to dose. Therefore, volume of distribution can be calculated as the following:

$$V_d = \frac{Dose}{C_0} \qquad\qquad [1\text{-}9]$$

Based on the above equation, a drug's volume of distribution can be estimated if we know the dose and initial concentration value. Equation 1-9 can be rearranged to calculate initial concentration and dose. For example, when a dose is given, if we know V_d of that drug, we can predict the initial concentration ($C_0 = \frac{Dose}{V_d}$). Similarly, if we know the value of V_d and the desired target concentration, we can determine the dose required to achieve the desired concentration ($dose = C_0 \times V_d$).

It is important to understand that V_d is a hypothetical volume, and it does not correspond to any specific physiological volume of body fluid or tissue spaces. To explain this concept, let's imagine the body as a tank filled with water. Figure 1-7 shows an example of two tanks of the same size, both of which filled with water and received the same dose of a drug. However, the drug concentrations in the second tank are much lower due to sequestration. Accordingly, the V_d values are different between these two tanks, with the V_d of the drug in the second rank being much larger than the actual water volume.

In general, hydrophilic drugs (i.e., water loving) tend to have smaller volume of distribution than lipophilic drugs (i.e., lipid loving), because the former cannot pass through cell membrane easily, while the latter can readily across cell membrane and enter tissue cells. For example, many antibiotics drugs are hydrophilic and are confined within the extracellular space. A typical case is aminoglycosides, which

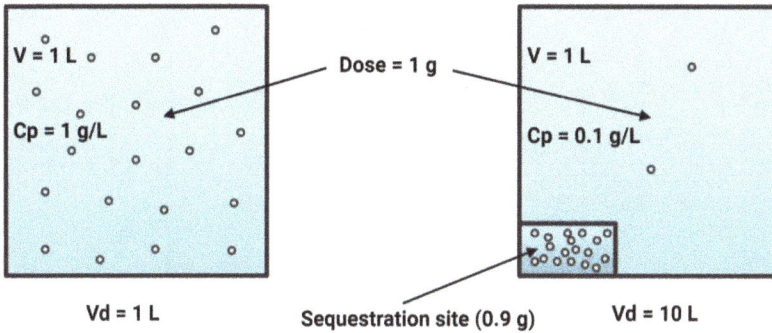

Figure 1-7. A dose of 1 g is added in each tank filled with one liter water. Drug concentration is 1 g/L in the left tank and 0.1 g/L in the right tank due to sequestration. The value of V_d of this drug is 1 L in the left tank and 10 L in the right tank.

cannot penetrate tissue cells and have a small volume of distribution that is close to the volume of extracellular space; the V_d of aminoglycosides is about 18 L for a 70 kg adult (i.e. 0.25 L/kg).

On the other hand, many anticancer agents are lipophilic and often have large volume of distribution. For example, many anthracycline drugs, including doxorubicin, mitoxantrone, and idarubicin, have large volume of distribution, with V_d values larger than 1000 L! This value means that if the drug concentration in tissues is the same as plasma concentrations, we would need 1000 L tissue volume. Do we have that large physical volume to accommodate the drug? Of course, no. The physical volume of a 70-kg adult is about 70 L, assuming the density of 1 between mass (kg) and volume (L). Therefore, V_d is just a hypothetical volume, and it does not correspond to the physiological tissue space; the value of 1000 L just indicates that the anthracycline drugs mentioned above have extensive tissue distribution, with tissue concentrations much higher than plasma concentrations.

1.5.4. Clearance (CL)

In addition to volume of distribution, another fundamental pharmacokinetics parameter is clearance (CL). Clearance is a measure of the removal of a drug from plasma. It does not indicate the amount of a drug being eliminated. Clearance may be viewed as the volume of plasma from which the drug is removed over a specified time (unit is volume/time). We can imagine our body as a tank filled with water and clearance is the volume of water that is drained out of the tank over a specific time (e.g. per hour) by an open outlet valve (Figure 1-8).

Clearance can be calculated using the following equation:

$$CL = \frac{Dose}{AUC}$$ [1-10]

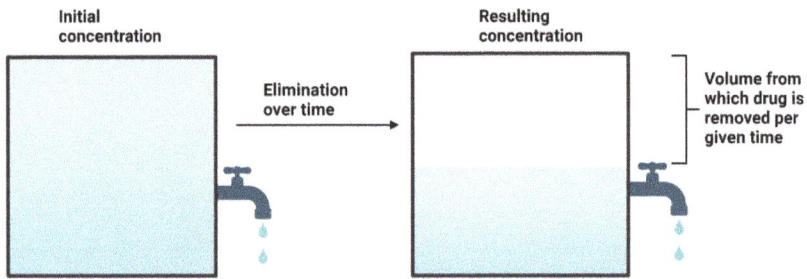

Figure 1-8. Clearance may be viewed as the volume of plasma from which drug is removed over a specified time.

Where AUC represents the area under the concentration-time curve. The calculation of AUC is provided in the next section.

Drugs can be eliminated from the body through different pathways, such as hepatic metabolism, urinary excretion, and biliary excretion. CL represents the total body clearance, which is the sum of all individual elimination pathways. Detailed information on hepatic clearance and renal clearance will be covered in Chapter 4.

1.5.5. Relationship among pharmacokinetic parameters

For the parameters discussed in this section, namely k_e, $t_{1/2}$, V_d, and CL, they remain unchanged regardless of the level of doses and drug concentrations (i.e., dose- and concentration-independent). They are all key pharmacokinetics parameters as they play a central role in predicting drug concentrations and guiding dose regimen selection. It is important to understand the relationship among these parameters. Followings are several key messages:

- *V_d and CL are primary pharmacokinetics parameters.* V_d is the hypothetical volume of plasma, and CL is the hypothetical volume of plasma being removed over a specific time. V_d and CL together determine k_e and $t_{1/2}$. We can image a water tank with an open outlet valve on the bottom. The size of the tank (i.e., capacity of water), the efficiency of the outlet valve, and the water in the tank can be viewed as V_d, CL, and the drug, respectively. The size of the tank (i.e., V_d) and the efficiency of the open outlet valve (i.e., CL) together determine how long it would take to drain all the water out of the tank (i.e., k_e and $t_{1/2}$).

- *V_d and CL are independent from each other.* Changing the size of the tank will not affect the efficiency of the open outlet valve. Changing the diameter of the valve will not affect the size of the tank. However, changing the size of the tank or the diameter of the valve will affect the time needed to drain out all the water (i.e., k_e and $t_{1/2}$).

- k_e *and* $t_{1/2}$ *are secondary pharmacokinetic parameters.* They are determined by V_d and CL with the following relationship:

$$k_e = \frac{CL}{V_d} \qquad\qquad [1\text{-}11]$$

$$t_{1/2} = \frac{0.693 \cdot V_d}{CL} \qquad\qquad [1\text{-}12]$$

- Equation 1-11 can be rearranged to calculate V_d and CL. If we know the values of ke and CL, V_d can be calculated as:

$$V_d = \frac{CL}{k_e} \qquad\qquad [1\text{-}13]$$

Similarly, if the values of k_e and V_d are known, CL can be calculated as:
$$CL = k_e \cdot V_d \qquad\qquad [1\text{-}14]$$

- The change of V_d or CL will *cause* the change of k_e and $t_{1/2}$. The change of k_e and $t_{1/2}$ is *due to* the change of V_d or CL. V_d and CL do not affect each other. In another word, V_d and CL are not dependent on other parameters, which is why they are considered primary pharmacokinetic parameters. On the other hand, k_e and $t_{1/2}$ are hybrid parameters, and their values are dependent on V_d and CL; that is why they are considered secondary pharmacokinetics parameters.
- The equation of $CL = k_e \cdot V_d$ means that if we know the values of k_e and V_d, we can use them to calculate CL. It does not mean CL is dependent on k_e and V_d. Similarly, the fact that V_d can be calculated by $\frac{CL}{k_e}$ does not mean V_d is dependent on CL and k_e.

For the bullet points listed above, many of them appear to be repetitive. I did this intentionally to ensure that readers have a fundamental understanding of these important pharmacokinetics parameters after receiving the same key messages multiple times.

1.6 Area Under the Curve (AUC)

AUC represents drug exposure over time. AUC can be used to assess how much drug entered the body. For example, the bioavailability of a drug (i.e. fraction of dose enters the body, F) can be estimated by calculating the ratio of AUC of reference dose and test dose; this part will be elaborated in Chapter 2. In addition, AUC can be used to assess how efficiently the body gets rid of the drug. For example, as shown in equation 1-10, CL can be calculated by dose over AUC.

AUC can be calculated by applying the trapezoidal rule. For the concentration-time plot, we can draw a line vertically to the x-axis from each measured concentration, then connect each of two adjacent concentrations and calculate the enclosed trapezoidal, piece by piece.

From time 0 to the last time point, each of the trapezoidal area is calculated using the following general formula:

$$AUC_{t_n - t_{n+1}} = (\frac{C_{n+1} + C_n}{2})(t_{n+1} - t_n)$$

AUC_{0-last} is the sum of each individual trapezoidal area.

In general, what we are interested in is $AUC_{0-\infty}$. Therefore, the residual area from the last time point to time infinity needs to be calculated as well. This terminal area can be calculated:

$$AUC_{last - \infty} = \frac{C_{last}}{k_e}$$

$AUC_{0-\infty} = AUC_{0-last} + AUC_{last-\infty}$, as shown in Figure 1-9.

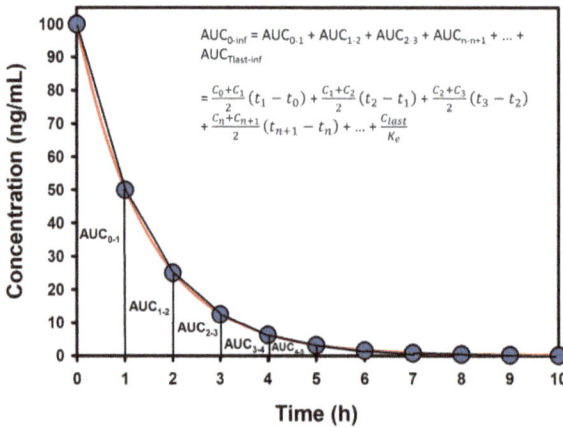

Figure 1-9. Calculation of AUC using the trapezoidal rule.

When AUC is calculated using the trapezoidal rule, the accuracy of the value is dependent on the number of data points. In general, the less the concentration data points, the bigger the error of AUC. This is because each of the two adjacent concentrations are connected using a straight line when we calculate the trapezoidal area. However, the concentration-time plot is curved. When there are limited data points, the calculated area tends to overpredict the actual area as shown in Figure 1-10. In clinical practice, it is rare to collect more than 3 samples after a dose. Therefore, in clinical practice, AUC is rarely used to determine clearance. AUC is used more frequently in clinical research or drug development, where pharmacokinetic samples are collected with a richer sampling schedule (usually >8 samples).

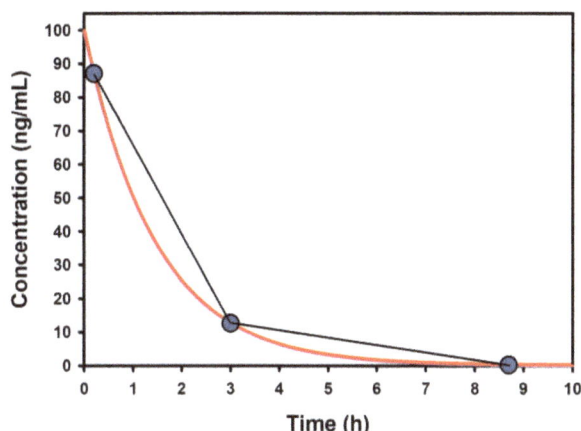

Figure 1-10. Caveat of using the trapezoidal rule to calculate AUC with limited data points.

1.7 Clinical Pharmacokinetics in Drug Development

Pharmacokinetics has about 100 years of history and it was primarily used as an academic tool in the early days. Over the years, the importance of pharmacokinetics has been recognized. In the 1990s, pharmacokinetics was no longer confined to academic research - it began to be used as an integral part of the industrial drug development process. Since then, general interest in pharmacokinetics has increased dramatically. Pharmacokinetics of new drug candidates are extensively studied in both preclinical and clinical phases.

When a drug candidate enters the clinical phase, the first clinical trial is known as the first-in-human (FIH) study where several doses, ranging from very low to high, are evaluated in healthy volunteers. Blood samples are collected at various time points over a specified period (usually 5-10 days) for pharmacokinetics evaluation. Typically, the FIH study is a single-ascending dose (SAD) study, and once the drug is demonstrated to be safe in a single dose setting, it is further evaluated in a multiple-ascending dose (MAD) study, where drug candidates are given multiple times (e.g., twice daily for 5 days). Both SAD and MAD studies have the same goal - to evaluate the pharmacokinetics, tolerability, and safety of the drug candidate.

After SAD and MAD studies are completed, depending on the drug ADME features, several other types of Phase 1 studies may be conducted where pharmacokinetics endpoints are the primary objective; these studies include food effect study, drug-drug interaction studies, and pharmacokinetic studies in special populations. Clinical pharmacokinetics information gained from these Phase 1 studies provides the scientific basis of dose selection for the next phase studies.

The efficacy and safety of the drug candidate are then evaluated in Phase 2 studies conducted in a small number of patients, followed by Phase 3 studies carried out in a large patient population. In these late phase studies, usually pharmacokinetics samples are still collected, but with a sparse sampling schedule (e.g. 1- 2 samples per subject). These sparse pharmacokinetic data can be pooled into the rich pharmacokinetics data collected in Phase 1 studies, and then linked to efficacy data obtained in Phase 2/3 studies to characterize the pharmacokinetic/pharmacodynamic relationship and inform dose selection.

Therefore, drug development builds on pharmacokinetics. Before a drug is approved, its pharmacokinetics has to be studied thoroughly and the pharmacokinetic results play an important role in dose regimen selection.

1.8 Clinical Pharmacokinetics in Clinical Practice

After a new drug is approved, the drug company issues a package insert, in which the recommended dose regimen is provided along with several other information, including pharmacokinetics, such as the drug's half-life, volume of distribution, clearance, pharmacokinetic linearity, pharmacokinetics in special populations, and drug-drug interactions, etc. If you are a PharmD student, you may feel that there is no point to learn the mathematical equations covered in this book - it seems that there is no need to study pharmacokinetics in clinical practice since it has been thoroughly evaluated already during the drug development phase.

So, why is pharmacokinetics still widely applied in clinical practice? The reason is because people differ and the "one-dose-for-all" approach is not applicable. Following the same dose, drug concentrations may vary substantially among different patients. For drugs with narrow therapeutic window, it is important to ensure that the plasma concentrations fall within the therapeutic range for each individual patient. This is because toxicity may occur when concentrations exceed the maximum effective concentration, while the drug may be ineffective when the level is below the minimum effective concentration. Therefore, while the doses recommended in the package insert can be used as the starting point, for some drugs, evaluating their pharmacokinetics in an individual patient is still needed to determine the right dose for that specific patient.

1.8.1. Source of drug variability

Drug variability can come from various sources:

- Variation in drug absorption. Factors that affect the rate and extent of absorption include variable gastric empty time, gastrointestinal fluid composition, food effect, etc.
- Variation in drug distribution due to difference in body weight and body fat composition among patients.
- Variation in drug metabolism. For example, the expression level and function of drug metabolizing enzymes in the liver varies among patients. This would lead to large variability in hepatic clearance (and bioavailability for drugs with significant first-pass metabolism).
- Variation in drug excretion due to age, and differences in the activity of drug transporters in the liver and kidneys, etc.

- Disease states that affect renal functions (e.g. kidney failure), liver functions (e.g. liver impairment), plasma protein levels (e.g. cirrhosis, myocardial infarction).
- Drug-drug interactions by competing for the same drug metabolism enzymes, drug transporters, as well as plasma proteins.
- Pharmacogenetics (e.g. polymorphism of drug metabolism enzymes and drug transporters).
- Variation in pharmacodynamics.

Pharmacokinetics variability arising from drug-drug interaction and pharmacogenetics is covered in Chapter 4. Detailed information on pharmacokinetics variability caused by age, disease, and other factors is provided in Chapter 11.

1.8.2 Therapeutic drug monitoring (TDM)

For some drugs, their pharmacokinetics information in each individual patient can be essential for dose regimen optimization. This is done by *therapeutic drug monitoring* (TDM), which is an integral part of personalized medicine. The steps of TDM are shown in Figure 1-11. First, a drug is selected based on the disease

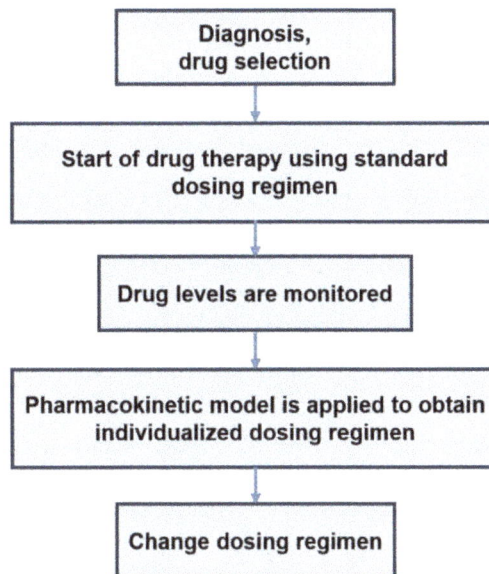

Figure 1-11. Steps of therapeutic drug monitoring and application of the pharmacokinetic modeling.

diagnosis, and therapy starts with a standard dose regimen. After the dose is given, 2 to 3 blood samples are collected, and plasma drug concentrations are measured. Based on the concentration values, a pharmacokinetics model is applied and pharmacokinetic parameters of the drug in the specific patient are obtained using relevant mathematical equations. Based on these pharmacokinetic parameters, concentrations at different times are predicted, and dose adjustments are performed to ensure drug concentrations fall within the therapeutic range.

TDM does not bring value for every drug. For drugs with a wide safety margin, there are no significant consequences associated with either too high or too low drug concentrations. Therefore, TDM may not be needed. In addition, TDM may have limited value for drugs with no well-defined therapeutic plasma concentration range.

TDM is valuable for the following types of drugs/situations:
- Drugs with narrow therapeutic windows. Monitoring drug concentrations is beneficial because the same dose may produce the desired effect in one patient but cause toxicity in another patient.
- Drugs with a good correlation between drug response and plasma concentration; this relationship allows for predicting therapeutic response or toxicity as drug concentrations change.
- Drugs with significant pharmacokinetics variability. Wide variation in drug concentrations among patients from a given dose.
- Drugs that are toxic but adverse drug reactions may be avoided by therapeutic drug monitoring.
- The drug's pharmacodynamic response cannot be assessed easily. There is a difficulty in interpreting therapeutic or low toxicity of a drug based on clinical evidence alone.
- When the drug is used in special populations, such as critically ill patients.

In clinical practice, TDM is routinely performed for:
- Antimicrobial agents (e.g. aminoglycosides, vancomycin, and antifungal agents).
- Cardiovascular drugs (e.g. digoxin, procainamide, and lidocaine).
- Anti-seizure drugs (e.g. phenytoin and phenobarbital).
- Immunosuppressive drugs (e.g. cyclosporine, tacrolimus, sirolimus).
- Drugs treating bipolar disorder (e.g. lithium and valproic acid).
- Cytotoxic anticancer drugs (e.g. methotrexate and busulfan).
- Other medications, such as anti- tuberculosis drugs.

Although I did not allocate separate chapters for the drugs with TDM, the pharmacokinetics and dose optimization of some of these drugs are covered in case studies and problem sets throughout chapters 1-11.

1.9 Miscellaneous Notes

❖ In mathematics, constants refer to names associated with values that never change. However, this is not the case for pharmacokinetics, a discipline that sits between mathematics and biology. For example, the pharmacokinetic parameter "elimination rate constant" having constant in its name does not mean that the value of k_e will never change. The value of k_e will change when the body's ability to handle the drug changes. For example, when a patient's kidneys do not function well (e.g. kidney injury), the body's ability to clear the drug decreases (i.e. CL decreases). Accordingly, the drug will stay in the body for a longer period of time, leading to a decreased k_e and a longer $t_{1/2}$.

❖ In this chapter, the concentration data points shown in Figure 1-6 are perfectly lined up. Plugging any of the two data points in Equation 1-6, you always get the same k_e value. In the real world, we rarely get such ideal data. The real data, almost always, have some "noises" due to the errors/variations introduced during sample collection, sample preparation, bioanalysis processes, instrumentation, etc. Although you still see a trend of straight line when you plot the data on a log scale (indicates first-order kinetics), the observed data points never sit exactly on the line. Because of the inherent "wiggle" in the data, you may get different k_e values when different data points are used for calculation. When you have multiple concentration time points, the best way to calculate k_e is to obtain the slope of the curve using linear regression analysis.

❖ After a drug is administered, usually a blood sample is collected into a tube with anticoagulant, then is centrifuged, and the supernatant is used for drug analysis. The supernatant is plasma, which includes both free drug molecules and drug molecules bound to plasma proteins, such as albumin and α1-acid glycoprotein. For small-molecule drugs, the drug concentration in plasma is commonly measured by a technique called liquid chromatography-mass spectrometry (LC-MS). LC-MS method is a robust and sensitive quantitative method. LC-MS method can measure drug concentrations at the ng/mL level (i.e., µg/L). Sometimes, a very sensitive LC-MS method can even detect drug concentrations as low as the pg/mL level. Usually, the plasma concentrations measured are total drug concentrations (i.e., free drug + bound drug).

1.10 Case Study

Patient IL (60 kg, female) received a single i.v. dose of gentamycin, an aminoglycoside antibiotic which is hydrophilic. The study nurse forgot to record the dose. Two blood samples were collected and sent to the bioanalytical lab for drug concentration measurement. The result showed that the plasma drug concentrations were 12 mg/L at 2 hours and 3.8 mg/L at 6 hours after the dose. Gentamycin, similar to other aminoglycosides, has limited volume of distribution, with a V_d value of 0.25 L/kg. To maintain the antibiotic effect of gentamycin, its plasma concentration should not be lower than 2 mg/L. Gentamycin follows first-order elimination and can be described by a 1-compartment model. Please calculate:

a) The half-life of gentamycin in this patient.
b) The dose of gentamycin used.
c) The initial concentration of gentamycin.
d) The clearance of the gentamycin in this patient.
e) What is the duration of antibiotic effect of gentamycin in Patient AG? [hint: you need to calculate how long would it take to drop the concentration below 2.0 mg/L]

I encourage you to first work on the above case example yourself before you look at the calculations that I provided below.

$$\sim \sim \sim$$

To solve this type of problem, my suggestion is to list all quantitative information on a scratch paper and see which parameter can be calculated first. The information we have includes bodyweight (BW, 60 kg), V_d in the unit of L/kg (which means that it is a bodyweight normalized value), as well as two data points. As V_d with the unit of L is required, we need to calculate that by multiplying BW. In addition, with two data points on hand, we can calculate k_e directly.

- $V_d = 0.25\ {}^{L}\!/_{kg} \times 60\ kg = 15\ L$
- $k_e = -slope = -\dfrac{\ln 3.8 - \ln 12}{6 - 2} = 0.288\ h^{-1}$ *(note: calculated based on equation 1-6)*

Once we get k_e, we can calculate $t_{1/2}$ based on equation 1-7:

- $t_{1/2} = \dfrac{0.693}{k_e} = \dfrac{0.693}{0.288} = 2.41\ h$ *(note: this answers question a)*

With the information of k_e and just one data point, we can calculate initial concentration C_0 using equation 1-4. You have two data points on hand. You can plug in any of these two.

- $12 = C_0 \cdot e^{-0.288 \cdot 2} \rightarrow C_0 = 21.3\ {}^{mg}\!/_{L}$ *(note: this answers question c)*

Since we know the values of V_d and C_0, we can calculate the dose based on equation 1-9:

- $Dose = V_d \cdot C_0 = 15 \times 21.3 = 320\ mg$ *(note: this answers question b)*

With information of ke and Vd, we can obtain CL based on equation 1-14:

- $CL = k_e \cdot V_d = 0.288 \times 15 = 4.32\ {}^{L}\!/_{h}$ *(note: this answers question d)*

The duration of antibiotic effect of gentamycin is determined by the time period of gentamycin plasma concentrations remain above 2 mg/L. We can use equation 1-4 to solve this problem:

- $2 = 21.3 \times e^{-0.288 \cdot t} \rightarrow t = 8.21\ h$ *(note: this answers question e)*

Problem Sets   *(Answers to study problems are in the appendix)*

1. The amount of drug eliminated per given time is defined as clearance.
   A. True
   B. False
2. When drug half-life changes, it affects drug clearance.
   A. True
   B. False
3. For a drug following zero-order kinetics, its half-life remains constant.
   A. True
   B. False
4. When an adult with 70 kg receives a drug, its volume of distribution should not exceed 70 L.
   A. True
   B. False
5. Volume of distribution and half-life are primary pharmacokinetics parameters, and they are independent of each other.
   A. True
   B. False
6. In the real world, most drugs undergo the first-order elimination process over therapeutic dose range.
   A. True
   B. False
7. For drugs following first-order kinetics, when V_d changes, for sure t1/2 will change.
   A. True
   B. False
8. The most commonly used model in clinical pharmacokinetic situation is the one-compartment model.
   A. True
   B. False
9. The peripheral compartment usually represents those highly perfused organs.
   A. True
   B. False
10. TDM is particularly valuable for drugs with narrow therapeutic windows.
    A. True
    B. False

Chapter 2.

Absorption

Learning Objectives

After reading this chapter, the reader shall be able to:

1. Understand the extent of absorption and rate of absorption.

2. List factors that can affect a drug's oral bioavailability.

3. Describe the first-pass metabolism; describe how drug transporters can affect a drug's absorption.

4. Define bioavailability F, and know how to use equations to calculate F.

5. Define drug absorption rate constant k_a. Define C_{max} and T_{max} and describe the pharmacokinetic curve following an oral dose.

6. List the pros and cons of immediate-release drugs and extended-release drugs. Understand the kinetics difference between sustained-release and controlled-release drugs.

7. Understand which parameters will change and what the concentration-time profiles look like when extent and/or rate of absorption change.

For drugs administered through extravascular routes, their pharmacokinetics starts with the absorption process. Regardless of the extravascular sites, drug absorption has two aspects: *how much* the drug is absorbed (i.e., *extent of absorption*) and *how fast* the drug is absorbed (i.e., *rate of absorption*). These two aspects are elaborated in section 2.1 and section 2.2, respectively. As oral administration is the most common extravascular route, plus it is more complicated than others, I will focus on oral drug absorption in the first two sections and only briefly talk about other routes in section 2.3. Changes in the extent and/or rate of absorption can affect drug exposure related parameters and the pharmacokinetic profiles; this will be discussed with examples in section 2.4. A few miscellaneous topics related to drug absorption are covered in section 2.5. Finally, this chapter ends with a case study (section 2.6) and problem sets.

2.1 Extent of Oral Absorption

2.1.1. Barriers and sites of loss during drug absorption process

For an orally administered drug, the absorption process starts in the gastrointestinal tract and is considered completed after the drug reaches systemic circulation. Moving from gastrointestinal tract to systemic circulation is not a small task for the drug, as there are multiple barriers along the way and drug loss could occur in any of these barriers (Figure 2-1). Only the drug molecules reaching systemic circulation are considered absorbed. The followings are barriers and factors that can affect drug absorption in each step:

- *Drug loss in the gastrointestinal lumen.*

If a drug is administered in a solid dosage form (e.g., tablets and capsules), it needs to be disintegrated first, then dissolved in gastrointestinal fluids, as solid particles cannot pass through membranes. For a drug with poor *solubility* and low dissolution rate, a considerable portion of the dose may go to feces directly instead of passing through the gut wall. In addition, drug may also be lost by degradation (i.e., decomposition) in the gastrointestinal lumen. Only drug molecules which are neither lost in feces nor degraded in the lumen have the chance to move to the next site: the gut wall.

- *Drug loss in the intestinal wall.*

When a drug moves across the intestinal epithelium without assistance from carrier proteins (e.g., transporters), it can diffuse through the membrane via either transcellular (through cell) or paracellular (around cell) routes. Drug *permeability* plays an important role in this process. Highly permeable drugs tend to be absorbed fast and to a greater extent. On the other hand, drugs with low permeability are likely to be poorly absorbed; this is particularly true for drugs that are polar and relatively large (e.g., molecular weight > 500 g/mol) because they are too polar to diffuse transcellularly and too big to transfer paracellularly through the tight junction of the gastrointestinal tract.

In addition to permeability, another factor that affects how much drug can pass through the gut wall is the *first-pass loss* caused by the drug metabolizing enzymes expressed in the intestine. Although the liver is the chief organ for drug metabolism, drug metabolizing enzymes are expressed not only in the liver, but also in other tissues, such as the intestine. Among the drug metabolizing enzymes expressed in human small intestine, cytochrome P450 3A4 (CYP3A4) is the dominant enzyme. For a drug that is a substrate of CYP3A4, some drug molecules may be metabolized in the gut wall during the absorption process, leading to *intestinal first-pass loss*.

Only drug molecules which can move across the intestinal epithelium and escape intestinal first-pass loss have the chance to move to the next site: the liver.

- *Drug loss in the liver.*

For a drug that successfully passes across the gut wall, it travels with the blood in gastrointestinal tissues and is drained into the liver via the hepatic portal vein; this means that the drug must pass through the liver before reaching systemic circulation. When passing through the liver, the drug is subject to *hepatic first-pass loss* if it is a substrate of a certain drug metabolizing enzyme (e.g., CYP3A4) that is expressed in the liver. Only drug molecules that escape hepatic first-pass loss can enter systemic circulation, the destination from the absorption perspective.

The extent of absorption is the product of the amount of the drug that remains at each of the above three sites. The pharmacokinetic parameter associated with the extent of drug absorption is *bioavailability*, which is expressed as F and represents the fraction of dose that reach systemic circulation. Bioavailability can be described by the following three factors:

$$F = F_{abs} \times F_G \times F_H$$

Where:

F_{abs} =fraction of drug that survives in the gastrointestinal lumen.

F_G =fraction that does not get lost in gut wall, and

F_H = fraction that escapes hepatic first-pass loss.

For example, if 50% of the drug is lost at each step, the value of F would be $0.5 \times 0.5 \times 0.5 = 0.125$, which means that 12.5% of the dose reaches systemic circulation.

When we calculate a drug's bioavailability, often it is difficult to estimate the extent of drug loss at each step. Among F_{abs}, F_G, and F_H, the parameter that may be calculated is F_H as it can be estimated from the hepatic extraction ratio; this will be covered in Chapter 4.

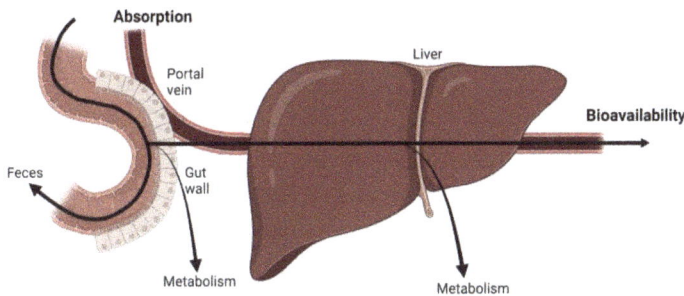

Figure 2-1. The potential barriers and sites of loss that a drug could encounter when it is administered orally. A fraction of the drug may go to feces directly if the drug has poor solubility and slow dissolution rate; a fraction may get lost while passing through the gut wall; a fraction may be metabolized in the liver.

2.1.2. Role of transporters in drug absorption

In section 2.1.1, for the movement of the drug across the gut wall and the liver, I only talked about passive diffusion, which is a non-carrier-mediated process. For some drugs, in addition to passive diffusion, they also move across the gut wall and the liver with the help of drug transporters. Both intestinal epithelium cells (i.e., enterocytes) and hepatocytes are polarized cells with two domains: apical and basolateral. The apical side faces intestinal lumen (for enterocytes) or bile (for hepatocytes), while the basolateral side of both types of cells faces the blood.

Drug transporters can be expressed on either side, as shown in Figure 2-2, and their role in drug absorption is dependent on the side they are localized and the direction in which they transport drugs (as indicated by the straight arrows). There are many transporters expressed in the intestine and the liver. These transporters can be categorized into two classes: efflux transporters and uptake transporters.

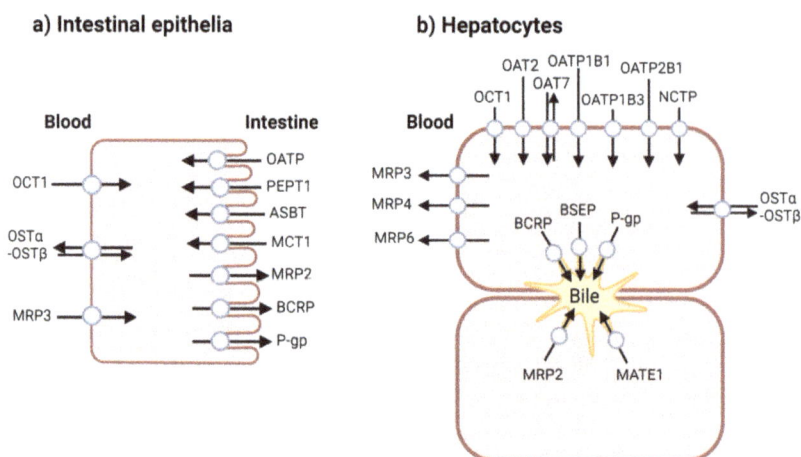

Figure 2-2. Drug transporters expressed in a) intestinal epithelia and
b) hepatocytes in human.

- *Role of efflux transporters in drug absorption.*

   Efflux transporters pump the drug out of the cell; this action explains why they are called "efflux" transporters and why the arrows for these transporters point out of the cell. Efflux transporters are usually localized on the apical side of the cells. To elaborate the role of efflux transporters in drug absorption, let's use P-glycoprotein (P-gp) as an example.

   P-gp is present in the intestinal side of the gut wall. For a drug that is a substrate of P-gp, when it enters the intestinal epithelia, some of its molecules will be pumped out the cells by P-gp and sent back to the intestinal lumen. This process may contribute to drug loss in the gut wall. Therefore, in addition to drug metabolism, efflux-transporter mediated drug efflux may also be a potential contributor to intestinal first-pass loss.

   P-gp is also expressed in the bile side of the liver. For a P-gp substrate, when it enters the hepatocytes, some drug molecules will be pumped out by P-gp and excreted into bile. This process may contribute to drug loss in the liver. Therefore, besides drug metabolism, drug efflux mediated by efflux transporters may also be a potential source of hepatic first-pass loss.

   Therefore, for drugs that are substrates of efflux transporters, their bioavailability could be low.

- *Role of uptake transporters in drug absorption.*

   Uptake transporters take the drug into the cells, which explains why they are called "uptake" transporters and why the arrows associated with them point into the cells (Figure 2-2). Different from efflux transporters which are localized in the apical side, uptake transporters can be expressed on either apical or basolateral side. To understand the role of uptake transporters in drug absorption, let's use two organic anion transporting polypeptides (OATP) isoforms, OATP2B1 and OATP1B1, as examples.

OATP2B1 is expressed on the apical side (facing the intestinal lumen) of the gut wall. OATP2B1 helps its substrate to enter the intestinal epithelia. Therefore, the bioavailability of an OATP2B1 substrate could be high.

OATP1B1 is present on the basolateral side (facing blood) of the liver. OATP1B1 takes the drug into hepatocytes. Some drugs are substrates of both OATP1B1 and P-gp, and these two transporters work in concert to move the drugs out of the body –OATP1B1 moves the drug into hepatocytes, and once the drug is in them, P-gp moves it into bile. For a drug that is a substrate of both an uptake transporter (on the basolateral side) and an efflux transporter (on the apical side), it could have poor bioavailability due to the joint effort of these two transporters in moving the drug into bile.

2.1.3. Calculation of bioavailability

As noted earlier, bioavailability (F) represents the fraction of the drug that reaches systemic circulation. F can be expressed as:

$$F = \frac{Amount\ of\ drug\ reaching\ systemic\ circulation}{Total\ amount\ of\ drug\ administered\ (i.e.,dose)}$$

If a drug is given through I.V. administration, F equals to 1 since 100% of the dose is available in systemic circulation. For an orally administered drugs, F has a value between 0 (no drug) to 1 (all of the administered drug). A drug's oral bioavailability can be calculated based on its dose and AUC information.

- *Absolute bioavailability*

Absolute bioavailability is the amount of drug from an oral dose that reaches systemic circulation relative to an I.V. dose. To determine a drug's absolute oral bioavailability, both an oral dose and an I.V dose need to be evaluated. After collecting blood samples at different time points (usually > 8 samples), drug concentrations are measured, and the AUC of the plasma concentration-time curve is calculated. The oral dose and I.V. dose used in the study could be the same or different. The absolute bioavailability of a drug can be calculated based on the dose and AUC information using the following equation:

$$F = \frac{AUC_{oral} \times Dose_{iv}}{AUC_{iv} \times Dose_{oral}}$$

Absolute bioavailability is often unavailable for drugs that are marketed for oral administration only. For those drugs, the I.V. formulation usually does not exist.

- *Relative bioavailability*

Relative bioavailability is the amount of drug from an oral formulation (i.e., test formulation) that reaches systemic circulation relative to a different non-IV formulation (i.e., reference formulation). The doses of the test formulation and reference formulation could be the same or different. The relative bioavailability of a drug can be calculated using the following equation:

$$F = \frac{AUC_{test} \times Dose_{reference}}{AUC_{reference} \times Dose_{test}}$$

Relative bioavailability is frequently evaluated during drug development. For example, the drug formulation used in a later phase study (e.g. Phase 2 and Phase 3 studies) may not be the same as the one used in the first-in-human (FIH) study. In this case, a relative bioavailability study needs to be conducted to make sure that the extent of drug absorption of the new formulation (i.e., test formulation) is comparable to that of the original formulation (i.e., reference formulation). Similarly, the food effect on drug pharmacokinetics is routinely evaluated during drug development, and the relative bioavailability of the drug is calculated to compare the extent of drug absorption between fasted (i.e., without food) and un-fasted/fed (i.e., with food) conditions.

Relative bioavailability is also closely related to bioequivalence. You may have heard of brand-name drugs (the innovator) and generic drugs (the "copycat"). Generic companies need to perform a bioequivalence study to prove that their product is equivalent to the innovator drug. Bioequivalence is determined based on the relative bioavailability of the innovator medicine versus the generic medicine. A certain criterion is used for bioequivalence evaluation. For example, the 90% confidence interval for the relative bioavailability should be within 0.80–1.25.

2.2 Rate of Oral Absorption

Different oral formulations of the same drug can vary substantially in their rate of absorption. For solid oral dosage forms, the conventional form is the immediate release (IR) dosage form. IR medications can be absorbed quickly just as their name indicates. Generally, an IR tablet or capsule instantaneously disintegrates after swallowing, making the drug quickly available for absorption into the systemic circulation. The advantage of an IR dosage form is that the drug can produce its pharmacological effect quickly; this can be important for diseases that require fast-acting medications (e.g. pain and insomnia). Another advantage of an IR dosage form, more from the manufacturing perspective, is that it is easier to formulate compared with other types of dosage forms.

While the IR formulation works quickly, the effect does not last long for drugs with a short half-life; this represents a disadvantage since patient compliance will be an issue if a medication needs to be taken multiple times a day. Therefore, for drugs with very short half-life, a slower rate of absorption with a stable effect over a longer time may be more desirable. Slow absorption can be achieved by manipulating the rate of drug release from the formulation. A common formulation for this purpose is the extended-release (ER) dosage form, usually labeled with "ER" or "XR" at the end of its name. The advantages of an ER dosage form include reduced frequency of drug administration, improved patient compliance, as well as less fluctuation in drug plasma concentrations across the course of the day. The disadvantages of an ER formulation include potential incomplete absorption and increased cost as it is usually more expensive than the IR dosage form.

There are two subtypes of ER dosage form: controlled-release (CR) formulation and sustained-release (SR) formulation. The CR dosage form releases the drug at a constant rate (e.g., 1 mg of the drug is released every minute). The SR dosage form releases the drug over a sustained period, and how much the drug is released per given time is dependent on the amount of drug remaining at the absorption site. Therefore, the absorption of CR dosage form is zero-order kinetics (behaves like Tom), while the absorption of SR form is first-order kinetics (behaves like Jerry).

Figure 2-3 summarizes the advantages and disadvantages of the immediate release (IR) and extended release (ER), as well as the features of controlled release (CR) and sustained release (SR) dosage forms.

	Immediate Release (IR)	Extended Release (ER)	
Advantage	➢ Produce drug effect quickly ➢ Easy to formulate	➢ Reduced frequency of drug administration ➢ Improved patient compliance ➢ Less fluctuation of drug levels	
Disadvantage	➢ May need to take multiple times a day for drugs with very short half-life; patient compliance issue	➢ Potential incomplete absorption ➢ Increased cost	
	Notes:	Subtypes	
		Controlled-release (CR)	Sustained-release (SR)
	Absorption is first-order kinetics	➢ Release the drug at a constant rate	Slow release over a sustained period but not at a constant rate
		➢ Absorption is zero-order kinetics	Absorption is first-order kinetics

Figure 2-3. Comparison of immediate release (IR) and extended release (ER), as well as the features of the controlled release (CR) and sustained release (SR) dosage forms.

The pharmacokinetic parameter associated with the rate of drug absorption is *absorption rate constant*, which is expressed as k_a. K_a is a zero-order rate constant for CR dosage forms and a first-order rate constant for both IR and SR formulations since they both undergo first-order absorption kinetics. For an IR dosage form, its absorption process usually is much faster than its elimination process. In contrast, the absorption process of an ER formulation could be slower than the drug's elimination rate. As a result, how fast the drug can be cleared is dependent on how fast the drug is absorbed, which means that an ER dosage form can artificially extend a drug's half-life; this is a phenomenon known as *flip-flop kinetics,* which will be discussed in Chapter 8.

2.3 Absorption from Other Extravascular Routes

In addition to oral administration, other common extravascular routes include intramuscular (I.M.) and subcutaneous (S.C.) administration. Regarding the extent of drug absorption, the bioavailability of a drug given via I.M. or S.C. injections usually is higher than the one given orally due to the following reasons:

- For I.M. or S.C. injections, the drug is prepared in a solution, instead of a solid dosage form. Accordingly, there is no drug solubility issue.
- There are minimal drug metabolizing enzymes and drug transporters expressed in muscle and subcutaneous tissues. Therefore, there is no first-pass loss as seen in orally administered drugs.
- The capillary membrane in muscle and subcutaneous tissues is much looser than the tight junction of the epithelial cells in gastrointestinal tract. As a result, there is less concern about potential drug permeability issue since even polar drugs with large molecular weight can easily pass through the capillary membrane.

Regarding the rate of drug absorption after I.M. and S.C. administrations, how fast the drug is absorbed is dependent on the local blood flow of the surrounding tissues. Muscle blood flow is higher than that of subcutaneous tissues. Accordingly, a drug given via I.M. injection is absorbed faster than that given through S.C. injection. When local blood flow changes, the rate of drug absorption could also change. For example, after a drug is given through I.M. administration, absorption is increased during exercise. Similarly, rubbing the area of injection can increase the absorption after a drug is given via S.C. injection.

2.4 Effect of Extent and Rate of Absorption on Pharmacokinetic Profiles

For a drug that is given via oral administration, its pharmacokinetics profile typically looks like what is shown in Figure 2-4. Plasma drug concentration is zero at the beginning since all drug molecules are still in the gastrointestinal site at that time. Then the absorption process starts. Accordingly, plasma concentration increases till it reaches the maximum concentration, which is expressed as C_{max}. The time needed to reach C_{max} is expressed as T_{max}. The rising portion of the curve is considered the *absorption phase*. This does not mean that the drug is not eliminated during this phase. On the contrary, the elimination process starts once the drug enters systemic circulation. It just means that the absorption process dominates during this phase. The moment the drug reaches its peak concentration is when the rate of absorption is identical to the rate of elimination. After that, the elimination process dominates, and accordingly drug concentrations decline in the body. The downward portion of the curve is known as the *elimination phase*.

When we have a concentration-time dataset for an orally administered drug, usually three parameters can be obtained relatively easily without performing compartment modeling: C_{max}, T_{max}, and AUC. C_{max} and T_{max} can be obtained from the dataset directly, they are also easy to spot from the concentration-time plot. AUC can be calculated using the trapezoidal rule introduced in Chapter 1. Do you know that these three parameters can provide valuable hints on the extent and rate of drug absorption? Following is the explanation:

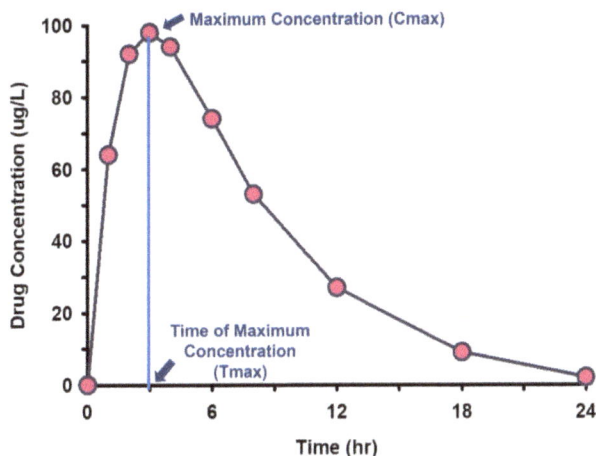

Figure 2-4. An example concentration-time profile after a drug is administered orally.

- When the amount of drug entering systemic circulation changes, C_{max} and AUC are affected. For example, when more drug molecules are absorbed (i.e., extent of absorption increases, F↑), the concentrations in blood are higher and the area under the curve is larger. In this case, both C_{max} and AUC increase.

- When the rate of drug absorption changes, T_{max} and C_{max} are affected. For example, when the same amount of the drug is absorbed faster (i.e., rate of absorption increases, k_a↑), the amount of drug absorbed per hour is increased and the absorption process is completed sooner. Therefore, the drug reaches its maximum concentration not only at a higher level but also more quickly. As a result, C_{max} increases and T_{max} decreases.

To elaborate on the above information, I use food/beverage – drug interactions as examples. Food can slow down gastric emptying, and accordingly will delay the time of drug arrival at the small intestine, the main site of drug absorption. Food is frequently found to change drug absorption by affecting the extent and/or rate of absorption. This is why food effect studies are often conducted during the drug development phase for new drugs intended for oral administration. Information on food-drug interactions usually is available in a drug's package insert. Let's look at the following four published reports, all of which involve food/beverage-drug interactions.

Example 1. Food- molnupiravir *interaction*

Molnupiravir is an anti-viral medication. Figure 2-5 shows the concentration-time profiles of molnupiravir under fasted (without food) and non-fasted (with food) conditions. As it shows, compared with fasted condition, C_{max} of molnupiravir is lower and T_{max} is longer when molnupiravir was administered with food. However, the AUC values are essentially the same between these two conditions. Based on the information of C_{max}, T_{max}, and AUC, we can conclude that food decreased the rate of molnupiravir absorption but had no impact on its extent of absorption.

Food- molnupiravir interaction

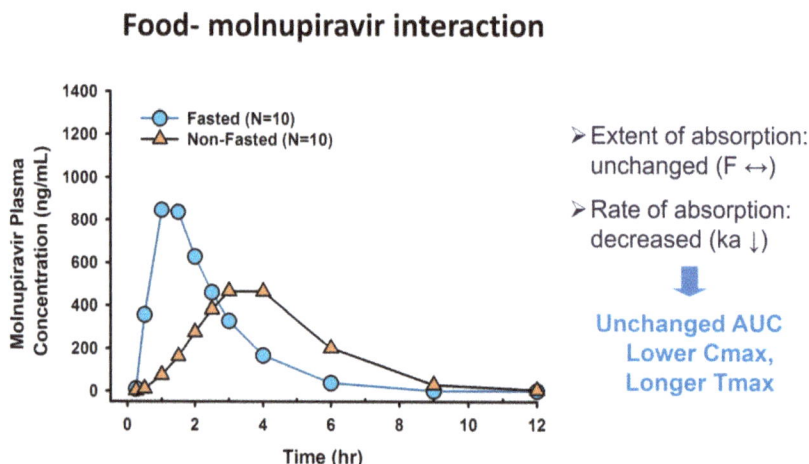

Figure 2-5. Molnupiravir pharmacokinetics under fasted (without food) and non-fasted (with food) conditions in 10 healthy subjects. *Adapted from: Painter WP, et al. Antimicrobial Agents and Chemotherapy 2021;65: e02428-20.*

***Example 2**. Food-aspirin interaction*

Aspirin is a nonsteroidal anti-inflammatory drug (NSAID) commonly used for reducing pain, fever, and/or inflammation. It is also used as a blood thinner. Figure 2-6 shows the concentration-time profiles of aspirin with and without food. From the plot we can clearly see that non-fasting group had a lower AUC, lower C_{max} and longer T_{max}, indicating that both the rate and extent of absorption of aspirin were affected. Food delayed gastric emptying, drugs entered small intestine slower, and accordingly decreased the rate of aspirin absorption. As the time that the drug stayed in the small intestine decreased, there wasn't enough time for drug absorption, leading to incomplete absorption (i.e. decreased extent of absorption, $F\downarrow$).

***Example 3**. Milk-ciprofloxacin interaction*

Ciprofloxacin is a fluoroquinolone antibiotic, a broad-spectrum antibiotic commonly used to treat different types of bacterial infections. Figure 2-7 shows the plasma concentration-time profiles of ciprofloxacin after administration with water or milk. As it shows, the curve from the milk group has the same T_{max}, lower C_{max}, and lower AUC compared to the water group, indicating that a less amount

Food-Aspirin Interaction

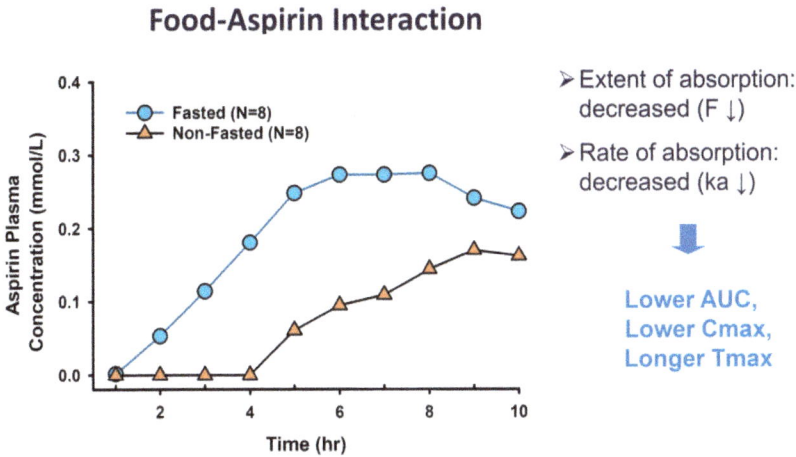

> Extent of absorption: decreased (F ↓)

> Rate of absorption: decreased (ka ↓)

**Lower AUC,
Lower Cmax,
Longer Tmax**

Figure 2-6. Plasma concentration-time profiles of aspirin under fasted (without food) and non-fasted (with food) conditions in 8 healthy male volunteers. *Adapted from: Bogentoft C, et al. European Journal of Clinical Pharmacology 1978;14(5):351-5.*

of drug got in the body in the presence of milk, albeit the drug was absorbed equally fast. Therefore, milk reduced the extent of ciprofloxacin absorption (F↓) but had no impact on the rate of absorption ($k_a \leftrightarrow$).

The mechanism of this example is different from the first two examples as milk does not affect gastric emptying. Milk contains high amounts of calcium, and calcium ions have a high affinity to ciprofloxacin. Therefore, milk reduces ciprofloxacin bioavailability because ciprofloxacin binds to calcium, forming insoluble chelates.

Milk-Ciprofloxacin Interaction

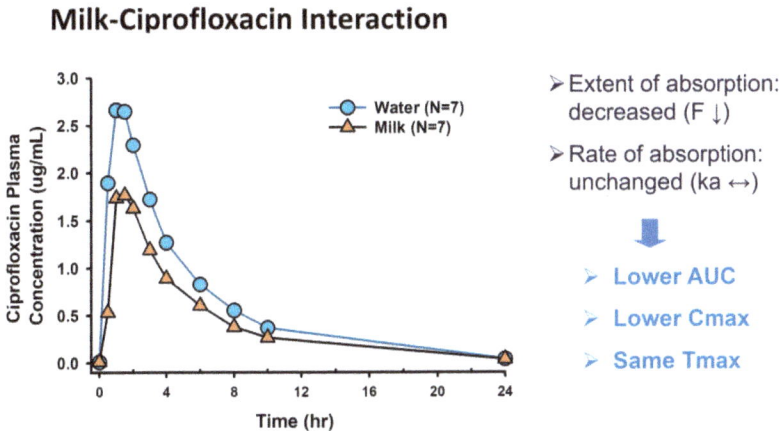

> Extent of absorption: decreased (F ↓)

> Rate of absorption: unchanged (ka ↔)

> **Lower AUC**

> **Lower Cmax**

> **Same Tmax**

Figure 2-7. Mean plasma concentration-time profiles of ciprofloxacin after administration of 500 mg ciprofloxacin with 300 ml of water or milk in 7 healthy volunteers.   *Adapted from: Neuvoren PJ et al. Clinical Pharmacology and Therapy 1991;50:498-502.*

Example 4. Green tea -nadolol interaction

Nadolol is a beta blocker medication that is used to treat high blood pressure. The effect of green tea on the pharmacokinetics of nadolol was investigated. As shown in Figure 2-8, when nadolol was taken with green tea, the curve has similar T_{max}, lower C_{max}, and lower AUC compared to the water group, suggesting that green tea reduced the extent of nadolol absorption ($F\downarrow$) but did not affect the rate of absorption ($k_a \leftrightarrow$).

Nadolol is a substrate of OATP1A2, an uptake transporter expressed in the apical side of the intestinal epithelial cells and facilitates the absorption of nadolol. Green tea is an OATP1A2 inhibitor. Therefore, green tea reduced the bioavailability of nadolol through OATP1A2 inhibition.

Green Tea- Nadolol Interaction

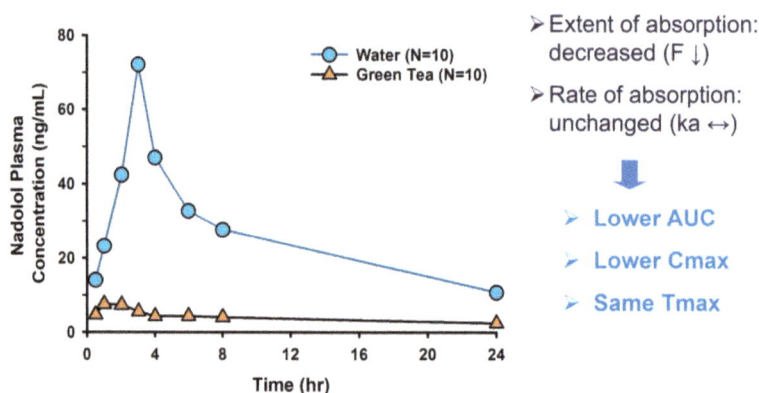

Figure 2-8. Plasma concentration-time profiles of nadolol after administration of 30 mg nadolol with water or green tea in 10 healthy volunteers.   *Adapted from: Misaka S, et al. Clinical Pharmacology and Therapeutics 2014;95(4):432-438.*

I hope the above examples give you a sense of which parameter(s) to consider when you suspect that there is a change in drug absorption. Although the above examples center on food/beverage-drug interactions, same principles can be applied to evaluate the interaction of a drug with another drug, herb, toxicant, or other types of xenobiotics.

2.5 Miscellaneous Notes

❖ *A story about efflux transporters:*

In addition to P-gp mentioned in section 2.1.2, another important efflux transporter is breast cancer resistance protein (BCRP). The name of BCRP may look strange at the first glance since we just learned that efflux transporters are expressed in normal tissues, such as the intestine and liver discussed in this chapter. Why is this transporter protein named "breast cancer resistance protein"? This is because it was first identified in 1998 in breast cancer cells that were resistant to anticancer drugs. BCRP, same as P-gp, is present in many different types of cancer cells. Many anticancer drugs are substrates of both BCRP and P-gp. Imagine, when an anticancer drug is trying to enter tumor cells to do its job, it keeps getting kicked out of the cells by BCRP and P-gp; this is NOT good. Therefore, efflux transporters, such as P-gp and BCRP, not only are present in normal tissues and play an important role in drug pharmacokinetics, but also are expressed in many types of cancer cells and represent an important mechanism of anticancer drug resistance.

❖ *Chemical form (S)*

Sometimes, the chemical form of a drug, expressed as S (i.e., salt factor), may also need to be considered when calculating bioavailability F. S represents the fraction of the dose that is the active drug. For example, aminophylline is the ethylenediamine salt of theophylline, the active moiety. For aminophylline, 80% to 85% by weight is theophylline. Therefore, the S for aminophylline is around 0.8. When you calculate the bioavailability of aminophylline tablets, the S of 0.8 should be included in the equation. Similarly, 300 mg of phenytoin sodium contains 276 mg of phenytoin, when means that the S is 0.92. Not all drugs need the incorporation of S during bioavailability evaluation as sometimes the manufacturers may have already labeled the amount of the active drug, resulting in S of 1. For example, valproate sodium tablets contain the sodium salt of valproic acid, and it is manufactured and labeled with the amount of valproic acid directly (i.e., S=1).

2.6 Case Study

This case study is based on the result of the oxfendazole food effect study published by my own group. Oxfendazole is an antiparasitic drug that is currently marketed for use against lungworms and enteric helminths in beef livestock. Due to its great efficacy and safety profiles in animals, FDA has granted fast track designation for the transition of oxfendazole from veterinary medicine to human antiparasitic treatment. Its pharmacokinetics, safety and tolerability have been evaluated in the FIH study. After the FIH study was completed, a food effect study was conducted to evaluate the effect of food on oxfendazole absorption. Figure 2-9 shows the concentration-time profiles of oxfendazole in humans with and without food (same dose was administered). The AUC, C_{max} and T_{max} information from both groups is presented in Table 2-1.

Table 2-1. Oxfendazole plasma exposure parameters under fed state versus fasted state

Parameter	Fasted state (mean value)	Fed state (mean value)
AUC_∞ (ng·h/mL)	36600	64500
C_{max} (ng/mL)	3010	4500
T_{max} (h)	1.99	8.90

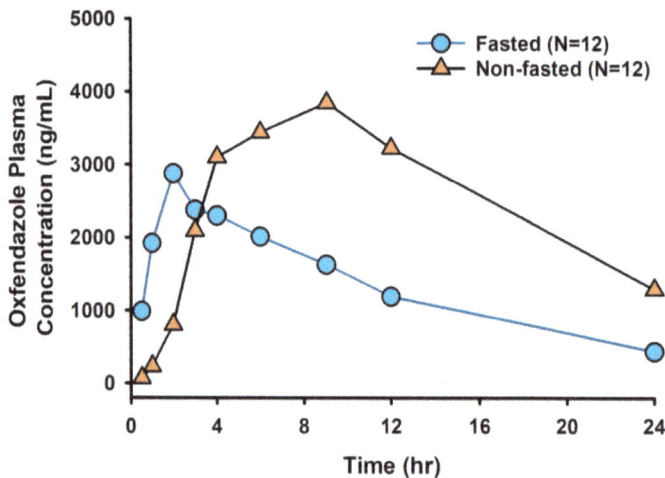

Figure 2-9. Plasma concentration-time profiles of oxfendazole in human after administration of 3 mg/kg oxfendazole under the fasted state and the fed state in 12 healthy volunteers. *Adapted from: Bach T, et al. Antimicrobial Agents and Chemotherapy 2020;64(1): e01018-20.*

Based on Figure 2-9 and Table 2-1, please answer the following questions:
  a) What is the effect of food on oxfendazole absorption?
  b) The potential mechanism of the observed food-oxfendazole interaction.
  c) Calculate the relative bioavailability of oxfendazole.
  d) Do you think oxfendazole under fed state is "bioequivalent" to the one under the fasted state (yes or no)? Please explain your answer.

I encourage you to first work on the questions yourself before you look at the answers provided below.

~ ~ ~

a) *Food increased the extent of oxfendazole absorption and reduced the rate of oxfendazole absorption.*

   Based on Table 2-1, the AUC of oxfendazole increased when the drug was given with food. This indicated that the amount of drug in the body was increased (i.e., F↑). T_{max} of oxfendazole also increased in the fed state, indicating that the drug was absorbed slower than that without food (ka↓). C_{max} is a parameter that can be affected by both the extent and rate of absorption. With the increase in F, C_{max} increases. With the decrease in K_a, C_{max} decreases. Therefore, when the extent of absorption increases but rate of absorption decreases, the direction of the change of C_{max} depends on which *side plays a bigger role. In this case, C_{max} increases, indicating that the extent of absorption has a bigger effect than the rate of absorption.*

b) *Food delayed the gastric emptying process and accordingly reduced the rate of oxfendazole absorption. Oxfendazole is a lipophilic drug with poor solubility. During fed state, the gallbladder releases bile into the intestine. It is well known that bile salts can enhance the solubility of a drug and function as drug absorption enhancers, especially for drugs with poor solubility. That is why food increased the extent of oxfendazole absorption.*

c) *The relative bioavailability of oxfendazole in the fed condition compared to the fast condition is 1.76.*

$$F = \frac{AUC_{test} \times Dose_{reference}}{AUC_{reference} \times Dose_{test}} = \frac{64500}{36600} = 1.76$$

d) *Oxfendazole under fed state will be "bioequivalent" only if the 90% confidence interval for the relative bioavailability is within 0.80–1.25. In Table 2-1, 90% confidence interval of the relative bioavailability is not provided. However, based on the mean ratio of 1.76, which is much higher than the upper limit of 1.25, oxfendazole under fed condition is unlikely to be bioequivalent to that under fast condition.*

Problem Sets   *(Answers to study problems are in the appendix)*

1. When a drug is absorbed more slowly, T_{max} will be longer, however C_{max} will remain unchanged.
   A. True
   B. False
2. When a drug is given via non-oral extravascular routes, in general, it is impossible for the manufacturer to make a sustained release product, but making a controlled release product may be possible.
   A. True
   B. False
3. When a drug is given at 100 mg via I.V. bolus, the AUC is 500 mg*h/L. When 200 mg dose of drug is given orally, and the AUC is 750 mg*h/L. Please calculate the absolute oral bioavailability of this drug.
       The bioavailability is _____
4. When the extent of drug absorption is changed, which of the following parameters will be affected (choose all that apply)?
   A. C_{max}
   B. T_{max}
   C. AUC
   D. All of the above

5. As uptake transporters help the drug enter the cells, the bioavailability of their substrates must be reduced when the drug is co-administered with an inhibitor of the same uptake transporter.
   A. True
   B. False
6. Followings are some of the factors that can potentially affect drug bioavailability (choose all that apply)
   A. Drug solubility.
   B. Drug permeability.
   C. Drug absorption rate.
   D. Drug stability in gastrointestinal lumen.
   E. First-pass metabolism
7. The relative bioavailability of a drug can be obtained without the need of using I.V. dose as the reference.
   A. True
   B. False
8. During the drug absorption phase, no drug molecules will be eliminated from the body.
   A. True
   B. False
9. For a drug with ER dosage form, how fast the drug can be cleared is dependent on how fast the drug is absorbed. An ER dosage form often can artificially extend a drug's half-life.
   A. True
   B. False
10. Hepatic clearance determines CL and plays no role in bioavailability.
    A. True
    B. False

Chapter 3.

Distribution

Learning Objectives

After reading this chapter, the reader shall be able to:

1. Understand the extent of distribution and rate of distribution.

2. List the factors that affect drug distribution.

3. Calculate volume of distribution based on drug protein binding data.

4. Define the terms "fraction unbound" and "plasma protein binding".

5. List the major plasma proteins and the major factors that affect drug protein binding.

6. Understand the relationships between tissue and plasma protein binding, the accessible tissue volume, and the volume of distribution.

7. Define perfusion limited distribution and permeability limited distribution.

8. Judge whether for a certain drug a change in protein binding will affect the free drug levels.

Regardless of the route of administration, once a drug reaches systemic circulation, the distribution process starts. The general considerations of drug properties and membrane characteristics that affect drug distribution are discussed in section 3.1. Drug distribution has two aspects: *how much* the drug is distributed into tissues (i.e., *extent of distribution*) and *how fast* the drug is distributed into tissues (i.e., *rate of distribution*). These two aspects are elaborated in section 3.2 and section 3.3, respectively. Several miscellaneous topics, including the practical consideration of estimating volume of distribution, are covered in section 3.4. Then this chapter ends with problem sets. I did not allocate a separate section for case study because there are 3 case studies embedded in sections 3.2 and 3.3.

3.1 Drug Properties and Membrane Characteristics that Affect Drug Distribution

3.1.1 Properties of the drug and the membrane that are important for transmembrane passage of drugs.

Once a drug enters the bloodstream, it will follow the circulatory path of the blood. While it travels in systemic circulation, drug molecules move across endothelial membranes and enter tissues. For drugs that transport via passive diffusion (i.e., non-carrier-mediated process), the movement of drugs across the membrane occurs by passive transcellular (through cell) and paracellular (around cell) pathways, as shown in Figure 3.1. Some drugs readily move across a membrane, while others do not. The ability of a drug to pass through the membrane is defined as drug *permeability*. The following are three major drug properties that determine permeability:

- *Lipophilicity* In general, the more lipophilic ('lipid-loving') the drug, the higher is its permeability, and accordingly the easier for the drug to pass through the membrane. A common way to evaluate the lipophilicity of a drug is to measure the ratio of its concentration between a nonpolar phase (n-octanol) and an aqueous phase (water), a parameter known as *partition coefficient*. The higher the partition coefficient, the greater the drug's lipophilicity. The logarithm of the partition coefficient is known as LogP.

- *Charge (or degree of ionization)* Charged (i.e., ionized) drugs are difficult to move across the membrane. Based on the pH partition hypothesis, only the un-ionized nonpolar form of a drug can penetrate the membrane. Please note that this hypothesis mainly applies to drugs moving through the membrane via passive transcellular pathway; it may not be suitable to those involving transporters, or small-sized drugs that can pass through the membrane via paracellular pathway. Nevertheless, charge remains a major constraint to transmembrane passage. Accordingly, the degree of ionization is an important factor in determining permeability. The percentage of a drug in its unionized form can be calculated based on the drug's pKa and the environment pH.

- *Size* For hydrophilic ("water loving") drugs that cannot permeate through the lipid membrane via the transcellular pathway, some of them may be able to pass across the membrane through the paracellular route. Whether a drug can move paracellularly is dependent on the size of the drug as well as the intercellular space between the cells (i.e., the tightness of the intercellular junctions). Examples of drugs utilizing the paracellular route include the β-receptor antagonist atenolol and the H_2-receptor antagonists cimetidine, both of which are hydrophilic and have small size (molecular weight within 250–270 g/mol).

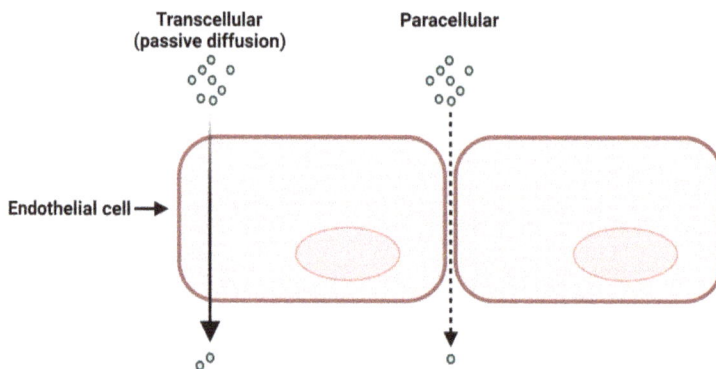

Figure 3-1. For the drug that transport via passive diffusion, the movement of drugs across membrane occurs by passive transcellular (through cell) and/or paracellular (around cell) pathways.

In addition to the drug properties mentioned above, namely, lipophilicity, charge, and size, the characteristics of the membrane could also affect the transmembrane passage of drugs. Some membranes, such as blood capillaries in most tissues, are loosely knit and are highly permeable to molecules up to 5000 g/mol in size. In these cases, even hydrophilic or charged drugs with relatively large molecular weight (e.g. >500 g/mol), can readily pass through paracellularly via large fenestrations ("pores") in the membrane. On the other hand, some membranes are more tightly knit (e.g. gastrointestinal membranes, blood brain barrier) and are more difficult for hydrophilic drugs to pass through.

Other than the tightness of the intercellular junctions, other factors that can affect the transport of drug include membrane thickness and surface area. In general, the thinner the membrane, the shorter the distance and the higher the permeability. Similarly, the larger the surface area, the higher the drug penetration rate.

3.1.2. Role of transporters in drug distribution

In Section 3.1.1, I only mentioned passive diffusion, through which the drug moves across the membrane via a passive transcellular pathway or a paracellular pathway. Passive diffusion represents the dominant route for many drugs, but not all. For some drugs, in addition to passive diffusion, they also move across the membrane with the help of drug transporters. In Chapter 2, under section 2.1.2, we have learned that drug transporters are expressed in the intestine and the liver and can play an important role in the absorption of orally administered drugs that are substrates of the transporters. The presence of drug transporters is not limited to the intestine and the liver; they are also expressed in several other tissues and can play a role in drug distribution. A typical example is the blood-brain barrier (BBB), a physiological interface hosting many drug transporters, including both efflux transporters and uptake transporters (Figure 3-2).

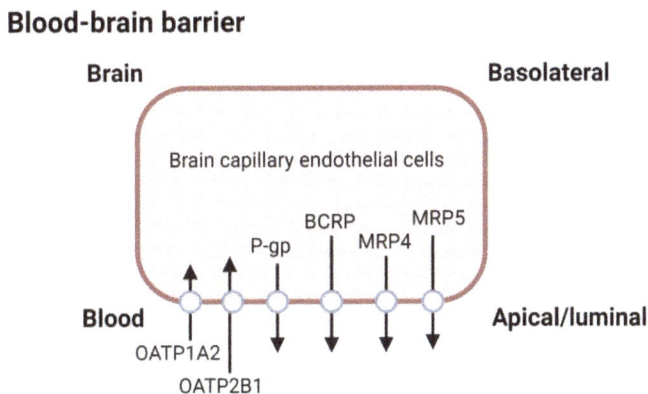

Figure 3-2. The presence of drug transporters in the blood-brain barrier.

The brain capillary endothelial cells forming the BBB are polarized cells, which means that they have an apical/luminal side (facing blood) and a basolateral side (facing brain). Drug transporters are expressed on the apical side of the BBB. The role of these transporters in drug distribution into brain is dependent on the direction in which they transport drugs (as indicated by the straight arrows). Efflux transporters pump the drug out of the brain endothelial cells and the drug is "kicked" back into the blood. Therefore, efflux transporters limit the brain distribution of their substrates. On the other hand, uptake transporters facilitate a drug's distribution in the brain by taking the drug from the blood into the cells. The major efflux transporters located in the BBB include P-glycoprotein (P-gp), breast cancer resistance protein (BCRP), and multi-drug resistance proteins (MRPs). The major uptake transporters present in the BBB include organic anion transporting polypeptides (OATPs).

Among all drug transporters, P-gp is the most studied due to its broad substrate spectrum - numerous drugs have been found to be transported by P-gp. When the site of action is in the brain, P-gp poses a big issue for drugs that are its substrates. A well-known case is the use of anticancer drugs to treat brain tumors, including primary brain tumors and brain metastases (cancer cells spread from other places to brain). Many anticancer drugs, including both conventional cytotoxic chemotherapies (e.g., mitoxantrone, doxorubicin) and the newer targeted therapies (e.g., tyrosine kinase inhibitors), have poor brain distribution due to P-gp mediated drug efflux. Accordingly, anticancer drugs that are P-gp substrates are largely ineffective against brain tumors.

Being a substrate of P-gp is not always a bad thing. In certain situations, researchers may intentionally design a compound to be transported by P-gp to avoid its brain penetration. An interesting example is antihistamines. The first-generation antihistamines, such as chlorpheniramine and diphenhydramine, can cause drowsiness due to their ability to pass through the BBB. The second-generation antihistamines, including azelastine, cetirizine, and fexofenadine, are all good substrates of P-gp. As a result, these second-generation antihistamines all have poor brain distribution and accordingly have no side effect of drowsiness.

3.2 The Extent of Drug Distribution

3.2.1 The concept of volume of distribution (V_d)

The extent of drug distribution (i.e., how much the drug gets into tissues) can be reflected by the volume of distribution V_d, a fundamental pharmacokinetic parameter that we have learned a little bit in Chapter 1 (see section 1.5.3). Let's briefly refresh the definition of V_d. V_d is the "apparent" volume of the body if a drug is present throughout the body at the same concentration as it is in plasma:

$$Volume\ of\ distribution\ (V_d) = \frac{Amount\ of\ drug\ in\ the\ body}{plasma\ concentration} \qquad [3\text{-}1]$$

For drugs given via I.V. bolus dose, their volume of distribution can be calculated using the dose and the initial plasma concentration C_0:

$$V_d = \frac{Dose}{C_0}$$ [3-2]

When I taught the drug distribution session during my PharmD course *"Pharmacokinetics and Dose Optimization"*, many students were confused at the beginning about the volume of distribution and mistakenly thought that V_d should not exceed the body size. As already elaborated in Chapter 1, I would like to emphasize again that V_d is a hypothetical volume, and its value can be higher than the volume of our total body weight (e.g., 70 L for a 70-kg adult assuming the density of 1 between mass and volume).

Figure 3-3 shows the volume of distribution of several representative drugs. Clearly, the value of V_d varies widely among drugs. As shown, many antibiotics, such as ampicillin, meropenem, and aminoglycosides (e.g., amikacin, gentamicin, tobramycin), have a small volume of distribution because they are hydrophilic and are difficult to partition into tissue cells. As a result, their volume of distribution is close to the extracellular space, which is about 18 L for a 70-kg adult. The small V_d values of antibiotics indicate that they have limited tissue distribution. On the other hand, many anticancer drugs shown in Figure 3-3, including both conventional cytotoxic agents (e.g., paclitaxel, mitoxantrone, and doxorubicin) and targeted therapies (e.g., tyrosine kinase inhibitor imatinib), have a volume of distribution greatly exceeding the body size, with $V_d > 400$ L. These large V_d values indicate that these anticancer drugs distribute extensively to tissues.

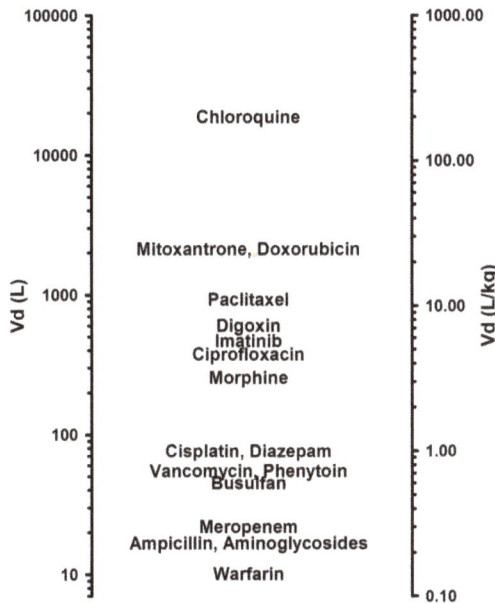

Figure 3-3. The volume of distribution of several representative drugs. The value of V_d among these drugs vary widely.

3.2.2 Plasma protein binding and tissue binding

After a drug reaches systemic circulation, a portion of the drug interacts with plasma proteins. As the drug-protein complex (i.e., bound drug) is too big to pass through the capillary walls, only the free drug (i.e. unbound drug) can diffuse out of the plasma and enter tissues. Similarly, the drug in tissues can interact with tissue components (e.g. proteins, lipids, DNA), and only the free drug can move back to plasma. Free drug in the plasma is in equilibrium with free drug in tissue. Therefore, there are two factors that influence the extent of drug distribution: binding to proteins in the plasma and binding to tissue components. Plasma protein binding is relatively easy to monitor due to easy access, while tissue binding usually cannot be measured directly. This section focuses on plasma protein binding since there is rich literature information on this topic.

Plasma proteins that interact with drugs: There are two different types of plasma proteins that interact with drugs:

- _Low-affinity, high-capacity binding proteins_

There are three major proteins in this category: _albumin, α_1-acid glycoprotein, and lipoproteins_. Albumin is the most abundant, with levels ranging from 3.4 to 5.4 g/dL in the blood (i.e., 34 to 54 g/L). α_1-acid glycoprotein and lipoproteins also have high concentrations, albeit less abundant than albumin. General information for these three proteins is presented in Table 3-1. Due to their high levels in the blood, these proteins are considered _high-capacity_ proteins, and they can rarely be saturated when drugs are given within therapeutic dose ranges (usually in mg dose range). They are also considered _low-affinity_ proteins because the affinity of drugs with these proteins is low, and drugs are associated with and dissociated from these proteins easily. This type of proteins is the one that drugs commonly interact with. Acidic drugs commonly bind to albumin, while basic drugs tend to bind to α_1-acid glycoprotein. Neutral lipophilic drugs often interact with lipoproteins.

This case can be viewed as a huge classroom (i.e., plasma protein) with numerous seats in the room (i.e. numerous binding sites on protein). When students (i.e., drugs) enter the room, they choose to sit on a chair and can stand and leave the room easily (i.e., low affinity). Because the room is so huge, students rarely can occupy all the seats (i.e., cannot saturate the protein).

- _High-affinity, low-capacity binding proteins_

In contrast to the proteins mentioned above, there are proteins with opposite features. Their levels in the blood are low (i.e., low capacity) and they can bind the drug tightly (i.e., high affinity). This type of protein binds specific compounds. Examples of such proteins include cortisol-binding globulin and sex-hormone binding globulin. This type of protein can be saturated relatively easily and the dissociation of the drug from the protein is a slow process.

This case can be viewed as a small classroom with limited seats. Once students sit on the chairs, either because there is glue on them or some other reason, students get stuck there and cannot get up and leave the room easily. Due to the limited number of seats, the room can be easily occupied.

Table 3-1. Major plasma proteins that interact with drugs.

Protein	Molecular weight (g/mol)	Normal Conc.	Types of Drugs Bound	Example
Albumin	67,000	34-54 g/L	Anionic; cationic; Acidic	Phenytoin, Diazepam
α₁-acid glycoprotein	42,000	0.4-1.0 g/L	Cationic; Basic	Quinidine
Lipoproteins	200,000-2,400,000	Variable	Lipophilic	Cyclosporine

Percentage of protein binding among drugs   Plasma protein binding varies widely among different drugs. As shown in Figure 3-4, protein binding can range from nearly 0 (e.g., metformin) to more than 99% (e.g., ibuprofen). Hydrophilic drugs, such as antibiotics, tend to have low plasma protein binding. In general, the higher the lipophilicity, the higher the percentage of protein binding.

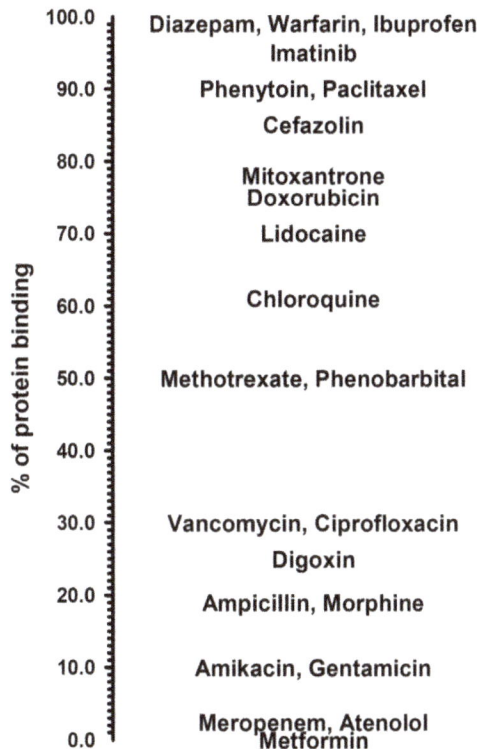

% of protein binding

100.0	Diazepam, Warfarin, Ibuprofen
	Imatinib
90.0	Phenytoin, Paclitaxel
	Cefazolin
80.0	Mitoxantrone Doxorubicin
70.0	Lidocaine
60.0	Chloroquine
50.0	Methotrexate, Phenobarbital
40.0	
30.0	Vancomycin, Ciprofloxacin
	Digoxin
20.0	Ampicillin, Morphine
10.0	Amikacin, Gentamicin
0.0	Meropenem, Atenolol Metformin

Figure 3-4. Percentage of plasma protein binding of several representative drugs.

Calculation of % protein binding and fraction of unbound drug   The percentage of plasma protein binding can be calculated based on total and free drug concentrations in plasma using the following formula:

$$\% \ protein \ binding = \frac{[total \ drug \ ]-[unbound \ drug]}{[total \ drug]} \times 100\%$$ [3-3]

It is generally agreed that only free drug can interact with its target, which means that only free drug is pharmacologically relevant. Therefore, there is a natural interest in estimating fraction of unbound drug (f_u) in plasma. f_u can be calculated using the following two equations:

$$f_u = \frac{(100 - \% \ protein \ binding)}{100}$$ [3-4]

$$f_u = \frac{[free \ drug \ concentration]}{[total \ drug \ concentration]}$$ [3-5]

Therefore, f_u can be calculated if % protein binding is known, and vice versa (i.e., % protein binding = $(1-f_u)\cdot 100\%$). The % of plasma protein binding of a drug is often provided in the package insert.

The fraction of unbound drug is associated with an associate constant and plasma protein level. Following is the expression of the relationship:

$$f_u = \frac{1}{1 + K_a \bullet f_{up} \bullet P_t}$$ [3-6]

Where:

f_u= fraction of unbound drug in the plasma,

K_a = associate constant,

f_{up} = fraction of free binding sites on the protein, and

P_t = total level of the plasma protein that interacts with the drug.

For albumin and other low-affinity high-capacity proteins, usually f_{up} is close to 1 because there are numerous binding sites, and the drug only interacts with a tiny portion of it. Therefore, based on equation 3-6, fraction of unbound drug remains relatively constant at a given protein concentration and *f_u is dose- and concentration-independent.*

Situations that may affect fraction of unbound drug   As noted above, for drugs that bind to high-capacity plasma proteins, their f_u remains constant within the therapeutic concentration ranges. However, the fact that f_u is dose- and concentration-independent does not mean that this value will never change. Following is the two situations that can affect the fraction of unbound drug:

- *Disease state*   Disease state can change the level of plasma proteins and subsequently affect f_u. For example, albumin concentration decreases with several diseases, including cirrhosis, burns, renal failure. Albumin level also decreases in pregnancy. Similarly, α_1-acid glycoprotein levels also change under disease conditions. For example, α_1-

acid glycoprotein concentrations are increased with surgery, myocardial infarction, Crohn's disease, and arthritis. These disease states affect the protein concentration, and P_t changes accordingly. Based on Equation 3-6, when P_t changes, f_u changes in the opposite direction. For instance, when albumin level drops, P_t decreases, f_u increases, indicating that there will be more free drugs available in plasma.

- *Drug-drug interaction*   When two drugs, which are known to be able to highly bind to the same protein, are co-administered, changes in the plasma protein binding of the drug of interest can occur. For example, both phenytoin and valproic acid have a high percentage of binding (~90%) to albumin. When these two drugs are administered concomitantly, valproic acid functions as a displacer and as such it displaces some of the phenytoin from the albumin, leading to a reduction in the protein binding of phenytoin (e.g. reduced from 90% to 80%) and an increased free fraction of unbound phenytoin. The change in f_u can also be predicted mathematically. When the displacement of a drug from protein occurs by a displacer, the associate constant K_a decreases. Based on Equation 3-6, when K_a decreases, f_u increases, indicating that there will be more free drugs available in plasma.

When the fraction of unbound drug changes, it may affect the volume of distribution and the free drug concentration level. These changes might have a significant impact on therapeutic and toxic effects, and dose adjustment may be necessary in some situations. The influence of changes in protein binding on the volume of distribution and free drug levels will be discussed in section 3.2.4.

3.2.3 Physiologic model – a conceptual perspective of the volume of distribution

While the volume of distribution V_d is a hypothetical volume and does not correspond to any specific tissue spaces, several factors discussed in the previous section, including plasma protein binding and tissue binding discussed, can influence a drug's volume of distribution. These factors can be incorporated into a physiological model to provide a conceptual perspective of the volume of distribution. Following is the equation:

$$V_d = V_p + V_t \cdot \frac{f_u}{f_{u,t}} \qquad\qquad [3\text{-}7]$$

Where:

V_d = volume of distribution,

V_p = plasma volume,

V_t = tissue volume,

f_u = fraction of unbound drug in the plasma, and

$f_{u,t}$ = fraction of unbound drug in the tissue.

Based on this equation, a drug's volume of distribution is dependent on the volume of the plasma, the volume of the tissue, the fraction of unbound drug in the plasma, and the fraction of unbound drug in the tissue. Change in any of these factors can affect a drug's volume of distribution. In the previous section, we learned how to calculate f_u and the factors (e.g. disease state, drug-drug interaction) that affect f_u. Tissue binding, as noted in the previous section, is difficult to measure, and $f_{u,t}$ often cannot be obtained directly. How about the plasma volume V_p and the tissue volume V_t? Can these two be estimated with physiological values? The answer is yes. To address this question, let's first look at the water in the human body, as drugs cannot move without water.

Up to 60% of the human adult body is water. As shown in Figure 3-5, for a 70-kg adult, the total body water is about 40 -42 L. Based on where the water is found within the body, total body water can be further categorized into extracellular water (i.e. outside of cells), which is about 18 L, and intracellular water (inside the cells), which is about 23 L. The extracellular water can either be in plasma or interstitial space. The plasma water and interstitial fluid are about 3 L and 15 L, respectively.

Based on Figure 3-5, for a 70-kg adult, the V_p of a drug is approximately 3 L. Regarding V_t, it is the accessible tissue volume, and its value is dependent on the properties of a drug. Most hydrophilic drugs may have hard time to enter tissue cells but will be able to distribute within the extracellular fluid, unless they are too big. Therefore, the V_t of a hydrophilic drug is approximately 15 L (i.e. the interstitial space). Lipophilic drugs can distribute throughout the body (entire extra- and intracellular space), and their V_t is about 38 L (i.e., 15 L interstitial fluid + 23 L intercellular fluid).

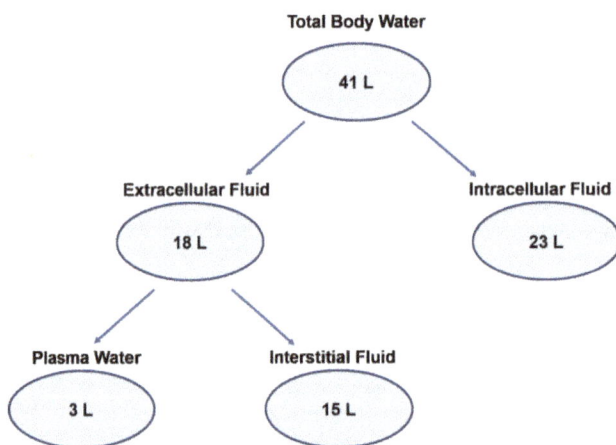

Total Body Water

41 L

Extracellular Fluid

18 L

Intracellular Fluid

23 L

Plasma Water

3 L

Interstitial Fluid

15 L

Figure 3-5. A picture of 70-kg human with respect to how much water and where is the water.

The definitions of V_p and V_t are straightforward, and their values are easy to get. In addition to V_p and V_t, as shown in equation 3-7, the volume of distribution is also dependent on the ratio of f_u and $f_{u,t}$, which means that both plasma protein binding and tissue binding matter. As shown in Figure 3-6, the extent of drug distribution is dependent on the result of a tug of war between plasma protein binding and tissue binding: if plasma protein binding is more pronounced than tissue binding (i.e. plasma wins; $\frac{fu}{fut}$ <1), more drug molecules are retained in the plasma; accordingly, V_d will be small. On the other hand, if tissue binding is more pronounced than plasma protein binding (i.e. tissue wins; $\frac{fu}{fut}$ >1), more drug molecules stay in the tissue, and the value of V_d could be big.

Binding in plasma   **Binding in tissue**

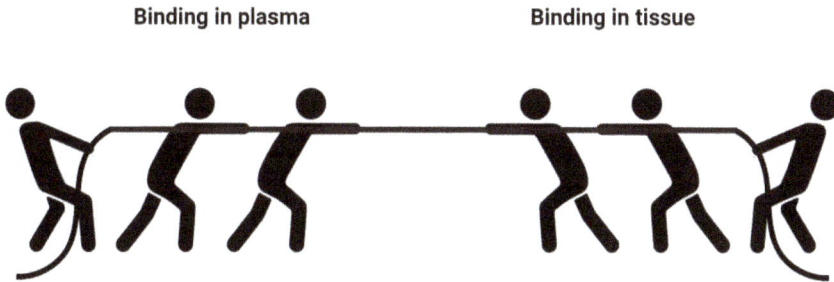

Figure 3-6. The extent of drug distribution is dependent on the result of a tug of war between plasma protein binding and tissue binding.

Case Example 3-1.

When I teach the distribution session in the class, every year I ask students the following true/false question:

Statement: "If a drug has extensive plasma protein binding, this drug must have small volume of distribution."

True or False?

If you like to make a judgment based on intuitive thinking, you may say this statement is true, since extensive plasma protein binding means more drug molecules will be retained in plasma, and accordingly V_d will be small.

During the class, I often encouraged my PharmD students to stop intuitive thinking and build a quantitative mindset, which means that they need to build a habit of solving problems using equations. Now back to the above T/F question. If we can find one example that a drug with extensive plasma protein binding has a large V_d value, we can confidently say that the above statement is "False".

~ ~ ~

Example: Drug A is a lipophilic drug, and it has extensive plasma protein binding (% of protein binding = 90%). Its tissue binding is 99%.

The V_d of Drug A can be calculate based on the following numbers:
$V_p = 3\ L$;
$V_t = 38\ L$ since it is a lipophilic drug;
$f_u = 0.1$ since plasma protein binding is 90%,
$f_{ut} = 0.01$ since tissue binding is 99%.
Based on the above numbers and equation 3-7, the V_d of Drug A is:

$$V_d = 3 + 38 \cdot \frac{0.1}{0.01} = 383\ L$$

Therefore, the statement made earlier is "False". In this example, Drug A has a large volume of distribution (i.e., 383 L), albeit it has extensive plasma protein binding. This is because its binding in tissue is even higher, which means that tissue wins the "tug of war" (see Figure 3-6).

The outcome of the example I showed here also occurs commonly in the real world. For example, paclitaxel has high plasma protein binding (90%) and its volume of distribution is more than 700 L. Similarly, imatinib, a drug with 98% oral bioavailability, has extensive plasma protein binding (95%) and large volume of distribution (370-470 L).

3.2.4 The impact of change in plasma protein binding in the volume of distribution and free drug levels.

Among the factors that determine a drug's volume of distribution, most of them, including plasma volume (V_p), accessible tissue volume (V_t) and fraction of unbound in tissue (f_{ut}), usually do not change. The one that we may need to pay attention is f_u, because the plasma protein binding of a drug may change during certain situations as discussed in section 3.2.2. When f_u changes, it may affect V_d according to equation 3-7 ($V_d = V_p + V_t \cdot \frac{f_u}{f_{u,t}}$). The change in V_d may subsequently affect initial drug concentration C_0 based on the following equation (for a drug given through I.V. bolus):

$$C_0 = \frac{Dose}{V_d} \tag{3-8}$$

As noted earlier, free drug is the one that is pharmacologically relevant. Change in f_u may affect the initial free drug concentration based on the following equation:

$$free\ C_0 = f_u \cdot \frac{Dose}{V_d} \tag{3-9}$$

Therefore, a change in plasma protein binding will affect f_u, which may subsequently influence V_d, total drug levels (e.g. C_0), and free drug levels (e.g. free C_0). Do we need to adjust the dose when a drug's f_u changes? How are V_d and free drug concentration affected by f_u among drugs with different percentage of protein binding? Let's look at the following case example and do some calculations. The result will naturally address the above questions.

Case Example 3-2.

Patient AG, 70-kg bodyweight, was administered 1000 mg Drug B via I.V. bolus. Drug B is a lipophilic drug with the following known information: V_p=3 L, V_t= 38 L, f_{ut}=0.1. In plasma, Drug B binds exclusively to albumin. Patient AG was diagnosed with cirrhosis recently, his albumin level dropped significantly. Accordingly, Drug B's f_u in this patient increased by 2-fold.

Scenario 1. Drug B has moderate plasma protein binding (50%). $f_u = 0.5$ under normal condition, f_u=1 under liver disease.

Scenario 2. Drug B has extensive plasma protein binding (99.5%). $f_u = 0.005$ under normal condition, f_u=0.01 under liver disease.

Please calculate V_d, C_0, and free C_0, and compare their values between normal and liver disease conditions in each scenario. Discuss if dose adjustment is needed in each scenario.

I encourage you to first work on the above case example yourself before you look at the calculations that I provide below.

$$\sim \sim \sim$$

Based on equations 3-7, 3-8, and 3-9, following is the calculations and results:

Scenario 1. V_p=3 L, V_t= 38 L, f_{ut}=0.1, fu = 0.5 under normal condition, fu=1 under liver disease.

$V_d = 3 + 38 \cdot \frac{0.5}{0.1} = 193\ L$ *(normal condition) vs* $V_d = 3 + 38 \cdot \frac{1}{0.1} = 383\ L$ *(liver disease)*

$C_0 = \frac{1000}{193} = 5.2\ mg/L$ *(normal condition) vs* $C_0 = \frac{1000}{383} = 2.6\ mg/L$ *(liver disease)*

free $C_0 = 0.5 \cdot \frac{1000}{193} = 2.6\ mg/L$ *(normal condition) vs free* $C_0 = 1 \cdot \frac{1000}{383} = 2.6\ mg/L$ *(liver disease)*

Scenario 2. V_p=3 L, V_t= 38 L, f_{ut}=0.1, fu = 0.005 under normal condition, fu=0.01 under liver disease.

$V_d = 3 + 38 \cdot \frac{0.005}{0.1} = 4.9\ L$ *(normal condition) vs* $V_d = 3 + 38 \cdot \frac{0.01}{0.1} = 6.8\ L$ *(liver disease)*

$C_0 = \frac{1000}{4.9} = 204\ mg/L$ *(normal condition) vs* $C_0 = \frac{1000}{6.8} = 147\ mg/L$ *(liver disease)*

free $C_0 = 0.005 \cdot \frac{1000}{4.9} = 1.0\ mg/L$ *(normal condition) vs free* $C_0 = 0.01 \cdot \frac{1000}{6.8} = 1.5\ mg/L$ *(liver disease)*

Conclusion: *With an increase in fu, the volume of distribution increases, and total drug concentrations will decrease. However, free drug levels may not change significantly for drugs with low or moderate plasma protein binding. In contrast, free drug level may increase greatly for drugs with extensive plasma protein binding (relative to tissue binding). Dose adjustment is not needed for scenario 1.*

Dose needs to be reduced in scenario 2 to avoid drug toxicity if Drug B has a narrow therapeutic window.

In the real world, a typical example that is analogous to scenario 2 is phenytoin. Phenytoin is an anticonvulsant drug used for seizure disorders. It binds to albumin extensively (90%) and is a narrow therapeutic window drug. When serum albumin level decreases, phenytoin's % plasma protein binding ↓, f_u↑, V_d↑ total concentration↓, and free phenytoin concentration↑. Free phenytoin concentrations are associated with efficacy/toxicity. Therefore, when albumin level drops, free phenytoin concentrations increase, toxicity may occur if dose adjustment is not performed. This is exactly the case as shown in Figure 3-7 – with a decrease in serum albumin, the percentage of patients with adverse effects of phenytoin increased.

Side effects of phenytoin can also occur when it is given together with valproic acid, an anticonvulsant drug that binds to albumin extensively. When these two drugs are given together, valproic acid competes for albumin binding and functions as a displacer. As a result, phenytoin % plasma protein binding ↓, f_u↑, V_d↑ total concentration↓, and free phenytoin concentration↑. Therefore, the side effect of phenytoin can occur if dose adjustment is not performed.

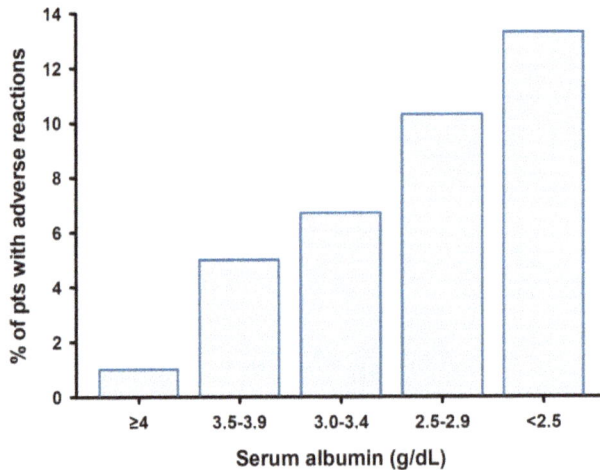

Figure 3-7. Adverse reactions to phenytoin as a function of serum albumin levels. *(adapted from Table 1 of Boston Collaborative Drug Surveillance Program. Clin Pharmacol Ther 14:529-532, 1973)*

3.3 The Rate of Drug Distribution

In addition to *how much* the drug is distributed into tissues (i.e., extent of distribution) discussed in section 3.2, drug distribution has another aspect - *how fast* the drug is distributed into tissues (i.e., rate of distribution). There are two scenarios for the rate of distribution: *perfusion rate limited distribution* and *permeability rate limited distribution*.

3.3.1 Perfusion rate limited distribution

In this scenario, the tissue membrane presents essentially no barrier, either because the drug is highly lipophilic and can pass through the membrane very fast, or because the membrane is loosely knit, allowing drugs to readily move across it. How fast the drug enters tissues depends on how much blood gets pumped through specific organs per given time (i.e., organ blood flow). Therefore, distribution is rate-limited by perfusion in this case.

Blood flow varies widely among different organs. The blood flow of several major organs in a standard 70-kg healthy adult is presented in Table 3-2. For drugs with perfusion-rate limited distribution (e.g. small lipophilic drugs), they will reach highly perfused organs (e.g. heart, liver, lung, kidneys, spleen) faster than poorly perfused organs (bone, skin, adipose).

Table 3-2. Blood flow of 10 representative organs in a standard 70-kg healthy adult.

Organ	Percent of body weight (%)	Blood flow (ml/min)	Perfusion rate (mL/min per g of tissue)
Bone	16	250	0.02
Brain	2.0	700	0.5
Adipose	15	200	0.025
Heart	0.4	200	0.6
Kidney	0.5	1100	4.0
Liver	2.3	1350	0.8
Lung	1.6	5000	10
Muscle	43	750	0.025
Skin	11	300	0.04
Spleen	0.3	77	0.4
Total body	100	5000	0.071

I noticed that students sometime are not sure if brain and muscle are highly perfused organs or poorly perfused organs. The brain is a high perfused organ since it has a high perfusion rate per g of tissue (i.e., 0.5 mL/min per g tissue). However, the tricky part is, for most drugs, their distribution into the brain is not rate-limited by perfusion due to the presence of BBB. On the other hand, although muscle blood flow is similar to brain blood flow (750 ml/min vs 700 ml/min), muscle is a poorly perfused organ because the perfusion rate is quite small after tissue weight normalization (0.025 mL/min per g of tissue). Propofol is a small lipophilic drug (MW=178 g/mol) and can pass through BBB easily. Therefore, propofol enters the brain much more rapidly than in muscle; this is expected considering that the brain has a much higher perfusion rate than muscle (0.5 mL/min g brain tissue vs 0.025 mL/min g muscle tissue).

3.3.2 Permeability rate limited distribution

In this scenario, the tissue membrane presents a barrier, either because the drug is hydrophilic and has difficulty in passing through the membrane, or because the membrane has tight junction so the drug cannot cross it easily. How fast the drug enters tissue is dependent on the drug's permeability, instead of organ blood flow. In this case, distribution is rate-limited by permeability. Permeability rate limited distribution often occurs for hydrophilic drugs diffusing across tightly knit membranes.

For permeability rate limited distribution, the physicochemical properties of a drug determine how fast the drug can enter the tissue. To elaborate the impact of physicochemical properties of drugs on permeability and distribution rate, a great example is the result of an old study that was published in 1960, which is more than 60 years ago. I use it as a case study here.

Case Example 3-3.

In this study, how fast several drugs, including thiopental, pentobarbital, barbital, salicylic acid, and sulfaguanidine, can enter the brain was evaluated. As shown in Table 3-3, the time to reach 50% equilibrium, a parameter reflecting the rate of brain distribution, ranges from the shortest for thiopental to the longest for sulfaguanidine (see circled column). Can you look at the physicochemical properties of these drugs listed in this table and explain why their rate of distribution are different? Please work on it yourself before looking at the explanations.

Table 3-3. Impact of physicochemical properties of drugs on permeability and rate of drug distribution (from: *J Pharmacol Exp Ther 1960; 130: 20-25*)

Drug	Time to reach 50% equilibrium (min)	Molecular weight (g/mol)	pKa	Fraction un-ionized at pH 7.4	Partition coefficient of un-ionized form	Effective partition coefficient at pH 7.4
Thiopental	1.4	264	7.6	0.6	3.3	2.0
Pentobarbital	4	232	8.1	0.8	0.05	0.042
Barbital	27	184	7.5	0.6	0.002	0.012
Salicylic acid	115	138	3.0	0.004	0.12	0.005
Sulfaguanidine	231	214	>10	1.0	0.001	<0.001

~ ~ ~

As shown in the third column in Table 3-3, these 5 drugs all have small molecular weight (130-270 g/mol). Therefore, size is not the factor contributing to the difference of their rate of brain distribution. There are two factors that are important in this case:

- Degree of ionization. For drugs that undergo passive diffusion, their ionized form cannot pass through the membrane. Therefore, the fraction of un-ionized form is an important factor. The higher the fraction of un-ionized form, the more drug molecules get the chance to pass through the membrane. The fraction of un-ionized

form of a drug is determined by the drug's pKa (the 4th column) and the environment pH (7.4 in this case). For example, thiopental has pKa of 7.6; this means that at pH 7.6, 50% of thiopental presents as the ionized form and 50% presents as the un-ionized form. When the environmental pH is 7.4, the fraction of thiopental in un-ionized form is 0.6 (i.e. 60% drug molecules are uncharged).

- Partition coefficient of un-ionized form   A drug with a high fraction of un-ionized form is not guaranteed an easy membrane passage. If the un-ionized form is polar, the drug still faces the difficulty in crossing the membrane. Therefore, the partition coefficient of the un-ionized form matters (the 6th column). The higher the partition coefficient, the more lipophilic of the un-ionized form, the easier the drug passes through the membrane.

Therefore, how fast a drug can pass through a tightly knit membrane (BBB in this case) depends on how much the drug remains as the un-ionized form and how lipophilic the un-ionized form is (assuming only passive diffusion and no involvement of drug transporters). The product of these two factors is effective partition coefficient, which is calculated as fraction of un-ionized form multiplied by partition coefficient of un-ionized form (see the last column of the table). The higher the value of effective partition coefficient, the shorter the time needed for a drug to move across the membrane. Based on this information, you can easily understand why the rate of distribution is quite different among thiopental, pentobarbital, barbital, salicylic acid, and sulfaguanidine.

3.4 Miscellaneous Notes

❖ When you calculate the volume of distribution based on the information of drug amount and concentration, pay attention to where the drug is measured. Drug concentration is usually measured in plasma. This may not be appropriate for drugs that are extensively partitioned into red blood cells. For those drugs, their concentrations in plasma may be low since the drug in the blood cells is removed during centrifugation. As a result, the calculated volume of distribution may be high using plasma concentration, albeit the drug may not have extensive distribution. For example, tacrolimus is extensively taken up by red blood cells. The apparent volume of distribution based on plasma concentrations (about 30 L/kg) is a lot higher than the value obtained using blood concentrations (1.0 to 1.5 L/kg). Similarly, chloroquine, an antimalarial drug, binds to red blood cells extensively. Using plasma concentration, the V_d value of chloroquine is higher than it should be.

❖ In Figure 3-3, I provided the V_d values of many representative drugs, all of which are I.V. administered. For orally administered drugs, their absolute bioavailability F is often unavailable. As a result, the calculated volume of distribution of an orally administered drug actually is V_d/F, instead of V_d. For an orally administered drug with poor bioavailability (e.g. F<0.1), a large apparent volume of distribution (i.e. V_d/F) could result from a small F, instead of a large V_d. Therefore, a large V_d/F does not necessarily mean that the drug (orally administered) for sure will have extensive tissue distribution.

Problem Sets   *(Answers to study problems are in the appendix)*

1. Due to the nature of biological membranes, drugs that are non-ionized and hydrophilic are more likely to cross most membrane barriers.
    A. True
    B. False
2. The larger the volume of distribution of a drug, the more drug is outside of plasma and the higher the clearance.
    A. True
    B. False
3. If a drug has extensive tissue protein binding, this drug must have large volume of distribution.
    A. True
    B. False
4. A hydrophilic drug with 80% plasma protein binding and 90% tissue binding is administered to a 70-kg human adult. The V_d of this drug is approximately _____ L.
5. For a drug that binds to high-affinity and low-capacity plasma proteins, its f_u is independent of drug concentrations.
    A. True
    B. False
6. Anionic drugs and weak acids are more likely to bind to:
    A. Globulin
    B. Albumin
    C. Lipoprotein
    D. $\alpha 1$-acid glycoprotein
7. Drugs that are very hydrophilic tend to distribute poorly into tissues.
    A. True
    B. False
8. Drug M is a lipophilic drug with a Vd of 41 L. What is the resulting V_d if the plasma protein binding decreased by 50%? V_d will be _____ L.
9. For a drug that binds to low-affinity and high-capacity plasma proteins, its f_u may be affected by:
    A. Drug concentrations.
    B. Doses.
    C. Drug-drug interactions.
    D. Disease states.
10. Change in plasma protein binding may affect the drug's half-life.
    A. True
    B. False

Chapter 4.
Elimination

Learning Objectives

After reading this chapter, the reader shall be able to:

1. Gain basic understanding of drug metabolizing enzymes and drug transporters.

2. Understand hepatic clearance, high and low extraction drugs.

3. Understand the effects of blood flow, intrinsic clearance, and protein binding on hepatic clearance for high and low extraction drugs.

4. Predict oral bioavailability based on hepatic clearance.

5. Define glomerular filtration, tubular secretion, and tubular reabsorption as processes of renal elimination.

6. Determine the relationship between pH (or urine flow) and renal clearance.

7. Estimate renal function based on creatine clearance using Cockcroft and Gault Method

8. Predict how physiological changes may affect pharmacokinetic parameters (CL, V_d, k_e, $t_{1/2}$) and change pharmacokinetics profiles.

Pharmacokinetics can be viewed as a drug's journey through the body, and it includes the processes of ADME. The phases of A (i.e., absorption) and D (i.e., distribution) have been discussed in Chapter 2 and Chapter 3, respectively. The M (i.e., metabolism) and E (i.e., excretion) represent different ways for our body to remove the drug. Therefore, both processes belong to *elimination*, which is the topic of this chapter. The basic background information of drug metabolizing enzymes and transporters, as well as their respective roles in drug metabolism and excretion, are provided in section 4.1. Drug elimination mainly occurs in two organs: liver and kidney. The removal of a drug through the liver is expressed as *hepatic clearance*, which is elaborated in section 4.2. The removal of a drug via the kidney is described as *renal clearance*, which is covered in section 4.3. Changes in physiological conditions affect pharmacokinetics parameters; these effects are discussed in section 4.4. Several case examples are provided throughout sections 4.1-4.4. A few miscellaneous notes are provided in section 4.5, then this chapter ends with problem sets.

4.1 General Information on Drug Metabolism and Excretion

4.1.1 Drug metabolizing enzymes and their role in drug metabolism

4.1.1.1 Phase 1 and Phase 2 metabolism

As shown in Figure 4-1 (left column), among the top 200 small-molecule drugs, about three-quarters are eliminated through metabolism. Metabolism is often divided into the following two phases of biochemical reaction:

- *Phase 1 metabolism*   Phase 1 reactions include oxidation, reduction, and hydrolysis. These reactions can either unmask or insert a polar function group (e.g., -OH, -SH, -NH2) in the drug. As a result, a drug undergoing phase I reaction is converted to one or more different substances, which generally are more polar (water soluble) and are easier excreted out of the body. Usually we call the drug "parent drug" and the converted substances "metabolites". Although there are several families of phase 1 drug metabolizing enzymes (e.g. flavin monooxygenase (FMO), alcohol dehydrogenase (ADH), aldehyde dehydrogenase (ALDH)), the cytochrome P450 (CYP) superfamily is by far the most important. As shown in Figure 4-1 (middle column), among the drugs cleared by metabolism, around three-quarters are metabolized by members of the CYP superfamily.

- *Phase 2 metabolism*   Phase 2 reactions include glucuronidation, acetylation, and sulfation. These reactions are also called ""conjugation reactions" because the parent drug is conjugated ("attached") with endogenous polar groups, such as glucuronate (MW=194 g/mol), acetate (MW=59 g/mol), and sulfate (MW=96 g/mol). As a result, the parent drug is converted to a metabolite that is more polar, bulkier, and easier to be excreted out of the body. Phase 2 drug metabolizing enzymes not only conjugate the parent drug, but also often conjugate the phase 1 metabolites to facilitate their elimination. Among phase 2 drug metabolizing enzymes, the major one is the UDP-glucuronosyltransferases (UGTs) superfamily, which is estimated to be responsible for the elimination of more than 10% of the drugs cleared by metabolism (Figure 4-1, middle column).

The names of "Phase 1" and "Phase 2" metabolism are sort of misleading and sound like any drug undergoing metabolism will have to go through these two phases of reactions. This is not the case - some drugs may undergo just phase 1 without phase 2 metabolism; some other drugs may do the opposite (i.e., phase 2 only without phase 1 metabolism). However, many drugs do undergo both phases, with phase 1 metabolism then phase 2 sequentially.

4.1.1.2 The Cytochrome P450 enzyme system

CYP enzyme system is responsible for around 50% of small-molecule drugs used clinically. Considering its important role in drug elimination, I allocated this stand-alone subsection to further discuss this superfamily.

CYP consists of a superfamily of isoforms that plays a key role in the oxidative metabolism of drugs. The clinically important isoforms include CYP1A2, CYP2B6, CYP2C19, CYP2C8, CYP2C9, CYP2D6, and CYP3A4. Among these isoforms, CYP3A4 is the most abundant one and is responsible for the metabolism of more drugs than any other CYP enzymes. As shown in Figure 4-1 (right column),

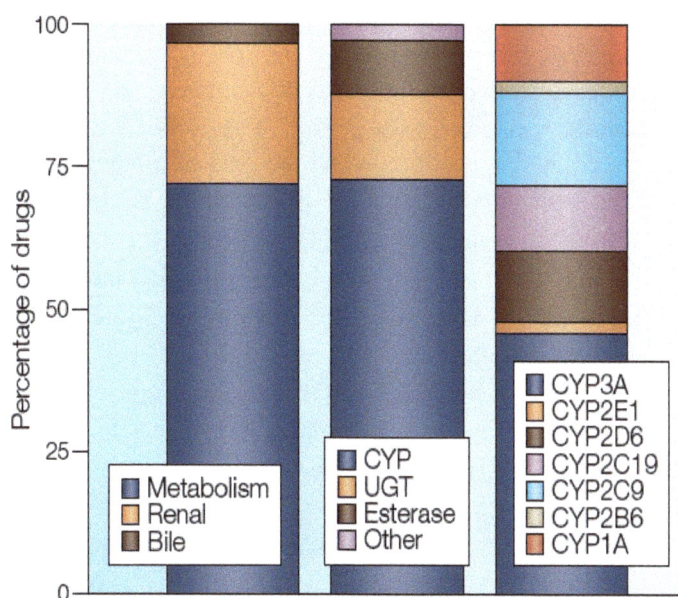

Figure 4-1. Among the top 200 small-molecule drugs, the major elimination pathways include metabolism, renal excretion, and biliary excretion (left); Major drug metabolizing enzymes involved in metabolism (middle); Major CYP isoforms involved in drug metabolism (right). *From: Nature Reviews Drug Discovery 4:825, 2005.*

the CYP3A system handles approximately 50% of CYP-mediated metabolism. The expression level of an isoform does not always correlate with its importance in drug metabolism. For example, the expression level of CYP2E1 accounts for 20% of total hepatic CYP but has little role in the metabolism of drugs. On the other hand, while the expression of CYP2D6 is low (about 2% of total hepatic CYP), it represents a major CYP isoform and plays an important role in many drugs' elimination.

Other than metabolizing drugs, CYP enzymes can be induced and inhibited by drugs. Drugs that are metabolized by, induce, and inhibit CYP enzymes are called "*substrates*", "*inducers*", and "*inhibitors*". In the presence of an inducer, the expression level of the enzyme is increased, leading to an increase in the rate of hepatic metabolism. Therefore, with an inducer, the enzyme can metabolize more of its substrates. Inhibitors act the opposite. In the presence of inhibitors, usually enzyme activity (not enzyme expression level except for the relatively rare suicidal inhibitors) is reduced. As a result, the rate of hepatic metabolism decreases.

When a substrate of an enzyme is co-administered with an inducer or inhibitor, drug-drug interaction may occur, and the pharmacokinetics of the substrate may change due to increased (caused by inducer) or decreased (caused by inhibitor) elimination. When such drug-drug interaction happens, the substrate is called "*victim drug*" and the inducer/inhibitor is called "*perpetrator drug*".

A drug is considered a *sensitive substrate* of an enzyme if >80% of its elimination is mediated by that enzyme. When the drug is co-administered with a strong inhibitor of the same enzyme, its AUC can increase ⩾5-fold. A drug is considered a *moderate sensitive substrate* of an enzyme if 50%-79% of its elimination is mediated by that enzyme; when the drug is co-administered with a strong inhibitor of the same enzyme, its AUC can increase ⩾2-fold to <5-fold.

A drug is considered a *strong inhibitor* if it increases the AUC of sensitive substrates of a given metabolic pathway ⩾5-fold. A drug that increases the AUC of sensitive substrates of a given metabolic pathway ⩾2-fold to < 5-fold is considered as a *moderate inhibitor*.

A drug is considered a *strong inducer* if it decreases the AUC of sensitive substrates of a given metabolic pathway by ⩾80%. A drug that decreases the AUC of sensitive substrates of a given metabolic pathway by ⩾50% to <80% is *moderate inducer*.

Table 4-1 lists representative sensitive substrates, strong inhibitors, and strong inducers of seven clinically important CYP isoforms. This information was obtained from the FDA website (https://www.fda.gov/drugs/drug-interactions-labeling/healthcare-professionals-fdas-examples-drugs-interact-cyp-enzymes-and-transporter-systems; access date: Feb 7, 2024). If you are a healthcare professional, I highly recommend you check the FDA website, which provides a more comprehensive list of substrates, inducers, and inhibitors of the CYP enzymes.

Whether a drug-drug interaction is clinically significant depends on the victim drug's therapeutic range. For drugs with wide therapeutic range, they can tolerate large change in drug exposure without clinical consequence. On the other hand, for a drug with a narrow therapeutic window, modest change in pharmacokinetics exposure may lead to drug ineffective (with an inducer) or toxicity (with an inhibitor) and require dose adjustment. A typical example is digoxin, where dose adjustment may be warranted with moderate increase of digoxin AUC of 36% by ritonavir. Similarly, the increase in the exposure of simvastatin (AUC increases 1.3- to 1.6-fold) by amlodipine is rather modest but is significant enough to increase the risk of muscle myopathy, a well know side effect of simvastatin.

4.1.1.3 CYP enzyme-mediated drug-drug interactions

Given the fact that there are numerous CYP substrates, inducers, and inhibitors, it is not surprising that there are rich documents on CYP enzyme-mediated drug-drug interactions. In this subsection, I only provide two literature reported CYP3A-mediated drug-drug interactions, with alprazolam being the victim drug in both reports. In one article, carbamazepine, a strong CYP3A inducer, was the perpetrator, while in another report, ketoconazole, a strong CYP3A inhibitor, was

Table 4-1. Representative sensitive substrates, strong inhibitors, and strong inducers of seven clinically important CYP isoforms. *(For enzymes that have no sensitive substrates or strong inhibitors/inducers, moderate sensitive substrates and moderate inhibitors/inducers are provided instead (see footnote of the table). Information from the FDA website (access date: Feb 7, 2024)*

Enzyme	Sensitive substrates	Strong inducers	Strong inhibitors
CYP1A2	alosetron; caffeine; duloxetine; melatonin; ramelteon; tasimelteon; tizanidine	phenytoin#; rifampin#; teriflunomide#; tobacco (smoking)#	ciprofloxacin; fluvoxamine
CYP2B6	efavirenz*	carbamazepine	
CYP2C19	omeprazole; S-mephenytoin	rifampin	fluconazole; fluoxetine; fluvoxamine; ticlopidine
CYP2C8	repaglinide	rifampin#	gemfibrozil
CYP2C9	celecoxib	enzalutamide#; rifampin#	amiodarone^;fluconazole^; miconazole^; piperine^
CYP2D6	atomoxetine; desipramine; dextromethorphan; eliglustat; nebivolol; nortriptyline; perphenazine; R-venlafaxine; tolterodine	Not inducible	bupropion; fluoxetine; paroxetine; quinidine; terbinafine
CYP3A4	alfentanil; avanafil; budesonide; buspirone; conivaptan; darifenacin; darunavir; dasatinib; dronedarone; eletriptan	apalutamide; carbamazepine; enzalutamide; ivosidenib; lumacaftor; ivacaftor; mitotane; phenytoin; rifampin; St. John's wort	ceritinib; clarithromycin; cobicistat; elvitegravir and ritonavir; idelalisib; indinavir and ritonavir; itraconazole; ketoconazole; lopinavir and ritonavir; nefazodone

*moderate sensitive substrate; # moderate inducer; ^ moderate inhibitor

the perpetrator. I hope these two case examples could 1) give you a sense of how the pharmacokinetics profile of a victim drug might look like when it is given with an inducer/inhibitor, and 2) strengthen your quantitative mindset by evaluating which pharmacokinetic parameters of the victim drug have changed using the mathematic equations covered in Chapter 1. Let's look at these two case examples.

Case Example 4-1.

CYP3A-mediated carbamazepine-alprazolam interaction

Alprazolam belongs to the class of benzodiazepines and is used to treat anxiety and panic disorders. Alprazolam is mainly metabolized by CYP3A. When alprazolam is given via oral administration, it is absorbed not only very fast (T_{max} can be reached within 1 hour) but also almost completely (bioavailability > 90%). Carbamazepine is an anticonvulsant and used to treat epilepsy and bipolar disorder. Carbamazepine is a well-known strong CYP3A inducer.

In this study, the effect of carbamazepine on the single oral dose pharmacokinetics of alprazolam was evaluated. Figure 4-2 shows the concentration-time profiles of alprazolam in the control group and the carbamazepine group.

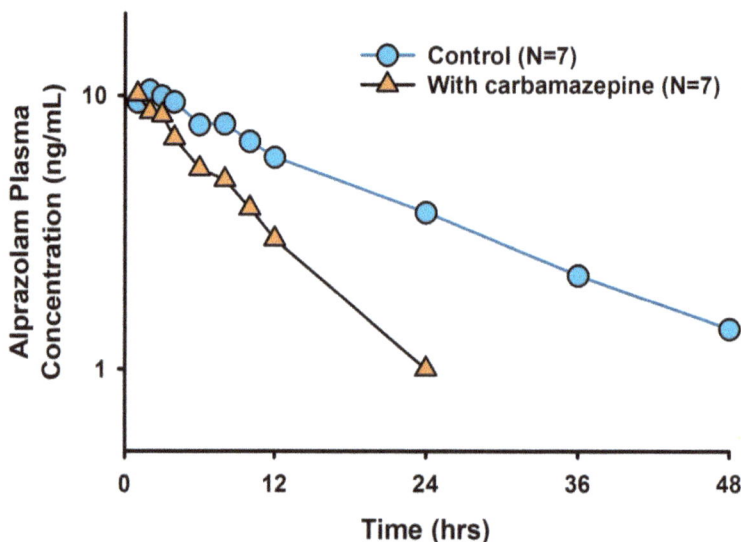

Figure 4-2. The mean concentration-time profiles of alprazolam in human following a single oral dose alone or with carbamazepine. Seven healthy male subjects took carbamazepine 300 mg/day or matched placebo orally for 10 days, and on the 8th day they took a single oral 0.8 mg dose of alprazolam. *Adapted from: Furukori H, et al. Neuropsychopharmacology 1998;18:364-369.*

To evaluate the impact of carbamazepine on the pharmacokinetic parameters of alprazolam, the following assumptions and modifications were made to simplify the situation:

- First-order kinetics. This is supported by the figure. Please note that Y-axis is a log scale.

- Considering the fast and complete absorption of alprazolam, let's assume that we can use I.V. models learned in Chapter 1 for describing alprazolam pharmacokinetics.
- To simplify the situation, alprazolam concentration at the first time point (i.e. 0.5 h) was not included. Only concentrations at ≥ 1 h time points were digitized from the original paper and provided in Figure 4-2. Let's assume the initial concentration is obtained at 1 h post dose.

Based on the above assumptions, please evaluate the effect of carbamazepine on the key pharmacokinetic parameters of alprazolam, namely CL, V_d, k_e, $t_{1/2}$.

Please work on it yourself before looking at the answers I provide below.

$\sim \sim \sim$

To address this type of question, first we need to look at what information we can get directly from the figure. Looking at those two curves, we see immediately that, with Carbamazepine, the concentration-time plot of alprazolam had 1) lower AUC; 2) steeper slope; and 3) same initial concentration. Based on these data, we can draw the following conclusion:

- *k_e=-slope, and the slope is steeper in carbamazepine co-administration group. Therefore, carbamazepine increased k_e of alprazolam*
- *$t_{1/2}=\dfrac{0.693}{k_e}$. Since k_e increased, $t_{1/2}$ of alprazolam decreased.*
- *$CL=\dfrac{Dose}{AUC}$, and the AUC is lower in carbamazepine co-administration group. Therefore, carbamazepine increased CL of alprazolam.*
- *$V_d=\dfrac{Dose}{C_0}$, and the initial concentration remains unchanged. Therefore, carbamazepine did not affect V_d of alprazolam.*

In summary, the effects of carbamazepine on alprazolam pharmacokinetics include $CL\uparrow$, $V_d \leftrightarrow$, $k_e\uparrow$, and $t_{1/2}\downarrow$. With carbamazepine, there is a risk of lost efficacy for alprazolam.

Case Example 4-2.

CYP3A-mediated ketoconazole-alprazolam interaction

In this study, the effect of ketoconazole on alprazolam pharmacokinetic was evaluated. Ketoconazole is an antifungal and is used to treat a number of fungal infections. Ketoconazole is a strong CYP3A inhibitor, while alprazolam, as noted earlier, is a substrate of CYP3A. Figure 4-3 shows the concentration-time profiles of alprazolam when 1.0 mg of alprazolam was given with placebo (i.e., control group) or 200 mg ketoconazole (i.e., ketoconazole group).

Same as case example 1, let's assume that the absorption of alprazolam is so fast and complete, so that we can use I.V. models learned in Chapter 1 for describing alprazolam pharmacokinetics following an oral dose. What is the effect of carbamazepine on the key pharmacokinetic parameters of alprazolam, namely CL, V_d, k_e, $t_{1/2}$?

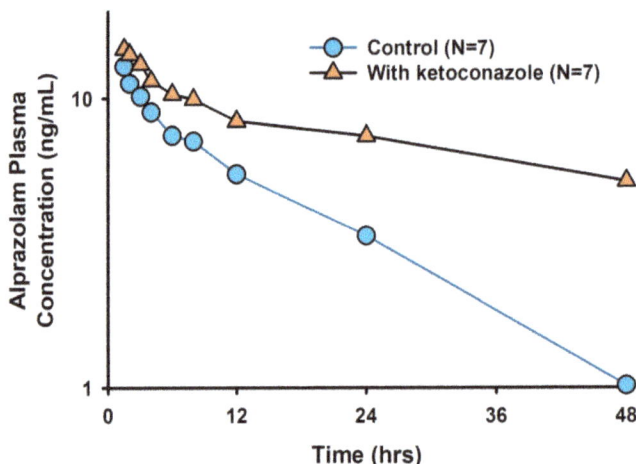

Figure 4-3. The mean concentration-time profiles of alprazolam in healthy subjects (N=7) following a single 1 mg oral dose of alprazolam with placebo or with 200 mg ketoconazole. *Adapted from: Greenblatt DJ, et al. Clinical Pharmacology and Therapeutics 1998;63(3):237-247.*

I will not provide detailed calculation steps for this case example since you could use the same thinking flow as you did in case example 1 to address the above question. Please work on it and compare your results with the conclusion I provide here:

The impact of ketoconazole on alprazolam pharmacokinetics includes $CL\downarrow$, V_d $\leftrightarrow$, $k_e\downarrow$, and $t_{1/2}\uparrow$. With ketoconazole, there is a risk of toxicity for alprazolam.

4.1.2. Drug transporters and their role in drug excretion.

4.1.2.1 Role of drug transporters in renal and biliary excretion

We have learned that transporters can affect drug absorption (Chapter 2) and drug distribution (Chapter 3). Considering the expression of various transporters in the two major drug eliminating organs in the body, namely liver and kidney, it is not surprising that transporters are involved in drug elimination as well. Among the processes of ADME, transporters could affect the phases of A (absorption), D (distribution), and E (excretion) of a drug; they do not play a role in the M (metabolism) part.

The presence of drug transporters in hepatocytes and renal proximal tubule epithelial cells is shown in Figure 4-4. Both hepatocytes and renal proximal tubule epithelial cells are polarized cells, with the apical side facing bile (hepatocytes) or urine (renal proximal tubule epithelial cells) and the basolateral side facing the blood. Drug transporters can be expressed on both sides. The role of a transporter in drug excretion depends on the side it locates as well as the direction of the transport (indicated by an arrow).

In Chapter 2, I have used OATP1B1, an uptake transporter, and P-gp, an efflux transporter, as examples and explained how these two transporters work in concert to transfer their substrates from blood into bile, a process known as biliary excretion. Since it has been discussed already, I will not provide further examples here. Biliary excretion represents not only a potential source of hepatic first-pass loss affecting the bioavailability of an orally administered drug, but also an elimination pathway after the drug reaches systemic circulation.

Similarly, uptake transporters and efflux transporters also work together in moving drugs from blood into urine, a process know as urinary excretion. Let's use organic anion transporter 1 (OAT1) and P-gp as examples and see how they affect urine excretion of a drug that is a substrate of both transporters.

As shown in Figure 4-4, OAT1 is present in the basolateral side (facing blood) of the kidney proximal tubules, and it takes the drug from blood into the tubule epithelial cells. After the drug is taken up into the cells, P-gp, expressed in the apical side (facing urine), pumps it into urine. Therefore, these two transporters work in concert to eliminate the drug via renally excreting the drug in its unchanged form. When a drug that is a substate of OAT1 and P-gp is co-administered with an inhibitor of these two transporters, the renal excretion of the drug will decrease.

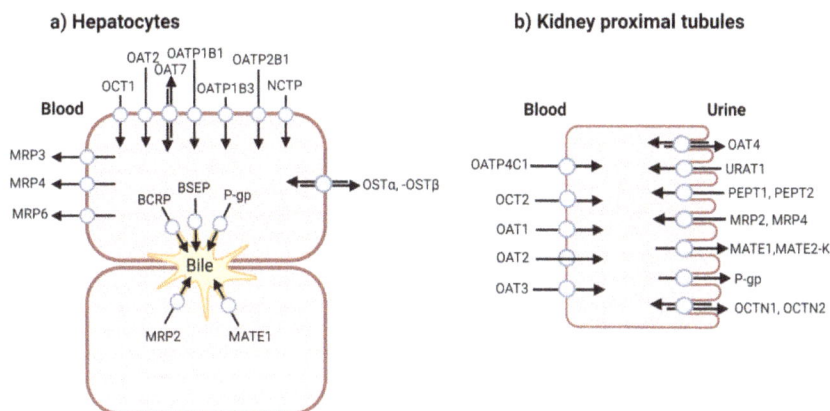

Figure 4-4. The presence of drug transporters in a) hepatocytes, and b) kidney tubules.

4.1.2.1 Transporter-mediated drug-drug interactions

Many drugs are substrates of transporters, but very few of them are eliminated exclusively via transporters. In addition, many transporters have overlapping substrate spectrum (i.e., drugs are often transported by multiple transporters). As a result, there are not many sensitive substrates that are specific to a certain transporter. Similarly, while there are many transporter inhibitors, it is difficult to make a clear classification of strong/moderate/weak inhibitors due to the lack of sensitive substrates. Table 4-2 lists representative substrates and inhibitors of clinically important drug transporters. This information was obtained from the FDA website (https://www.fda.gov/drugs/drug-interactions-labeling/healthcare-professionals-fdas-examples-drugs-interact-cyp-enzymes-and-transporter-systems; access date: Feb 7, 2024).

Table 4-2. Representative substrates and inhibitors of clinically important drug transporters. *Information from the FDA website (access date: Feb 7, 2024)*

Transporter	Substrates	Inhibitors
P-gp	dabigatran etexilate; digoxin; edoxaban; fexofenadine	amiodarone; clarithromycin; cobicistat; cyclosporine; dronedarone; erythromycin; itraconazole; ketoconazole; lapatinib; lopinavir and ritonavir; propafenone; quinidine; ranolazine; saquinavir & ritonavir; sofosbuvir & velpatasvir & voxilaprevir; verapamil;
BCRP	rosuvastatin; sulfasalazine	curcumin; cyclosporine; darolutamide; eltrombopag; febuxostat; fostamatinib; rolapitant; sofosbuvir and velpatasvir and voxilaprevir; teriflunomide
OATP1B1 & OATP1B3	atorvastatin; bosentan; docetaxel; elagolix; fexofenadine; glyburide; lovastatin; paclitaxel; pitavastatin; pravastatin; repaglinide; rosuvastatin; simvastatin	atazanavir and ritonavir; clarithromycin; cyclosporine; darolutamide; eltrombopag; gemfibrozil; lopinavir and ritonavir; rifampin; sofosbuvir and velpatasvir and voxilaprevir
OAT1	adefovir; ciprofloxacin; furosemide; tenofovir	probenecid
OAT3	baricitinib; bumetanide; cefaclor; ceftizoxime; ciprofloxacin; famotidine; furosemide; methotrexate; oseltamivir carboxylate; penicillin G;	gemfibrozil; probenecid; teriflunomide
OCT2	metformin	cimetidine; dolutegravir; isavuconazole; ranolazine
MATE1 & MATE2K	metformin	cimetidine; isavuconazole; pyrimethamine; ranolazine; trimethoprim; vandetanib

A classic example of clinically relevant drug-drug interaction involving renal drug transporters is the P-gp-mediated quinidine-digoxin interaction, which has been observed in several clinical studies. Digoxin is a narrow-therapeutic window drug, and it is used to treat congestive heart failure. Digoxin does not undergo extensive metabolism and it is a substrate of P-gp. Quinidine, an antiarrhythmic agent, is an inhibitor of P-gp. As shown in Figure 4-5, the plasma concentrations of digoxin increased when it was co-administered with quinidine. In this drug-drug interaction, quinidine acted as the perpetrator and it inhibited P-glycoprotein (P-gp)–mediated efflux of digoxin (the victim), resulting in decreased renal excretion of digoxin. As a result, digoxin had higher plasma exposure and increased risk of toxicity in the presence of quinidine.

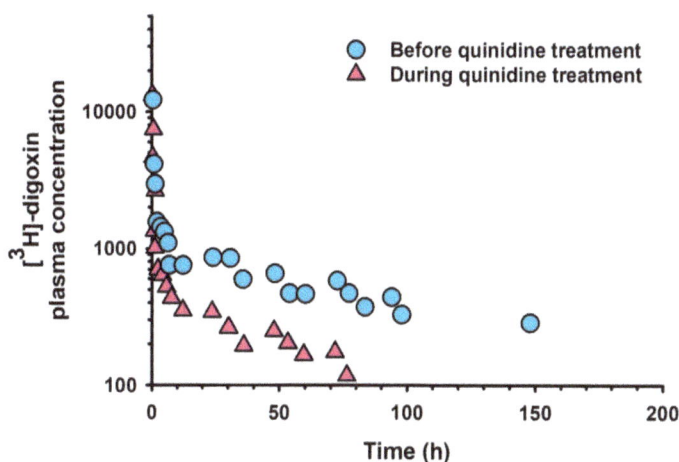

Figure 4-5. Concentration of [^{3}H]-digoxin in plasma after a single i.v. dose before quinidine treatment and during quinidine treatment in a representative patient. Adapted *from: Schenck-Gustafsson K& Dahlqvist R. British Journal of Clinical Pharmacology 1981;11:181-186.*

4.1.3. Pharmacogenetics of drug metabolizing enzymes and drug transporters

For the drug metabolizing enzymes in sections 4.1.1, the activity of many of them is under genetic control. *Polymorphism* refers to the occurrence of two or more variations in the DNA sequences at a given locus of a gene with a frequency greater than 1% in the population. The polymorphism of CYP enzyme system was first noticed about 50 years ago when a small portion of subjects receiving debrisoquine, an antihypertensive drug, had abnormally high plasma drug concentrations and extreme falls in blood pressure. This phenomenon stimulated extensive investigations, and it has subsequently been found that debrisoquine and more than 70 other drugs are metabolized by CYP2D6, a highly polymorphic enzyme. In addition to CYP2D6, the clinical significance of the polymorphism of CYP2C9 and CYP2C19 is also well recognized. In addition to drug metabolizing enzymes, polymorphism is also seen in drug transporters, including some subfamilies of OATPs, OATs, and OCTs.

Genetic polymorphism in CYP enzymes results in the change of enzyme activity, and subjects can be divided into several groups based on their enzyme activities:

- Normal metabolizer (NM) – enzyme has normal function.
- Intermediate metabolizer (IM) – enzyme has decreased function.
- Poor metabolizer (PM) – enzyme has no function.
- Rapid metabolizer (RM) – enzyme has increased function.
- Ultrarapid metabolizer (UM) – enzyme has highly increased function.

As shown in Figure 4-6, for a drug with narrow therapeutic window, it may reach plasma concentrations higher than the maximum effective concentration in patients who are intermediate or poor metabolizers and may result in plasma concentrations lower than the minimum effective concentration in patients who are rapid or ultrarapid metabolizers. As a result, toxicity or treatment failure may occur if dose adjustment is not done.

The polymorphism of drug metabolizing enzymes and transporters represents an important source of variability in drug pharmacokinetics. For a drug which has narrow therapeutic window and meanwhile is a sensitive substrate of certain highly polymorphic enzyme, such as CYP2D6, CYP2C9, and CYP2C19, running an enzyme genetic test (i.e., pharmacogenomics test) in an individual patient could be beneficial as the test result can help the doctor to personalize the patient's medication. Pharmacogenomic tests of CYP2C19 for clopidogrel, thiopurine methyltransferase (TPMT) for thiopurine drugs, and UGT1A1 for irinotecan are routine clinical practice. Other tests with considerable data include CYP2C9 for warfarin, and CYP2D6 for tamoxifen and codeine.

4.1.4 Concept of clearance

As noted earlier, the major drug elimination pathways include hepatic metabolism, renal excretion, and biliary excretion. This does not mean that every drug will be embolized by these three pathways. Some drugs may be eliminated exclusively through metabolism via a specific enzyme, albeit it is more common that drugs are metabolized by more than one enzyme. Some drugs may undergo minimal metabolism and mainly be cleared via renal excretion or biliary excretion. Therefore, each drug has its own elimination mechanism.

We have learned the concept of clearance as well as the equations to calculate CL in Chapter 1. When we estimate the clearance of a drug using the observed concentration-time profile, the parameter of CL represents the total elimination of that drug, which is the sum of each individual pathway involved in the elimination of the drug. For a drug that undergoes all major elimination pathways mentioned above plus a few other minor pathways, its elimination can be expressed as:

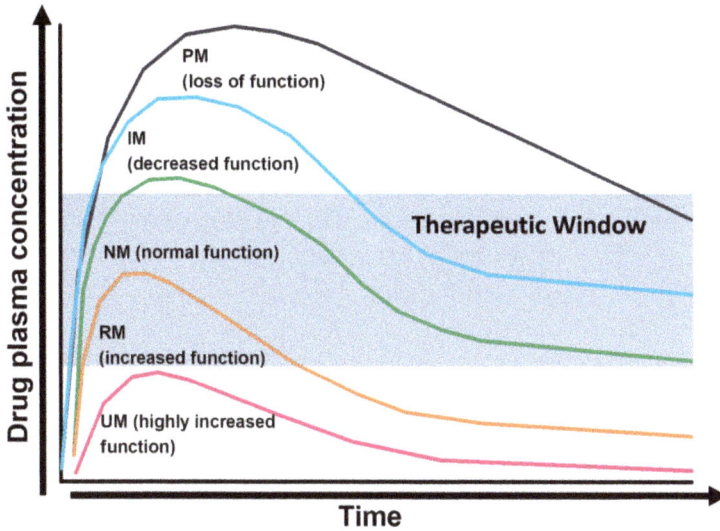

Figure 4-6. Effect of CYP enzyme polymorphism on the metabolism and pharmacokinetics of an example drug with narrow therapeutic window.

$$CL = CL_{H,m} + CL_{H,b} + CL_R + CL_{other} \qquad\qquad [4\text{-}1]$$

Where:

CL   = total clearance

$CL_{H,m}$ = eliminated by the liver *via* hepatic metabolism

$CL_{H,b}$ = eliminated by the liver *via* biliary excretion

CL_R = eliminated by the kidney *via* renal excretion

CL_{other} = clearance from other minor pathways in other organs

If a drug is exclusively eliminated through hepatic metabolism, $CL=CL_{H,m}$, If a drug is exclusively eliminated through renal excretion, $CL = CL_R$. And so on. $CL_{H,m}$ and $CL_{H,b}$ are often hard to separate, so, usually we estimate CL_H, which is the total hepatic clearance ($CL_{H,m}$ + $CL_{H,b}$).

Considering the critical role of the liver and kidney in drug elimination, I will go through hepatic clearance and renal clearance in the next two sections.

4.2 Hepatic Clearance

4.2.1. Liver blood flow (Q_H) and extraction ratio (E)

For a drug that is eliminated via hepatic metabolism, let's have a rough estimate of its hepatic clearance based on a few simplified scenarios.

Scenario 1. All the drug entering the liver is eliminated by the liver.

As shown in Figure 4-7, all drug molecules entering the liver are eliminated. In this case, what would be the hepatic clearance of this drug?

If you recall, we learned in Chapter 1 (section 1.5.4) that clearance may be viewed as the volume of plasma (or blood) from which drug is removed over a specified time (unit is volume/time). In this scenario, since all the drug is metabolized in the liver, its hepatic clearance would be related to how much blood is pumped to the liver per hour since all drug molecules present in this volume of blood are cleared per hour. The volume of blood supplied to the liver every hour is the hepatic blood flow, which is approximately 1450 ml/min (or 87 L/h) for a 70-kg adult.

Therefore, when all the drug entering the liver is eliminated, its hepatic clearance is identical to the hepatic blood flow (Q_H): $CL_H = Q_H$

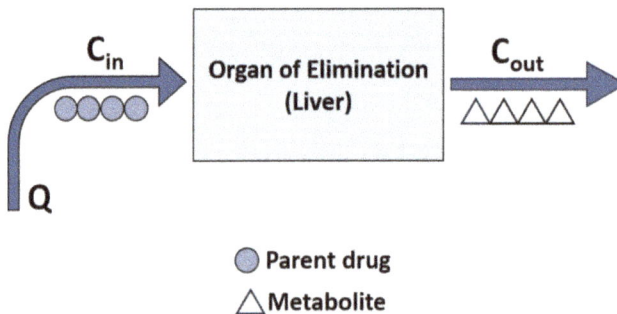

Figure 4-7. A drug entering the liver with a concentration C_{in} and leaving the liver with a concentration C_{out}. In this example, all the drug entering the liver is cleared. Therefore, $C_{out} = 0$.

Scenario 2. 50% of the drug entering the liver is eliminated by the liver.

As shown in Figure 4-8, among drug molecules entering the liver, 50% of them are eliminated. In this case, what would be the drug's hepatic clearance?

Intuitively, you can easily make a guess that the hepatic clearance of this drug would be half of the hepatic blood flow. The answer is correct. Let's find a mathematical way to estimate the hepatic clearance. For the fraction of the drug that is metabolized in the liver, we can call it "extraction ratio (E_H)" which is calculated as:

$$E_H = \frac{C_{in} - C_{out}}{C_{in}} \qquad [4\text{-}2]$$

In this scenario, 50% of the drug is eliminated, which means that the concentration of the drug coming out of the liver is half of the concentration entering in the liver (i.e. $C_{out} = 0.5 \cdot C_{in}$). Therefore, E = 0.5. Therefore, when 50% of the drug entering the liver is eliminated, its hepatic clearance is $CL_H = Q_H \cdot 0.5$, where 0.5 is the extraction ratio.

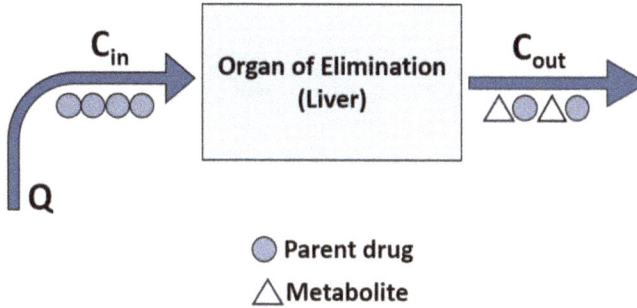

Figure 4-8. A drug entering the liver with a concentration C_{in} and leaving the liver with a concentration C_{out}. In this example, 50% of the drug entering the liver is cleared. Therefore, $C_{out} = 0.5 \cdot C_{in}$.

Based on these two scenarios, we can come up with the following general description of the hepatic clearance:

$$CL_H = Q_H \cdot E_H \qquad\qquad [4\text{-}3]$$

Extraction ratio E_H reflects the innate ability of the liver to metabolize the drug, which is associated with how much the drug metabolizing enzyme is available for metabolism as well as how active the enzyme is. The ability of the liver to metabolize the drug is described as *intrinsic clearance*, which is explained in the next subsection.

Before we end this subsection, let's look at the rate of drug extraction. For example, if we know $C_{in} = 10$ mg/L, $C_{out} = 1$ mg/L, and liver blood flow is 87 L/h. What is the amount of drug eliminated by the liver per hour (i.e., rate of drug extraction)?

First, let's calculate the amount of drug entering the liver per hour. Since there is 10 mg drug every liter of blood (i.e., $C_{in}=10$ mg/L), and there are 87 L blood pumped to liver every hour, we can easily calculate that the rate of drug input is 10 mg/L x 87 L/h = 870 mg/h. Using the same logic, we can get the rate of drug output (i.e., amount of drug leaving the liver per hour) is 1 mg/L x 87 L/h = 87 mg/h. Therefore, the rate of drug extraction (i.e., the amount being metabolized per hour) is 870 mg/h – 87 mg/h = 783 mg/h. The general description of rate of drug extraction can be expressed as:

$$Rate\ of\ extraction = Q_H \cdot (C_{in} - Q_{out}) \qquad\qquad [4\text{-}4]$$

Based on Equations 4-2 and 4-3, the above equation can be rearranged as:

$$Rate\ of\ extraction = Q_H \cdot E_H \cdot C_{in} \quad \rightarrow \quad Rate\ of\ extraction = CL_H \cdot C_{in}$$

Therefore:

$$CL_H = \frac{Rate\ of\ extraction}{C_{in}} \qquad\qquad [4\text{-}5]$$

4.2.2. Intrinsic clearance (CL$_{int}$)

Intrinsic clearance (CL$_{int}$) describes the liver's innate ability to clear drug. Intrinsic clearance reflects "intrinsic" efficiency of elimination, which is the hepatic clearance that would occur if there were no limitation due to liver blood flow. Intrinsic clearance can take any value (i.e., not limited to liver blood flow).

I know, the description of intrinsic clearance mentioned above is so dry, and I have successfully confused you. When I taught the PharmD PK course for the first few years, many students got confused about intrinsic clearance as well. Later, I came up with an example that helped the students to comprehend the concept of intrinsic clearance. I would like to share the same example here.

Case Example 4-3.

A Squirrel Story

Imagine that a squirrel lives in an animal kingdom, and he goes to his favorite cafeteria in the forest one day.

Scenario 1. He has a good appetite and can eat 500 acorns per hour (Figure 4-9, upper). The cafeteria serves acorns on a conveyor belt at the rate of 100 acorns per hour. In this case, how many acorns will this squirrel eat per hour?

Scenario 2. He ate a few poisonous mushrooms the day before and lost his appetite. Although he loves acorns, he can only eat 10 acorns per hour (Figure 4-9, lower). The conveyor belt in the cafeteria still delivers 100 acorns per hour. In this case, how many acorns will this squirrel eat per hour?

Please address the questions yourself and link them to what we have learned before looking at my explanations provided below.

$\sim \sim \sim$

In scenario 1, this squirrel will eat 100 acorns per hour. Although he has the ability to eat 500 acorns per hour, he won't get a chance to eat that many because the conveyor belt only delivers 100 acorns per hour. In this case, how many acorns he eats is rate limited by the conveyor belt delivery rate.

In scenario 2, this squirrel will eat 10 acorns per hour. Although the conveyor belt delivers 100 acorns per hour to him, his ability to eat acorns is only 10 acorns per hour. In this case, how many acorns he eats is rate limited by his innate ability.

Now, let's link this case example to what we just learned:

- *Conveyor belt delivering 100 acorns per hour = Liver blood flow (Q_H=87 L/h)*
- *Squirrel's ability to eat acorns per hour (i.e., 500 acorns/h in scenario 1 and 10 acorns/h in scenario 2) = Intrinsic clearance (CL$_{int}$)*
- *Number of acorns this squirrel actually eats per hour (i.e., 100 acorns/h in scenario 1 and 10 acorns/h in scenario 2) = Hepatic clearance of a drug (CL$_H$)*

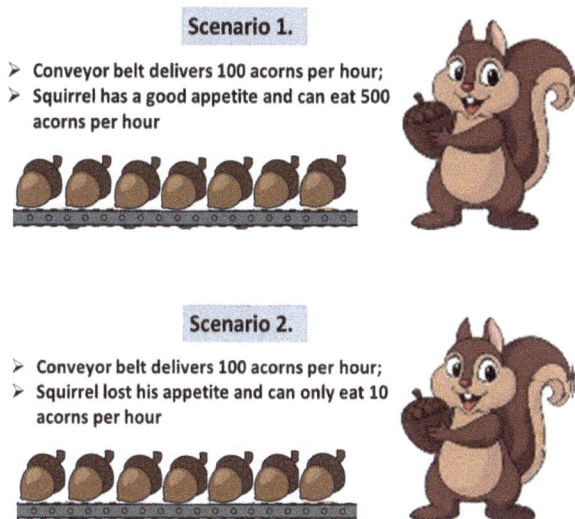

Scenario 1.
- Conveyor belt delivers 100 acorns per hour;
- Squirrel has a good appetite and can eat 500 acorns per hour

Scenario 2.
- Conveyor belt delivers 100 acorns per hour;
- Squirrel lost his appetite and can only eat 10 acorns per hour

Figure 4-9. A squirrel lives in an animal kingdom, and goes to his favorite cafeteria in the forest one day…

Now, let me copy & paste the paragraph on intrinsic clearance mentioned earlier, and I hope you understand the concept now. "Intrinsic clearance (CL_{int}) describes the liver's innate ability to clear drug. Intrinsic clearance reflects "intrinsic" efficiency of elimination, which is the hepatic clearance that would occur if there were no limitation due to liver blood flow. Intrinsic clearance can take any value (i.e., not limited to liver blood flow)."

I hope this case example is useful to you. By the way, this squirrel has a name. In Spring 2023, when I taught the Class of 2026, 5 PharmD students gave me a special gift - a toy of a squirrel holding an acorn, and they named him "Clint".

Intrinsic clearance can be described as:

$$CL_{int} = \frac{V_{max}}{K_m}$$
[4-6]

Where V_{max} is the maximum capacity of the reaction, while K_m corresponds to the concentration associated with 50% V_{max}. The higher the expression level of drug metabolizing enzymes, the higher V_{max}. The higher the affinity of the drug to the enzyme, the smaller the value of K_m.

You may wonder - why do we learn intrinsic clearance? I introduce this concept because intrinsic clearance, together with liver blood flow and fraction of unbound, can help us estimate hepatic clearance; this is the topic of the next subsection.

4.2.3. Estimation of hepatic clearance using a well-stirred model

Among several reported hepatic drug clearance models, the most widely used one is the well-stirred model, which was introduced by Rowland and colleagues in 1970s. The well-stirred model was built under several assumptions in order to simplify the complicated physiological processes. Since this book targets beginners, I will not go through the details of the model building process. All you need to be aware of is that the well-stirred model is not physiologic reality and may not be quantitatively accurate. The value of this model is that it allows us to predict the direction of change in hepatic clearance when one or more physiological factors are changed.

Following is the equation of the well-stirred model:

$$CL_H = \frac{Q_H \cdot f_u \cdot CL_{int}}{Q_H + f_u \cdot CL_{int}} \qquad [4\text{-}7]$$

Where Q_H is the hepatic blood flow; f_u is the fraction of unbound drug in plasma; and CL_{int} is the intrinsic clearance.

Based on Equation 4-7 and Equation 4-3, we can get the equation for extraction ratio E_H:

$$E_H = \frac{f_u \cdot Cl_{int}}{Q_H + f_u \cdot CL_{int}} \qquad [4\text{-}8]$$

Since the above equations look complicated, let's simplify them in two scenarios:

- **High extraction drug** where $f_u \cdot CL_{int} \gg Q_H$

[*Note: Scenario 1 of the squirrel story essentially describes the hepatic clearance of a high extraction drug*]

For a high extraction drug, the ability of the drug metabolizing enzyme to eliminate the drug is much higher than the liver blood flow, such that $f_u \cdot CL_{int} \gg Q_H$.

Therefore, $Q_H + f_u \cdot CL_{int} \approx f_u \cdot CL_{int}$

In this case, Equation 4-7 can be simplified as:

$$CL_H = \frac{Q_H \cdot f_u \cdot CL_{int}}{Q_H + f_u \cdot CL_{int}} \;\rightarrow\; CL_H = \frac{Q_H \cdot f_u \cdot CL_{int}}{f_u \cdot CL_{int}} \;\rightarrow\; CL_H = Q_H \qquad [4\text{-}9]$$

Accordingly, Equation 4-8 can be simplified as:

$$E_H = \frac{f_u \cdot Cl_{int}}{Q_H + f_u \cdot CL_{int}} \quad \rightarrow \quad E_H = \frac{f_u \cdot CL_{int}}{f_u \cdot CL_{int}} \quad \rightarrow \quad E_H = 1 \qquad [4\text{-}10]$$

Therefore, for high extraction drugs, their hepatic clearance depends on the hepatic blood flow, instead of fraction of unbound or intrinsic clearance. The extraction ratio is close to 1 and is not dependent on any of these three physiological factors.

- *Low extraction drug* where $f_u \cdot CL_{int} \ll Q_H$

[*Note: Scenario 2 of the squirrel story essentially describes the hepatic clearance of a low extraction drug*]

For a low extraction drug, the ability of the drug metabolizing enzyme to eliminate the drug is much lower than the liver blood flow, such that $f_u \cdot CL_{int} \ll Q_H$.

Therefore, $Q_H + f_u \cdot CL_{int} \approx Q_H$

In this case, Equation 4-7 can be simplified as:

$$CL_H = \frac{Q_H \cdot f_u \cdot CL_{int}}{Q_H + f_u \cdot CL_{int}} \quad \rightarrow \quad CL_H = \frac{Q_H \cdot f_u \cdot CL_{int}}{Q_H} \rightarrow \quad CL_H = f_u \cdot CL_{int} \qquad [4\text{-}11]$$

Accordingly, Equation 4-8 can be simplified as:

$$E_H = \frac{f_u \cdot Cl_{int}}{Q_H + f_u \cdot CL_{int}} \quad \rightarrow \quad E_H = \frac{f_u \cdot Cl_{int}}{Q_H} \qquad [4\text{-}12]$$

Therefore, for low extraction drugs, their hepatic clearance depends on the fraction of unbound and intrinsic clearance, instead of hepatic blood flow. The extraction ratio is affected by all three physiological factors.

In the real world, a drug eliminated mainly by the liver is considered a low extraction drug when $E_H < 0.3$, and a high extraction drug when $E_H > 0.7$. Table 4-3 shows the representative low, intermediate, and high extraction drugs.

For drugs with low or high extraction ratios, the simplified equations can be used to estimate the direction of change in their hepatic clearances when any of those three factors (i.e., Q_H, CL_{int}, and f_u) changes.

Figure 4-10 shows the effect of change in fraction unbound on the extraction ratio of propranolol and tolbutamide. The different behaviors of these two drugs can be explained using the simplified equations of E_H. Propranolol is a high extraction drug. Based on Equation 4-10, its E_H is close to 1 and is not affected by

Table 4-3. Hepatic extraction ratio of representative small-molecule drugs

Hepatic Extraction Ratio		
Low (<0.3)	**Intermediate (0.3-0.7)**	**High (>0.7)**
Alprazolam	Aspirin	Alprenolol
Carbamazepine	Quinidine	Cocaine
Diazepam	Codeine	Desipramine
Digitoxin	Cyclosporine	Lidocaine
Indomethacin	Nifedipine	Morphine
Phenobarbital	Nortriptyline	Propoxyphene
Phenytoin		Propranolol
Salicylic acid		Verapamil
Theophylline		
Tolbutamide		
Valproic Acid		
Warfarin		

f_u. On the other hand, the behavior of tolbutamide indicates that it is a low extraction drug. Based on Equation 4-12, the E_H of tolbutamide is positively affected by CL_{int} and f_u, and negatively affected by Q_H. With the increase in f_u, E_H of tolbutamide increases.

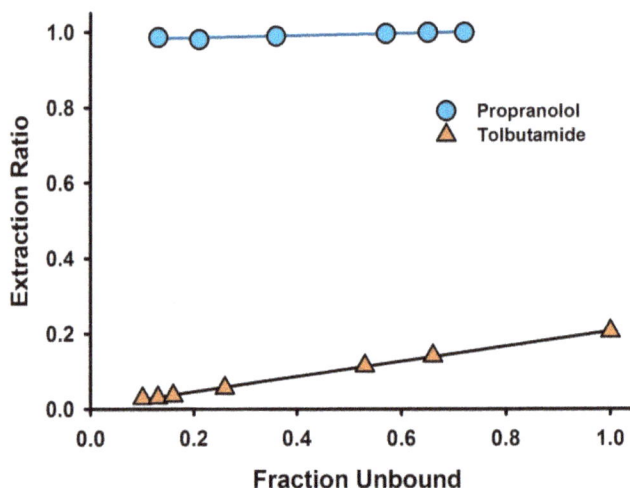

Figure 4-10. The effect of change in fraction unbound on the extraction ratio of propranolol and tolbutamide. Adapted from: 1) Schary WL & Rowland M. J Pharmacokinet Biopharm 1983;11:225-243. 2) Jones S, et al. Hepatology 1985;5:590-593.

Figure 4-11 demonstrates the effect of change in hepatic blood flow on the clearance of lidocaine and antipyrine. The different behaviors of these two drugs can be explained using the simplified equations of CL_H. Lidocaine is a high extraction drug. Based on Equation 4-9, its CL_H depends on Q_H, that is why we see the increase in lidocaine hepatic clearance with increase in hepatic blood flow. On the other hand, antipyrine is a low extraction drug. Based on Equation 4-11, its clearance depends on CL_{int} and f_u, but not Q_H. Therefore, with increase in hepatic blood flow, there is minimal change in antipyrine hepatic clearance.

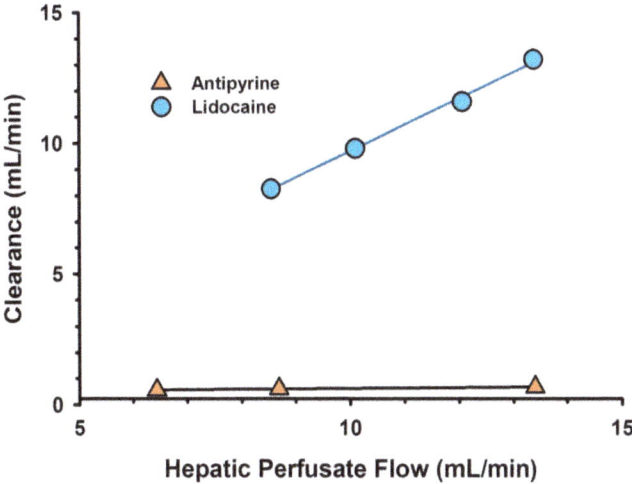

Figure 4-11. The effect of change in hepatic blood flow on the clearance of lidocaine and antipyrine. Adapted from: Pang KS & Rowland M. J Pharmacokinet Biopharm 1977;5:655-680.

4.2.4 Estimation of oral bioavailability based on the extraction ratio.

Liver is not only a major organ for drug elimination. As discussed in Chapter 2, liver also plays an important role in drug absorption because the orally administered drugs must pass through the liver before they reach systemic circulation. In Chapter 2 (section 2.1.1), we learned that $F = F_{abs} \times F_G \times F_H$. If we assume minimal drug loss in gastrointestinal lumen (i.e., $F_{abs} = 1$) and little intestinal first pass loss (i.e., $F_G = 1$), then the bioavailability of an orally administered drug is determined by the fraction of drug that escapes hepatic first-pass loss (i.e., $F = F_H$). Since the fraction of hepatic extraction is E_H, the fraction that escapes hepatic first-pass loss can be calculated as:

$$F = 1 - E_H \tag{4-13}$$

Based on Equation 4-8, the above equation can be expressed as:

$$F = 1 - \frac{f_u \cdot Cl_{int}}{Q_H + f_u \cdot CL_{int}} = \frac{Q_H + f_u \cdot CL_{int} - f_u \cdot Cl_{int}}{Q_H + f_u \cdot CL_{int}} \rightarrow F = \frac{Q_H}{Q_H + f_u \cdot CL_{int}} \tag{4-14}$$

For high extraction drug, since their $f_u \cdot CL_{int} \gg Q_H$, so that $Q_H + f_u \cdot CL_{int} \approx f_u \cdot CL_{int}$. Therefore, their bioavailability can be simplified as:

$$F = \frac{Q_H}{Q_H + f_u \bullet CL_{int}} \quad \rightarrow \quad F = \frac{Q_H}{f_u \bullet CL_{int}} \tag{4-15}$$

For low extraction drug, since their $f_u \cdot CL_{int} \ll Q_H$, so that $Q_H + f_u \cdot CL_{int} \approx Q_H$. Therefore, their bioavailability can be simplified as:

$$F = \frac{Q_H \bullet}{Q_H + f_u \bullet CL_{int}} \quad \rightarrow \quad F = \frac{Q_H}{Q_H} \quad \rightarrow \quad F = 1 \tag{4-16}$$

Equations 4-15 and 4-16 indicate that the oral bioavailability of a high extraction drug is positively correlated with hepatic blood flow and negatively associated with fraction of unbound and intrinsic clearance. The oral bioavailability of a low extraction drug is close to 1 and is not dependent on any of those three factors.

The simplified equations for CL_H, E_H, and F are useful, and we often need them in predicting the direction of their changes when any physiological factor changes. As a memory aid, I provide a "cheat sheet" below:

	Full Equation	High Extraction Drug ($f_u \cdot CL_{int} \gg Q_H$)	Low Extraction Drug ($f_u \cdot CL_{int} \ll Q_H$)
CL_H	$\dfrac{Q_H \bullet f_u \bullet CL_{int}}{Q_H + f_u \bullet CL_{int}}$	Q_H	$f_u \bullet CL_{int}$
E_H	$\dfrac{f_u \bullet Cl_{int}}{Q_H + f_u \bullet CL_{int}}$	1	$\dfrac{f_u \bullet Cl_{int}}{Q_H}$
F	$\dfrac{Q_H}{Q_H + f_u \bullet CL_{int}}$	$\dfrac{Q_H}{f_u \bullet CL_{int}}$	1

4.3 Renal Clearance

In addition to the liver, the kidney represents another major organ for drug elimination. Figure 4-12 shows nephron, the structural and functional unit of kidney. As it shows, when the blood from the renal artery enters the glomerulus, a portion of it is filtered into tubule (i.e., glomerulus filtration) and the rest of the blood exits the glomerulus into capillary network around the tubule. When the drug in the filtrate travels along tubule system, including the proximal tubule, loop of Henle, and the distal tubule, it can be reabsorbed into the capillary surrounding the tubule (i.e., tubular reabsorption). Similarly, the portion of drug that originally does not get filtered by the glomerulus travels along the capillary network and can be secreted into the tubule system (i.e., tubular secretion).

Therefore, there are three physiological processes determining the renal clearance of a drug: glomerular filtration, tubular reabsorption, and tubular secretion. The rate of renal excretion is the net result of the rate of these three processes:

Rate of excretion = rate of filtration + [rate of secretion − rate of reabsorption]

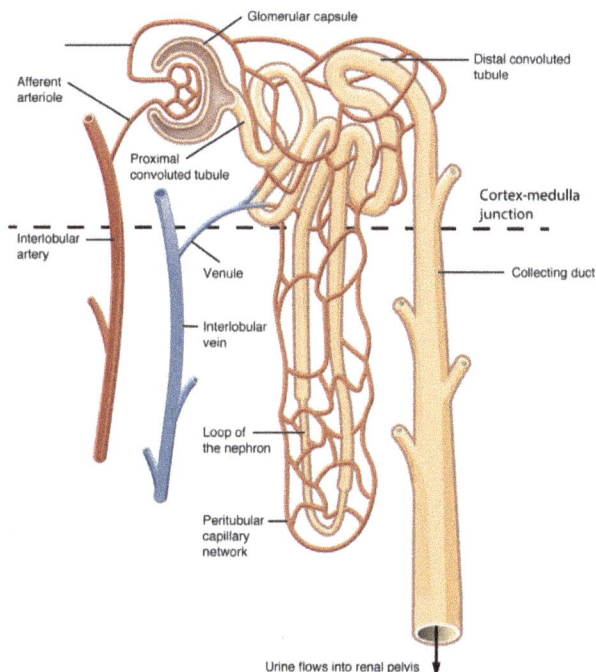

Figure 4-12. Nephron - the structural and functional unit of kidney.

4.3.1. Glomerular Filtration

The blood in the renal artery flows to the glomerulus at a rate of 1100 mL/min. Among this 1100 ml blood pumped into the glomerulus every minute, about 125 ml blood is filtered, and the rest of the 975 ml blood leaves glomerulus. Therefore, the glomerular filtration rate (GFR) is approximately 125 mL/min. During the glomerular filtration process, no large molecules are filtered. For drugs with molecular weight (MW) larger than 20,000 g/mol, filtration falls off sharply. Proteins with MW of 60,000 g/mol are not filtered at all.

Question 1: What is the maximum renal clearance of a small-molecule drug if only filtration goes on?

- *If there is only filtration step, the maximum clearance would be the situation when all the drug filtered through the glomerulus is removed from the body, which is the GFR (i.e., CL_R=GFR)*

Question 2: Can CL_R (based on filtration only) reach maximal CL_H?

- *The answer is no. As noted above, the maximum CL_R=GFR=125 mL/min if only filtration goes on. In contrast, the maximum hepatic clearance is hepatic blood flow (i.e., Q_H=1450 mL/min), which is a much larger number.*

Question 3: What is the maximum renal extraction ratio E (based on filtration only)?

- *Among all drug molecules in the volume of 1100 ml blood entering the glomerulus every minute, only those in the volume of 125 ml blood are filtered and subsequently eliminated. Therefore, if there is only filtration process, the maximum E is:*

$$E = \frac{GFR}{Renal\ blood\ flow} = \frac{125\ mL/min}{1100\ mL/min} = 0.11$$

Therefore, if a drug is renally eliminated only through glomerular filtration, by nature it is a low renal extraction drug.

For the 125 ml blood that is filtered every minute, so far, we assumed that all drug in this volume of blood is filtered. This is only true if the drug is present in free form. The drug bound to plasma proteins is too big to pass through the fenestration of the glomerular endothelial cells. Therefore, if we consider protein binding and only filtration going on, the renal clearance is:

$$CL_R = GFR \cdot f_u \qquad\qquad [4\text{-}17]$$

Question 4: How much urine will we produce everyday if only filtration goes on?

- $Total\ volume\ of\ urine = 125\,\dfrac{ml}{min} \times 60\,\dfrac{min}{h} \times 24\,\dfrac{h}{day} = 180\ L$

The math is simple, but the result is quite shocking. Imagine that if we produce 180 L urine every day, we will spend a lot of time in the restroom, and meanwhile we would need to keep drinking water to avoid dehydration. This is terrible. Luckily, our body is clever and actively reabsorbs most of the water via tubular reabsorption.

4.3.2. Tubular Reabsorption

Among the 180 L of water that is filtered by the glomerulus and enters the tubule, most of the water is reabsorbed when it passes down the tubule. As a result, the final volume of urine entering the bladder is only 1-2 L per day, with a urine flow of 1-2 mL/min. This is the fate of the water in the kidney.

Question 5: Would the fate of the water affect the fate of the drug in the filtrate?

- *The answer is yes. When the water in the filtrate is reabsorbed back to the blood, the filtrate is condensed. As a result, drug concentration in the filtrate is increased and is much higher than that in the blood. Therefore, when the water is reabsorbed, the drug tends to follow the water because of the concentration gradient. However, whether the drug can successfully follow the water or not depends on the drug's ability to pass through the tubular basement membrane. If you recall, in Chapter 3 (section 3.1.1), we learned the properties of the drug that are important for transmembrane passage. The same principle applies in passive drug reabsorption - only un-ionized nonpolar drugs can move across the tubular basement membrane and get reabsorbed (assuming passive diffusion is the only mechanism).*

<u>*Question 6:*</u> What is the renal clearance of a drug undergoing "full" passive reabsorption?

- *Among the 125 ml plasma water that is filtered into the tubule every minute, 99% of the water (i.e., around 123-124 ml) will be reabsorbed back; the final urine produced is 1-2 ml every minute (i.e., urine flow = 1-2 ml/min). For an un-ionized nonpolar drug, all drug molecules in that 99% of the water will be absorbed back. The concentration in the final filtrate (i.e. urine) is identical to the free drug concentration in the blood.*

Therefore, the renal clearance of a drug undergoing full passive reabsorption is calculated as:

$$CL_R = \frac{Rate\ of\ excretion}{C_P} \rightarrow CL_R = \frac{Urine\ flow \cdot Urine\ concentration}{C_P} \rightarrow$$
$$CL_R = \frac{Urine\ flow \cdot C_P \cdot f_u}{C_P}$$

Therefore, $CL_R = Urine\ flow \cdot f_u$ [4-18]

Equation 4-18 is for a lipophilic drug that is present in the filtrate with 100% un-ionized form. Generally speaking, if we assume only passive diffusion is involved, the completeness of a drug's reabsorption depends on the degree of ionization, which is determined by the drug's pKa and urine pH, as well as the lipophilicity of the drug's unionized form. For drugs that are partially ionized, if there are only glomerular filtration and passive tubular reabsorption, we would expect that their renal clearance is somewhere between $GFR \cdot f_u$ and urine flow $\cdot f_u$,

Case Example 4-4.

Methamphetamine renal excretion in urine with different pH

Methamphetamine, commonly referred to as meth, is a potent and highly addictive central nervous system stimulant and is a recreational drug. Figure 4-13 shows the amount of methamphetamine excreted in acidic urine (pH 4.9-5.3), alkaline urine (pH 7.8-8.2), or urine without pH control (around pH 6.4). Please look at this figure and explain why the renal elimination of methamphetamine behaves so differently in these three groups. Please work on it yourself before looking at the answer I provide below.

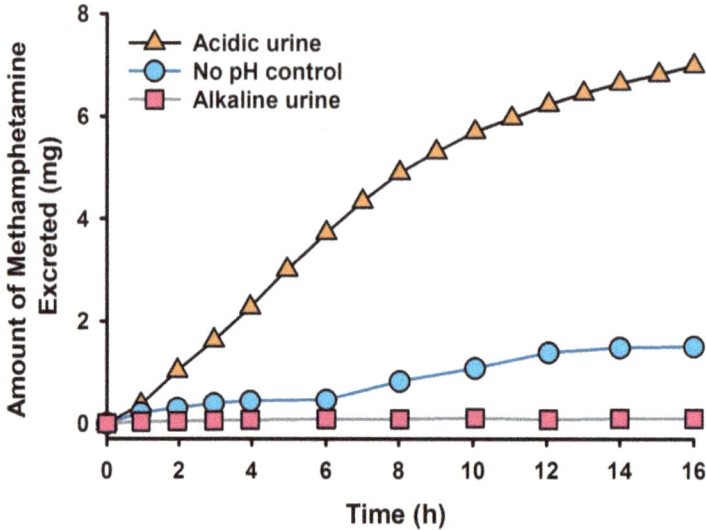

Figure 4-13. The impact of urine pH on the renal excretion of methamphetamine. *Adapted from: Beckett AH & Rowland M. Nature 1965;206:1260-1261.*

~ ~ ~

Methamphetamine is a weak and non-polar base (pKa 9.9). In alkaline urine, methamphetamine is mainly present in its un-ionized form, leading to full passive reabsorption and decrease in renal elimination. In contrast, methamphetamine is extensively ionized in acidic urine. As the ionized form cannot pass through the tubule basement membrane, the reabsorption of methamphetamine is close to zero, resulting in dramatic increase in the renal excretion of this drug. Therefore, for smart drug addicts, they would make their urine alkaline, so that the renal elimination of methamphetamine is reduced and the drug in the body can last longer. On the other hand, if a methamphetamine addict comes to the clinic, the doctor would make the patient's urine acidic to increase the renal elimination of methamphetamine.

Methamphetamine is just one example. In general, for a basic non-polar drug with pKa between 7 and 12, the extent of reabsorption may vary from close to zero to almost complete (equilibrium) with changes in urine pH. However, a basic drug that is polar in its un-ionized form will not be reabsorbed (assuming there is only passive diffusion), regardless of its ionization (e.g., gentamycin). On the other hand, a very weak basic nonpolar drug (pKa $\leq$7.0) is extensively reabsorbed regardless of urine pH (e.g. diazepam), because virtually 100% presents as un-ionized forms at different values of urine pH. Similar principles apply to acidic drugs.

As noted earlier, for drugs that undergo extensive passive reabsorption, their renal clearance is directly associated with the urine flow (see Equation 4-18). For these drugs, if there is a need to remove them from the body for detoxification purpose, one strategy is forced diuresis to increase the drug's renal elimination by increasing the urine flow.

So far, I have talked about *passive tubular reabsorption*. Tubular reabsorption can also occur against concentration gradient (i.e., *active tubular reabsorption*). As shown in Figure 4-4, there are many drug transporters expressed in the proximal tubules. Some transporters, such as peptide transporter 1 (PEPT1) and urate transporter 1 (URAT1), can actively move the drug in the filtrate to the blood. Therefore, for drugs that are substrates of that type of transporters, they can be reabsorbed back to the blood regardless of concentration gradient or ionization status.

Question 7: What would be the minimal renal clearance if a drug undergoes complete active reabsorption?

- *As noted earlier, the transporter can move drugs against concentration gradient and can transport not only non-polar unionized form, but also ionized form and polar unionized form. For a drug undergoing active tubular reabsorption with the help of the transporter, theoretically, all drug molecules present in the filtrate can be reabsorbed back to blood. Therefore, the renal clearance could be 0 for a drug undergoing complete active reabsorption ($CL_R=0$).*

Tubular reabsorption is indicated when CL_R is less than $GFR \cdot f_u$. Please note that while tubular reabsorption can occur either passively or actively, for exogenous compounds such as drugs, passive reabsorption is a more common pathway. Active reabsorption occurs more often for endogenous compounds, such as vitamins, electrolytes, glucose, amino acids, and uric acid; this makes sense since those are essential substances, and our body, which is clever, does not want to lose them and uses transporters to gain them back.

4.3.3 Tubular Secretion

We just talked about the transporters that can perform active tubular reabsorption. Some transporters can do the opposite task – they move the drug from the blood to the tubule system, a process known as tubular secretion. Tubular secretion is an active process, which means that the drug can be transported against concentration gradient and regardless of ionization status. As shown in Figure 4-4, many transporters, including P-gp, organic anion transporters (OATs) and organic cation transporters (OCTs), are involved in tubular active secretion process. Tubular secretion is indicated when CL_R is larger than $GFR \cdot f_u$.

Question 8: What would be the maximal renal clearance if a drug undergoes full active secretion?

- *As noted earlier, among the 1100 ml blood pumped into the glomerulus every minute, about 125 ml blood is filtered, and the rest 975 ml blood exits glomerulus. These 975 ml blood leaves glomerulus, but not the nephron – it travels in the capillary network which surrounds the tubule. Theoretically, for a drug that is a substrate of a transporter working on secretion, all drug in those 975 ml blood can be secreted into the tubule. This means that, after the drug enters the kidney, a portion of it is filtered into tubule via glomerular filtration, and the rest can be secreted into tubule by tubular secretion. Therefore, the maximal renal clearance could reach renal blood flow for a drug undergoing full active secretion (CL_R=Renal blood flow).*

4.3.4 Estimation of Renal Function

Renal excretion represents an important elimination pathway, and many drugs have been found to be eliminated mainly through the kidney. To name a few, many antibiotics, such as amikacin, ampicillin, cefazolin, gentamycin, penicillin, vancomycin, and cefepime, are mainly eliminated by the kidney.

Considering the important role of the kidney in drug elimination, there is a natural interest in finding a way to measure renal function. In 1960, Bricker proposed the 'intact nephron hypothesis', saying that if one part of the nephron is damaged, then function in the rest of the nephron is reduced to the same degree. This hypothesis provides the theoretical basis of using GFR as an overall measure of renal function since the renal clearance of drugs is reduced to the same degree regardless of the location of the disease.

Effort has been made to find markers of GFR. If we could make a wish list, the ideal marker of GFR should have the following features:

- Freely filterable at the glomerulus.
- No plasma protein binding
- Neither secreted nor reabsorbed by the tubules.
- No extra-renal route of excretion.
- Easily and accurately measured.

The marker that is close to this ideal situation is inulin, which is an exogenous marker. Inulin is freely filterable, no protein binding, does not undergo tubular secretion or reabsorption, and has no extra-renal route. Unfortunately, its measurement requires significant blood sample volume, assay to detect it is difficult, expensive, and time-consuming. Therefore, while inulin represents a gold standard for GFR, it is limited to investigational research or situations where accurate estimate of GFR is critical.

Creatinine as the GFR marker

Another marker for GFR is creatinine, which is an endogenous marker. Creatinine does not bind to plasma protein, is freely filtered by the glomerulus. However, it undergoes active tubular secretion, and has non-renal pathways. In addition, it is generated from muscle breakdown. Therefore, the level of creatinine is influenced by muscle mass and dietary intake of meat. While creatinine has several limitations, it still represents the most commonly used way to estimate GFR because it is easy to measure.

Creatinine clearance (CL_{Cr}) reflects GFR and can be determined using different ways. One way to calculate CL_{Cr} is based on the concentration of creatinine in urine and serum based on the following equation:

$$CL_{Cr} = \frac{Urinary\ excretion\ rate}{Serum\ concentration\ at\ midpoint\ of\ collection\ interval} = \frac{\frac{\Delta U}{\Delta t}}{C_{mid}}$$ [4-19]

Case Example 4-5.

Patient NY is admitted into the hospital. Urine is collected for 8 hours, and a total of 560 mg creatinine is excreted. The serum creatinine level after 4 hours, which is the midpoint of collection interval, is 1.0 mg/dL (i.e., 0.01 mg/mL). What is this patient's creatinine clearance?

~ ~ ~

For the unit of creatinine, usually mL/min is preferred so that the value can be easily compared with the GFR of 125 ml/min. During the calculation, please pay attention to the unit conversion. For example, 1 dL = 100 mL; 1 mg/mL = 1 g/L; 1 L/h= 1000 ml/60 min = 16.67 mL/min.

$$CL_{Cr} = \frac{\frac{\Delta U}{\Delta t}}{C_{mid}} = \frac{\frac{560\ mg}{8\ h}}{0.01\ g/L} = 7\ L/h = 117\ mL/min$$

Estimating creatinine clearance using both urine and plasma data is hard to implement in the clinic as the collection of urine samples is not convenient in every clinical setting. To overcome this issue, multiple methods, including the *Cockcroft and Gault method,* have been developed to estimate creatinine clearance using just one serum creatinine concentration, along with other routine clinical data such as patient age, gender, height, and weight.

Cockcroft and Gault method

FDA guidance recommends the use of the Cockcroft Gault equation to calculate CL_{Cr}, which represents the estimated GFR (eGFR), and estimate renal function using the following classifications:

- Normal renal function – $CL_{Cr} \geq 90$ mL/min
- Mild renal impairment - CL_{Cr} 60- 89 mL/min
- Moderate renal impairment - CL_{Cr} 30- 59 mL/min
- Severe renal impairment - CL_{Cr} 15-29 mL/min

- Kidney failure - $CL_{Cr} \leq 15$ mL/min

Following is the equations of *the Cockcroft and Gault method* for CL_{Cr} estimation in adults:

Equation for ***males***: $$CL_{cr} = \frac{(140 - age) \cdot BW}{CP_{cr} \cdot 72}$$ [4-20]

Equation for *females*: $$CL_{Cr} = \frac{(140 - age) \bullet BW}{Cp_{Cr} \bullet 72} \times 0.85$$ [4-21]

As creatinine does not reside in fat, following is the suggestion of the bodyweight used in the equation:

- Use actual body weight (TBW) when actual body weight is less than or equal to ideal bodyweight (IBW)
- Use IBW when actual body weight is greater than IBW by <25%
- Use adjusted body weight (ABW) when actual body weight is greater than IBW by 25% or more. ABW is calculated as:

    ABW = IBW + 0.4·(TBW-IBW)   [4-22]

IBW is calculate as:

    Males   IBW = 50 kg + 2.3 kg for each inch over 5ft   [4-23]
    Females   IBW = 45.5 kg + 2.3 kg for each inch over 5ft   [4-24]

For the CL_{Cr} calculated using Equations 4-20 and 4-21, the unit is mL/min, although the right side of the equation contains age in years, bodyweight in kg, and serum creatinine in mg/dL.

Case Example 4-6.

A 40 year-old female patient is hospitalized for a ruptured duodenal diverticulum. Before surgery you are asked to begin this patient on aminoglycosides. Other pertinent patient data include height 5ft, 4in, weight 60 kg, serum creatinine 1.7 mg/dL. Please estimate the creatinine clearance of this patient using the Cockcroft and Gault method.

~ ~ ~

As this is a female patient, Equation 4-21 should be used. But before we plug in the numbers provided, we need to first figure out which BW to use. Based on Equation 4-24, the IBW of this patient is:

- $IBW = 45.5 + 2.3 \times 4 = 54.7\, kg$

The difference between IBW and TBW of this patient is:

- $$\% \, difference = \frac{(TBW - IBW)}{IBW} \times 100\% = \frac{(60 - 54.7)}{54.7} \times 100\% = 9.7\%$$

Since TBW of this patient is greater than IBW by <25%, IBW is used to calculate CLcr using Equation 4-24:

$$CL_{Cr} = \frac{(140 - 40) \bullet 54.7}{1.7 \bullet 72} \times 0.85 = 38 \; mL/min$$

4.4 The impact of Change in Physiological Conditions in Pharmacokinetics Parameters and Pharmacokinetics Profiles

When certain physiological conditions are altered, they may affect one or several (or even all) key pharmacokinetics parameters. As a result, the pharmacokinetic profiles may change as well. In this section, I provide one case example below, and I hope it will help you to better understand the impact of change in physiological conditions in drug pharmacokinetics.

Case Example 4-7.

Iowa-001 is a lipophilic drug which is eliminated exclusively through liver metabolism. Iowa-001 is bound to albumin, and it is a low extraction drug. It follows the first-order kinetics, and its disposition can be described using a one-compartment model. Following are four scenarios in which physiological conditions change:
  A) Increase in liver blood flow.
  B) Decrease in drug metabolizing enzymes.
  C) Increase in the number of adipose cells.
  D) Increase in the plasma albumin binding.
      Based on the knowledge we have learned in Chapters 1, 3, and 4, please

1) predict the impact of each scenario on the key pharmacokinetic parameters of Iowa-001, namely, CL, V_d, k_e, $t_{1/2}$;

2) draw a figure for each scenario to illustrate the old and new pharmacokinetic profiles when Iowa-001 is given via I.V. bolus.

Please work on it yourself before looking at the answer I provide below.

$$\sim \; \sim \; \sim$$

To solve this type of problem, my suggestion is to list all relevant equations first. Iowa-001 undergoes hepatic elimination only, which means that the total clearance = hepatic clearance. As it is a low extraction drug, its clearance can be expressed using the simplified form as provided in Equation 4-11:

$$CL = CL_H = f_u \cdot CL_{int}$$

Based on what we learned in Chapter 3, V_d can be estimated using the following equation:

$$V_d = V_p + V_t \cdot \frac{f_u}{f_{u,t}}$$

The equations for k_e and $t_{1/2}$ are:

$$k_e = \frac{CL}{V_d} = \frac{f_u \cdot CL_{int}}{V_p + V_t \cdot \frac{f_u}{f_{u,t}}}$$

$$t_{1/2} = \frac{0.693}{k_e}$$

Now let's look at each scenario.

- *Increase in liver blood flow (scenario A) means that Q increases.*
- *Decrease in drug metabolizing enzymes (scenario B) will lead to decrease in intrinsic clearance (i.e., CL_{int} ↓)*
- *Since Iowa-001 is lipophilic, increase in the number of adipose cells (scenario C) will increase the binding of drug molecules to adipose cells, resulting in decrease in fraction of unbound drug in tissue (i.e., $f_{u,t}$ ↓).*
- *With increase in the plasma albumin binding (scenario D), fraction of unbound drug in plasma decreases (i.e., fu↓)*

Below table is provided to facilitate the comparison between your results and the one I provided here:

Table 4-4. *Impact of changes physiological factors on Iowa-001 pharmacokinetics parameters.*

Scenario	Physiological factor altered	CL	V_d	k_e	$t_{1/2}$
A	Q↑	↔	↔	↔	↔
B	CL_{int} ↓	↓	↔	↓	↑
C	$f_{u,t}$ ↓	↔	↑	↓	↑
D	fu↓	↓	↓	↓	↑

Figure 4-14 shows the impact of each scenario on Iowa-001 pharmacokinetics (note: solid black line is the original curve, and blue dashed line is the new curve).

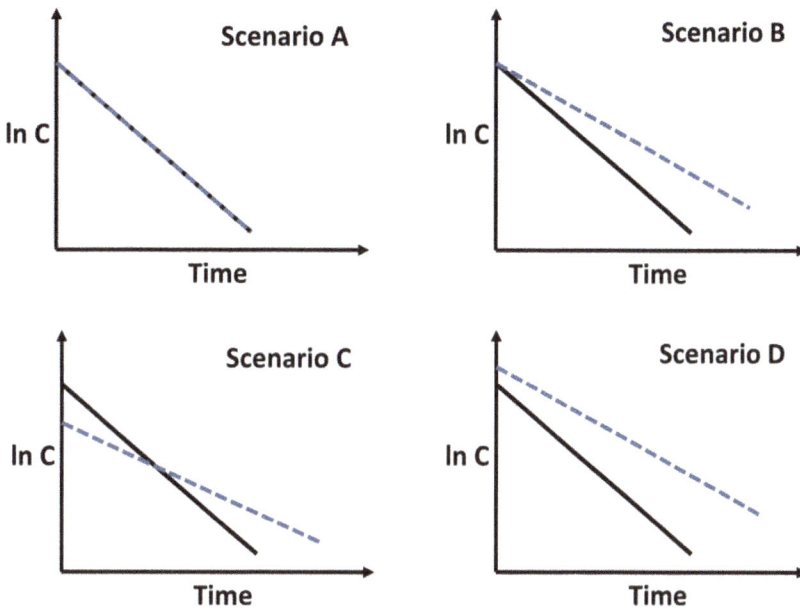

Figure 4-14. The effect of physiological changes on Iowa-001 pharmacokinetics. *Solid black line represents the original condition, and blue dashed line represents the new condition.*

4.5 Miscellaneous Notes

❖ *Enterohepatic circulation (EHC)*   For a drug undergoing biliary excretion, after it is secreted into the bile and then released into the small intestine, some drug molecules could be reabsorbed back to systemic circulation; this phenomenon is known as enterohepatic circulation (EHC). EHC can occur not only in parent drugs but also in conjugated metabolites. For example, after a glucuronide metabolite is released into the gut via biliary excretion, it can be converted back to the parent drug by glucuronidase, an enzyme found in the gut microbiota. Then the parent drug can be reabsorbed in systemic circulation. For a drug undergoing extensive EHC, its pharmacokinetic curve may show a second peak due to drug reabsorption.

Problem Sets   *(Answers to study problems are in the appendix)*

1. The renal clearance of a drug is 400 ml/min; this may suggest:
    - o The drug is only eliminated by glomerular filtration.   (True | False)
    - o The drug is eliminated by tubular secretion.   (True | False)
    - o Drug interactions in renal tubules are possible.   (True | False)
    - o The drug is likely to be un-ionized.   (True | False)
    - o The drug must not have tubular reabsorption.   (True | False)

2. For a high extraction drug, indicate which of the following parameters affects clearance (choose all that apply):
    A. Fraction bound in plasma.
    B. Liver blood flow
    C. Intrinsic clearance
    D. Tissue binding

3. When liver blood flow is increased in a patient taking a high extraction drug, the oral bioavailability of this drug will:
    A. Increase.
    B. Remain unchanged.
    C. Decrease.

4. When intrinsic clearance is increased in a patient taking a low extraction drug, the extraction ratio (E) of this drug will:
    A. Increase.
    B. Remain unchanged.
    C. Decrease.

5. When a high extraction drug undergoing CYP3A metabolism is co-administered with a CYP3A inhibitor (both given via I.V. route), its AUC will:
    A. Increase.
    B. Remain unchanged.
    C. Decrease

6. For a high extraction drug, indicate which of the following parameters affects its oral bioavailability (choose all that apply):
    A. Fraction bound in plasma.
    B. Liver blood flow
    C. Intrinsic clearance
    D. Tissue binding

7. A drug that is actively secreted must show a renal clearance larger than 125 mL/min (0.5 point)
    A. True
    B. False

8. Enzyme induction affects the hepatic clearance of low extraction drug.
    A. True
    B. False

9. The maximum value of renal clearance is that of the glomerular filtration rate.
    A. True

B. False
10. A drug with fu=0.01 and a renal clearance (CL_r) = 20 ml/min is:
   A. filtered only.
   B. filtered and reabsorbed.
   C. Filtered and actively secreted.

PART II

Utilize Compartment Models for Dose Optimization

Chapter 5.
Single IV Bolus (One-Compartment Model)

Learning Objectives

After reading this chapter, the reader shall be able to:

1. Predict the time course of drug concentration in the body using a one-compartment model.

2. Understand the relationship between dose, dosing regimen, clearance, and volume of distribution on drug concentration-time profiles. Apply these relationships for therapeutic drug monitoring (TDM).

3. Apply the model for dose optimization for drugs administered via I.V. bolus injection.

4. Familiar with formation-rate limited metabolism and elimination-rate limited metabolism.

So far, we have finished Part I of this book, which includes Chapters 1-4 and focuses on fundamental concepts. I have walked you through each individual process of pharmacokinetics, including **A**bsorption (Chapter 2), **D**istribution (Chapter 3), **M**etabolism and **E**xcretion (combined into Elimination in Chapter 4). The goal of Part II of this book, which includes Chapters 5-11, is to utilize compartment models to evaluate pharmacokinetics and perform dose optimization of drugs administered via different routes or in different populations. As the start of Part II, Chapter 5 covers the easiest situation - drugs following a single dose via I.V. bolus injection, whose pharmacokinetics can be characterized using a one-compartment model.

The good news is that most of the equations related to single I.V. bolus administration using a one-compartment model have already been covered in Chapter 1. We will refresh these equations in Section 5.1, then evaluate how changes in dose and primary pharmacokinetic parameters (i.e. CL and V_d) affect drug concentration-time profiles in Section 5.2. For drugs eliminated through metabolism, they are converted to different substances, namely metabolites, which undergo distribution and elimination processes as well. I will touch a little bit on the pharmacokinetics of drug metabolites in Section 5.3. We study pharmacokinetics not for fun; the ultimate goal is utilizing these mathematical equations for dose optimization to ensure safe and effective drug therapy. Section 5.4 provides a case example of applying the model for dose optimization. Additional case studies are provided in Section 5.5 before this chapter ends with problem sets.

5.1 Pharmacokinetic Equations for a Drug Following a Single IV Bolus Injection

For a drug administered via a single I.V. bolus injection, its pharmacokinetics can be described using a one-compartment model shown in Figure 5-1.

Based on this model, the rate of change of drug in the body (i.e., amount of drug changes in the body per given time) is described as:

$$\frac{dX}{dt} = -k_e \bullet X$$

$$X_0 = Dose$$

[5-1]

Where X represents drug amount in the body, k_e represents elimination rate constant, and X_0 represents initial amount in the body, which is dose for I.V. bolus injection. A negative sign is put in front of k_e since the amount of drug in the body decreases over time.

I.V. bolus dose

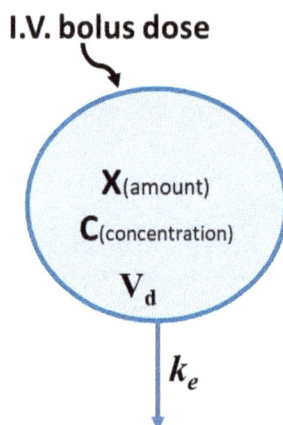

Figure 5-1. Schematic representation of a one-compartment model for a drug administrated via single I.V. bolus injection.

Equation 5-1 can be easily solved to get the following explicit equation:

$$X = Dose \bullet e^{-k_e \bullet t}$$

[5-2]

Since what we measure is drug concentration instead of drug amount, we would want an explicit equation for concentration C, which can be easily obtained since $C = \frac{X}{V_d}$:

$$\frac{X}{V_d} = \frac{Dose}{V_d} \bullet e^{-k_e \bullet t} \quad \rightarrow \quad C = C_0 \bullet e^{-k_e \bullet t}$$

[5-3]

Equation 5-3 contains the following two pieces:

- C_0, which determines the starting concentration and is dependent on dose and volume of distribution.
- $e^{-k_e \cdot t}$, a term ranges from 1 (when t=0) to 0 (when t =∞). This term describes how fast drug disappears from the body. The larger k_e, the faster the change from 1 to 0.

As noted in previous chapters, k_e is a secondary parameter and is determined by clearance and volume of distribution:

$$k_e = \frac{CL}{V_d} \quad\quad\quad [5\text{-}4]$$

In addition, k_e is inversely related to half-life ($t_{1/2}$), another secondary parameter, with the following relationship:

$$t_{1/2} = \frac{0.693}{k_e} \quad\quad\quad [5\text{-}5]$$

CL is a primary pharmacokinetics parameter, and it can be calculated as:

$$CL = \frac{Dose}{AUC} \quad\quad\quad [5\text{-}6]$$

Where AUC is the area of the concentration-time curve from time 0 to time infinity.

CL can also be obtained if the information k_e and V_d are available:

$$CL = k_e \bullet V_d \quad\quad\quad [5\text{-}7]$$

V_d is also a primary pharmacokinetic parameter, and it can be calculated based on the following equation:

$$V_d = \frac{Dose}{C_0} \quad\quad\quad [5\text{-}8]$$

If we know the information of CL and k_e, we can calculate V_d based on the following relationship:

$$V_d = \frac{CL}{k_e} \quad\quad\quad [5\text{-}9]$$

The information about AUC is useful as it reflects drug exposure. Unless specified, AUC refers to AUC from time 0 to time infinity. AUC can be calculated as follows:

$$AUC = \frac{Dose}{CL} \quad\quad\quad [5\text{-}10]$$

AUC can also be calculated based on the initial concentration and k_e:

$$AUC = \frac{Dose}{CL} \quad \rightarrow AUC = \frac{C_0 \bullet V_d}{k_e \bullet V_d} \quad \rightarrow AUC = \frac{C_0}{k_e} \quad\quad [5\text{-}11]$$

It is important to keep in mind that compartment models simplify the physiological processes and drug kinetics, and they are built under assumptions. The following are the assumptions for a one-compartment model:

- Immediate distribution, which means that once a drug is administered, it reaches the whole body simultaneously. This assumption allows us to use one compartment to represent our body.
- Elimination is the first-order process. As discussed in Chapter 1, most drugs follow first-order elimination within therapeutic dose ranges.
- Linear pharmacokinetics. Linear pharmacokinetics means that there is no saturation of binding sites, and no saturation of drug metabolizing enzymes and drug transporters. Therefore, under linear pharmacokinetics, CL and V_d are dose- and concentration- independent.

Drug concentration-time profiles are subject to change if there is a change in drug input (i.e., dose) or pharmacokinetics parameter. Let's examine these relationships in the next section.

5.2 Effect of Dose, Clearance, and Volume of Distribution on Drug Concentration-Time Profiles

In this section, I provide one case example below, which hopefully could help you to gain a good understanding on the impact of changes in drug input and pharmacokinetics parameters on drug concentration-time profiles.

> ### Case Example 5-1.

Iowa-001 is a new investigational drug with intended indication in alleviating last minute exam panic attacks. It follows the first-order kinetics, and its disposition can be described using a one-compartment model.

Scenario 1. A higher dose of Iowa-001 is administered.

Scenario 2. The clearance of Iowa-001 increases.

Scenario 3. The volume of distribution of Iowa-001 increases.

Please 1) evaluate the impact of each scenario on C_0, AUC, k_e and $t_{1/2}$ of Iowa-001 when it is administered via a single I.V. bolus injection; and 2) draw a figure for each scenario to illustrate the old and new pharmacokinetic profiles.

Please work on it yourself before looking at the answer I provide below.

~ ~ ~

To address this type of question, first we need to list the relevant equations.

- $C_0 = \dfrac{Dose}{V_d}$
- $AUC = \dfrac{Dose}{CL}$
- $k_e = \dfrac{CL}{V_d}$
- $t_{1/2} = \dfrac{0.693}{k_e}$

In scenario 1. The dose of Iowa-001 increases. Based on the above questions, the parameters that are affected by dose are C_0 and AUC. With an increase in dose, both C_0 and AUC of Iowa-001 increase proportionally. In contrast, k_e and $t_{1/2}$ are not affected by dose.

In scenario 2. Based on the above four equations, with an increase in clearance, C_0 stays the same; AUC decreases; k_e increases; and $t_{1/2}$ decreases.

In scenario 3. With an increase in V_d, C_0 decreases; AUC stays the same; k_e decreases; and $t_{1/2}$ increases.

The table below is provided to facilitate the comparison between your results and the one I provided here:

Table 5-1. Impact of changes in dose, CL, or V_d on Iowa-001 pharmacokinetics parameters.

	C_0	AUC	k_e	$t_{1/2}$
Increase in dose	↑	↑	↔	↔
Increase in CL	↔	↓	↑	↓
Increase in V_d	↓	↔	↓	↑

Figure 5-2 shows the impact of each scenario on Iowa-001 pharmacokinetics (note: solid black line is the original condition, and blue dashed line is the new condition).

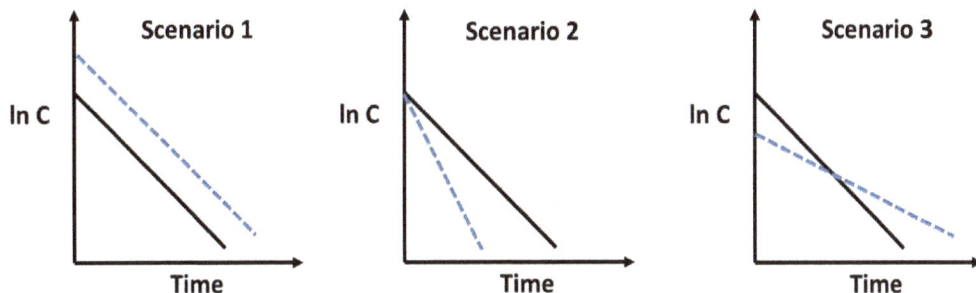

Figure 5-2. The effect of dose, CL, and V_d on Iowa-001 pharmacokinetics. *Solid black line represents the original condition, and blue dashed line represents the new condition.*

Please note that I drew Figure 5-2 using lnC instead of C, so that it directly shows straight lines, instead of curves. We can also plot C on a log scale, which will also show straight line, as I discussed in Chapter 1. To compare the pharmacokinetics profiles, illustrating the concentration-time profile using either lnC on a linear scale or C on a log scale is preferred; this is because we can examine the slope more clearly than that from a curve where C on a linear scale.

5.3 Pharmacokinetics of Drug Metabolites

As we have learned in Chapter 4, the major elimination pathways include hepatic metabolism, renal excretion, and biliary excretion. Drug excretion eliminates a drug in its unchanged form, while drug metabolism converts a drug to a metabolite (or several metabolites). Figure 5-3 (left panel) shows a model diagram of a drug undergoing multiple elimination pathways, including renal excretion, biliary excretion, and metabolism. X, U, B, M represent the drug in the body, drug excreted in urine, drug excreted in bile, and metabolite in the body, respectively. k_{ren}, k_{bil}, and k_{met} represent the elimination rate constant of urine excretion, biliary excretion, and drug metabolism, respectively.

When we look at the concentration-time profile on the right panel of Figure 5-3, we won't know the exact elimination mechanism of this drug. What we can get from the concentration-time profile is k_e, which is sum of each individual elimination rate constant:

$$k_e = k_{ren} + k_{bil} + k_{med} \qquad [5\text{-}12]$$

Accordingly, the clearance of this drug, calculated based on the concentration-time profile using the equation $\frac{Dose}{AUC}$, is the total clearance and is the sum of each individual elimination pathway:

$$CL = CL_{ren} + CL_{bil} + CL_{med} \qquad [5\text{-}13]$$

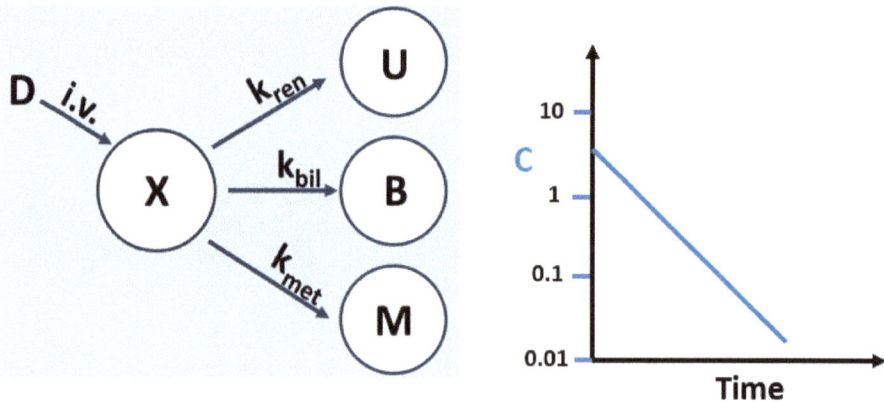

Figure 5-3. (left) Model diagram of a drug undergoing three parallel elimination pathways, namely renal excretion, biliary excretion, and metabolism. X, U, B, M represent the drug in the body, drug excreted in urine, drug excreted in bile, and metabolite in the body, respectively; (right) Concentration-time profile of the same drug.

Question 5-1: For the drug mentioned above, let's assume its renal clearance is 10 mL/min, its biliary clearance is 10 mL/min, and its clearance from metabolism is 80 mL/min. a) what is the total clearance? b) if we give a dose of 100 mg, how much of the dose would be metabolized?

- *Based on Equation 5-13, the total clearance is:*

$CL = CL_{ren} + CL_{bil} + CL_{med} = 10 + 10 + 80 = 100 \ mL/min.$

If we give a dose of 100 mg, the fraction of dose that is metabolized (f_m) is:

$$f_m = \frac{Cl_{med}}{CL_{ren} + CL_{bil} + CL_{med}} = \frac{80}{10 + 10 + 80} = 0.8$$

Accordingly, the amount of dose that is metabolized is:

$Dose \times f_m = 100 \times 0.8 = 80 \ mg$

The model diagram shown in Figure 5-3 illustrates the elimination pathways from the drug's perspective. To the parent drug, k_{met} represents the elimination rate constant resulting from drug metabolism. However, from the metabolite's perspective, k_{met} represents the formation rate constant of the metabolite. The metabolite is generated during drug metabolism, and once formed, it undergoes distribution and elimination processes as well. In most cases, metabolites are biochemically inactive compounds with neither a therapeutic nor toxic effect (i.e., inactive metabolites). In some situations, metabolites that are pharmacologically active are formed (i.e., active metabolites).

Since some drugs may have active metabolites, it is useful to understand the pharmacokinetics of metabolites. Let's touch a little bit on the equations that can be used to characterize metabolite disposition. I use the same example drug shown in Figure 5-3. Since the focus is on the metabolite now, let's update the model diagram by adding the elimination pathway of the metabolite (Figure 5-4).

Based on the model diagram of the metabolite, its rate of change in the body (i.e., the amount of metabolite change in the body per given time) can be described as:

$$\frac{dM}{dt} = k_{met} \bullet X - k_e^M \bullet M \qquad\qquad [5\text{-}14]$$

Where:

M = amount of the metabolite in the body

X = amount of the drug in the body

k_{met} = formation rate constant of the metabolite, which is also the elimination rate constant (metabolic pathway) of the drug.

k_e^M = elimination rate constant of the metabolite.

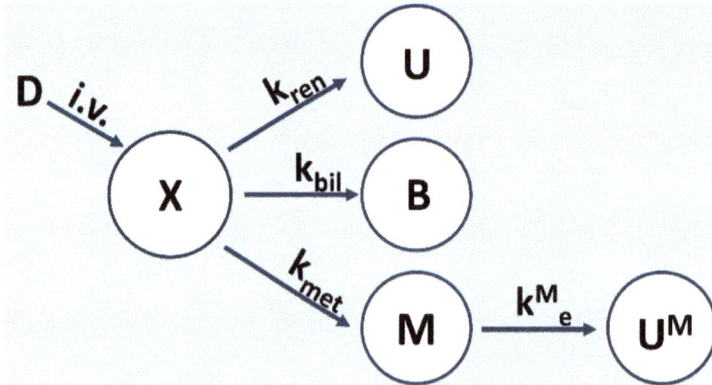

Figure 5-4. Model diagram of a drug undergoing three parallel elimination pathways, as well as the metabolite generated during drug metabolism.

In Equation 5-14, there two rate functions:

- $k_{met} \cdot X$ describes the amount of the metabolite generated per given time. It is a positive term since it represents the formation of the metabolite.
- $k_e^M \cdot M$ characterizes the amount of the metabolite eliminated from the body. A negative sign is put in front of this function since it represents the elimination of the metabolite.

Equation 5-14 can be solved to get the following explicit equation:

$$C_P^M = \frac{k_{met} \cdot D}{V_D^M \cdot (K_e^M - k_e)} \cdot (e^{-k_e \cdot t} - e^{-k_e^M \cdot t})$$ [5-15]

Where:

D   = dose of the drug.

C_P^M = concentration of the metabolite in plasma.

V_D^M = volume of distribution of the metabolite.

k_{met} = formation rate constant of the metabolite, which is also the elimination rate constant (metabolic pathway) of the drug.

k_e = total elimination rate constant of the parent drug.

k_e^M = elimination rate constant of the metabolite.

This is a long equation. To simplify it, let's call the first portion of the equation "Constant". Therefore:

$$C_P^M = Constant \cdot (e^{-k_e \cdot t} - e^{-k_e^M \cdot t})$$ [5-16]

Where constant $= \dfrac{k_{met} \cdot D}{V_D^M \cdot (K_e^M - k_e)}$

In equation 5-16, there are two e terms, one containing k_e and another containing k_e^M. The pharmacokinetics of metabolites often fall into the following two scenarios:

- *Formation-rate limited metabolism (k_e^M is much larger than k_e)*

In this scenario, because k_e^M is much larger than k_e, $e^{-k_e^M \cdot t}$ approaches zero first at later time points. Therefore, the concentration of the metabolite at later time points can be simplified as

$$C_P^M = Constant \cdot e^{-k_e \cdot t} \qquad\qquad [5\text{-}17]$$

Equation 5-17 indicates that the slope of the metabolite concentration-time profile reflects the elimination rate constant of the parent drug; this is because how fast the metabolite is cleared is rate-limited by how fast the metabolite is generated, a phenomenon known as *formation-rate limited metabolism.*

Figure 5-5, left panel shows the anticipated concentration-time profiles of a drug and its metabolite, with formation-rate limited metabolism (i.e., k_e^M is much larger than k_e).

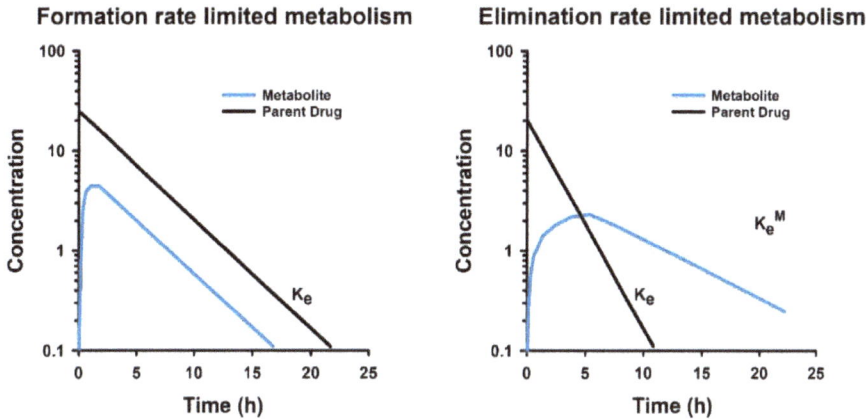

Figure 5-5. Anticipated concentration-time profiles of a drug and its metabolite when the drug undergoes formation rate limited metabolism (left) or elimination rate limited metabolism (right).

- *Elimination-rate limited metabolism (k_e is much larger than k_e^M)*

In this scenario, because k_e is much larger than k_e^M, $e^{-k_e \cdot t}$ approaches zero first at later time points. Therefore, the concentration of the metabolite at later time points can be simplified as

$$C_P^M = Constant \cdot e^{-k_e^M \cdot t} \qquad\qquad\qquad\qquad [5\text{-}18]$$

Equation 5-18 indicates that the slope of the metabolite concentration-time profile reflects its own elimination rate constant k_e^M since how fast the metabolite is cleared is rate-limited by its own elimination, a phenomenon known as *elimination-rate limited metabolism*.

Figure 5-5, right panel demonstrates the anticipated concentration-time profiles of a drug and its metabolite, with elimination-rate limited metabolism (i.e., k_e is much larger than k_e^M).

Based on Figure 5-5, we can conclude that regardless of different scenarios, the half-life of the metabolite will not be shorter than the half-life of the parent drug. Under the scenario of formation rate limited metabolism, the half-life of the metabolite is the same as the parent drug since the slopes of their concentration-time profiles parallel. Under the scenario of elimination rate limited metabolism, the half-life of the metabolite is longer than that of the parent drug since the slope of the plot of the metabolite is shallower than that of the drug.

We can easily tell whether a drug follows formation rate limited metabolism or elimination rate limited metabolism based on the concentration-time profiles of the drug and its metabolite. Before I joined academia, I worked at Abbott (now known as AbbVie) in Chicago for two and half years and worked on many interesting compounds. One particularly interesting compound is ABT-384, and I published several papers on this compound, including one drug-drug interaction study that is shown in Figure 5-6. In this study, the impact of ketoconazole, a potent CYP3A inhibitor, on the pharmacokinetics of ABT-384 and its two metabolites was evaluated. ABT-384 is a substrate of CYP3A, and its plasma exposure is greatly increased when it was co-administered with ketoconazole.

However, what I really want to show you is the pharmacokinetics of those two metabolites, namely A847082 and A1331480. Based on what we just learned, what is your comment on the concentration-time profiles of the metabolites shown in Figure 5-6?

The terminal slope of A1331480 concentration-time profile is in parallel to that of ABT-384, while the terminal slope of A847082 is shallower than that of ABT-384, indicating that A1331480 is the product of formation-rate limited metabolism and A847082 is the product of elimination-rate limited metabolism.

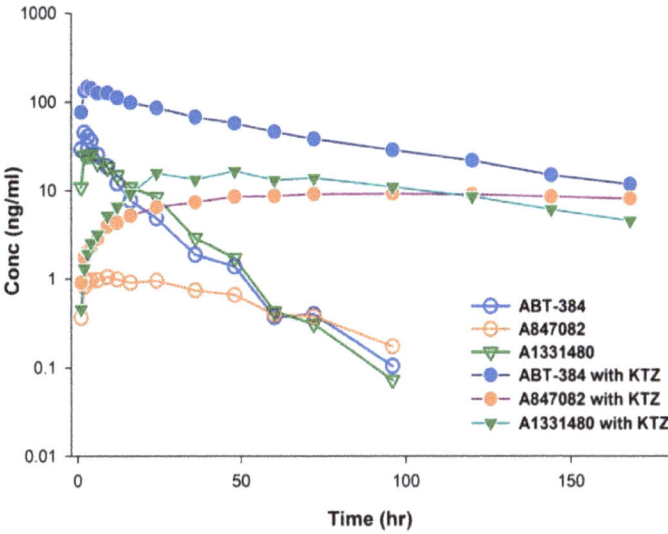

Figure 5-6. The pharmacokinetics of ABT-384 and its two metabolites, namely A847082 and A1331480, in healthy volunteers following a single oral dose of ABT-384 alone (open symbols) or with ketoconazole (filled symbols). *From: An G, et al. Drug Metabolism and Disposition 2013;41:1035-1045.*

5.4 Applying the Model for Dose Optimization

   As noted at the beginning, we make great efforts in learning pharmacokinetics and related equations because we need these tools in clinical practice (for pharmacists and professional practitioners in clinic), drug development (for pharmaceutical scientists in the industry), and pharmaceutical research (for researchers). This enables us to perform dose optimization for safe and effective drug therapy. In this section, I provide one case example so that you can practice applying the model for dose optimization based on what you have learned in this chapter.

Case Example 5-2.

Cefepime is a fourth-generation cephalosporin with activity against both Gram-positive and Gram-negative organisms. Cefepime is known to display time-dependent killing, which means that the duration of action is dependent on the length of time the plasma concentration above the minimum inhibitory concentration (MIC), which is the lowest concentration of cefepime that inhibits the growth of a given strain of bacteria. Because of its broad coverage, cefepime has been extensively used as an empirical therapy in critically ill patients with severe infections.

One day, a patient with sepsis was admitted to the ICU and you are the lead pharmacist making decision on the dose regimen of cefepime. You recommended a traditional dose regimen of cefepime as the initial therapy: 1 g cefepime every 12 hours via I.V. bolus injections. Right after the first dose, two blood samples were collected and the concentrations of cefepime were found to be 30.4 mg/L at 2 h and 7.2 mg/L at 6 h. The goal of the therapy is to keep the concentration of cefepime above the MIC of 2 mg/L for the entire dosing interval (i.e. 12 h for the current dose regimen) following the first dose. Cefepime has a good safety profile, so you don't need to worry about the toxicity of this drug.

- Calculate the plasma concentration of cefepime at 1 h and 10 h.
- What is the CL, V_d, k_e, and $t_{1/2}$ of cefepime in this patient?
- Calculate the duration of action of cefepime under the current dose regimen.
- Evaluate if the initial empirical dose regimen (i.e., 1 g every 12 h) of cefepime can meet the targeted goal (i.e. maintaining drug concentrations above MIC of 2 mg/L over the entire dosing interval).
- If the current dose regimen is not ideal. Based on the pharmacokinetic parameters of cefepime in this patient, design a new regimen that can meet the goal.

Please work on it yourself before looking at the answer I provide below.

$$\sim \sim \sim$$

Based on the information provided, the first pharmacokinetic parameter that we can calculate is k_e since we have two data points on hand:

$$k_e = - slope = - \frac{\ln C_2 - \ln C_1}{t_2 - t_1} = - \frac{\ln 7.2 - \ln 30.4}{6 - 2} = 0.360 \, h^{-1}$$

With k_e and Equation 5-3, we can plug in any of the two data points to obtain C_0:

$$30.4 = C_0 \cdot e^{-0.36 \cdot 2} \quad \rightarrow C_0 = 62.5 \, mg/L$$

With k_e an C_0, we can predict cefepime concentration at 1 h and 10 h using Equation 5-3:

$$C_{1h} = 62.5 \cdot e^{-0.36 \cdot 1} = 43.6 \, mg/L$$
$$C_{10h} = 62.5 \cdot e^{-0.36 \cdot 10} = 1.71 \, mg/L$$

Since k_e was obtained already, we can calculate $t_{1/2}$ based on Equation 5-5:

$$t_{1/2} = \frac{0.693}{k_e} = \frac{0.693}{0.360} = 1.93 \, h$$

V_d can be calculated based on the information of dose (1 g, which is 1000 mg) and initial concentration calculated earlier ($C_0 = 62.5$ mg/L) using Equation 5-8:

$$V_d = \frac{Dose}{C_0} = \frac{1000}{62.5} = 16.0 \, L$$

With information of V_d and k_e, we can obtain CL using Equation 5-7:
$$CL = V_d \cdot k_e = 16.0 \times 0.360 = 5.76\ L/h$$

Since cefepime will lose effect after its plasma concentration drops below MIC of 2 mg/L, the duration of cefepime action can be calculated using Equation 5-3:
$$2 = 62.5 \cdot e^{-0.36 \cdot t} \quad \rightarrow t = 9.56\ h$$
Therefore, under the initial empirical dose regimen (i.e., cefepime 1 g every 12 h), cefepime can be effective for 9.56 h, instead of the whole dosing interval (12 h), following the first dose. Therefore, dose regimen optimization is needed. There are two ways to optimize dose regimen:

- *Same dose (1 g) but different dosing interval:*

Since the effect of cefepime can be maintained for 9.56 h following 1 g dose, any dosing interval ≤9.56 h can meet the goal. To keep the regimen easy to be implemented in clinical practice, we can propose 8 h. Therefore, one treatment option is cefepime 1 g every 8 h.

- *Same dosing interval (12 h) but different dose:*

$$2 = C_0 \cdot e^{-0.36 \cdot 12} \quad \rightarrow C_0 = 150\ mg/L$$
$$Dose = C_0 \cdot V_d = 150 \times 16.0 = 2400\ mg = 2.4\ g$$

Therefore, the second treatment option is cefepime 2.4 g every 12 h.

I hope the above case example gives you the idea of how to apply the knowledge we learned in this Chapter in clinical practice. While you work on case example 5-2, you may realize the power of the pharmacokinetic model – we can use it to 1) predict drug concentrations at any time; 2) estimate the duration of drug action; 3) optimize the dose regimen to ensure effective therapy. To strengthen your quantitative skills, one more case example is provided in Section 5.5.

5.5 Case Study

Case Example 5-3.

Tobramycin is an aminoglycoside antibiotic with activity against Gram-positive and Gram-negative bacteria. A patient (70 kg male) with urinary tract infection was given a 100 mg I.V. bolus dose of tobramycin every 8 hrs. The desired peak level (i.e. the highest concentration after a dose) and trough level (i.e. the concentration of a sample collected right before next dose is given) are 6 and 0.5 mg/L, respectively, after the first dose. The half-life of tobramycin in this patient is 1.5 h. The volume of distribution of tobramycin is 0.25 L/kg. Please determine if the peak and trough after the current dose regimen meet the goal. If not, recommend a more appropriate dose regimen.

Please work on it yourself before looking at the answer I provided below.

$$\sim \sim \sim$$

Based on the half-life of 1.5 h, we can calculate k_e of tobramycin:

$$k_e = \frac{0.693}{1.5} = 0.462 \ h^{-1}$$

The volume of distribution of tobramycin in this patient is:

$$V_d = 0.25 \ L/kg \times 70 \ kg = 17.5 \ L$$

With the information of V_d, we can estimate the initial concentration following the dose of 100 mg:

$$C_0 = \frac{100}{17.5} = 5.71 \ mg/L$$

Following the original dose regimen (100 mg every 8 h), the trough concentration after the first dose is:

$$C_{8h} = 5.71 \cdot e^{-0.462 \cdot 8} = 0.141 \ mg/L$$

Thus, the original dose regimen did not achieve the therapeutic goal as the peak concentration (i.e., C_0 for I.V dose) and trough concentration (i.e., C_{8h}) do not meet the desired levels. If we want the peak level to be 6 mg/L and trough level to be 0.5 mg/L following the first dose, we need to propose a new dose regimen.

The desired dose should be:

Dose $= C_0 \cdot V_d = 6 \times 17.5 = 105 \ mg$

The desired dosing interval should be:

$$0.5 = 6 \cdot e^{-0.462 \cdot t} \quad \rightarrow \quad t = 5.38 \ h$$

Problem Sets　　*(Answers to study problems are in the appendix)*

After the I.V. bolus dose of Drug B (dose =100 mg), plasma concentration was found to be 8 mg/L at 1 h post dose and 2.5 mg/L at 9 h post dose. Drug B is mainly eliminated via CYP3A metabolism. Please estimate:

1) Drug B's elimination rate constant.
2) Drug B's half-life.
3) Drug B's clearance.
4) Drug B's AUC from zero to infinity.
5) Drug B's volume of distribution.
6) Drug B's initial concentration following the dose of 100 mg.
7) Drug B's hepatic extraction ratio (E).
8) Is Drug B a high extraction drug or low extraction drug?
9) When Drug B is co-administered with a CYP3A inducer, its AUC will a) increase; b) no change; c) decrease.
10) When Drug B is given orally together with a CYP3A inhibitor, its oral bioavailability will a) increase; b) no change; c) decrease.

Chapter 6.
Multiple IV Bolus (One-Compartment Model)

Learning Objectives

After reading this chapter, the reader shall be able to:

1. Understand the principle of superposition and how it applies to multiple drug dosing.

2. Understand terms related to multiple drug dosing, including accumulation, steady state, fluctuation, dosing interval, loading dose, maintenance dose, average steady state level.

3. Understand the impact of dose, dosing interval, clearance, and V_d on accumulation, average steady state levels, and fluctuation.

4. Understand the factors controlling the time to steady state and the average steady-state plasma concentration.

5. Calculate the peak and trough plasma concentrations after multiple I.V. bolus doses.

6. Design dosing regimens to achieve a certain average steady state level, and a certain fluctuation.

7. Perform individualized therapy using a multiple dose one-compartment model to ensure that drug concentrations are maintained within the desired therapeutic range for a drug with a narrow therapeutic window.

In Chapter 5, we have learned how to apply a one-compartment model to predict drug pharmacokinetics after a single I.V. bolus injection. While single dose administration happens in the clinic, a more commonly encountered situation is that drugs are given multiple times. Therefore, we need to be able to predict drug concentration-time profiles and perform dose optimization following multiple dose administrations. This chapter focuses on the least complex model: multiple I.V. injections using a one-compartment model.

I will introduce the principle of superposition and how it applies to multiple drug dosing in Section 6.1. The scenario of multiple dose regimens brings up many new terms, such as accumulation, steady state, fluctuation, dosing interval, loading dose, maintenance dose, and average steady state concentration; each of these terms will be discussed in Section 6.2. The impact of drug input and primary pharmacokinetic parameters on the accumulation, steady-state, and fluctuation of a drug is evaluated in Section 6.3. Dose regimen design centers on two questions: what dose should a drug be administered, and how frequently should a drug be taken? A road map of dose regimen design, along with case examples showing how to apply the model for dose optimization, is provided in Section 6.4. Additional case examples are provided in Section 6.5, then this chapter ends with problem sets.

6.1 Predicting Drug Concentrations After Multiple I.V. Dosing Based On Superposition Principle

The principle of superposition states that under linear pharmacokinetics conditions (i.e. dose- and concentration-independent clearance and volume of distribution), the total concentration of a drug in the body is the sum of the remaining concentrations from each administered dose at the time when the concentration is measured. The principle of superposition assumes that the drug remaining in the body from early doses does not affect the pharmacokinetics of subsequent doses.

While the superposition principle may seem complicated and fancy, it is nothing more than a simple addition. For example, let's assume a drug is given at a dose of 10 mg at 8AM, and the initial concentration is 10 ng/mL. At 4 hours after the first dose (i.e. 12 PM), the concentration drops to 2 ng/mL. At the meantime, we give a second dose of 10 mg at 12 PM. What would be the concentration of this drug at 12 PM? You can figure it out relatively easily that the total concentration at 12 PM will be 12 ng/mL, which is the sum of the remaining concentrations from each dose (i.e. 2 ng/mL from the first dose and 10 ng/mL from the second dose). Now let's use generalized equations to characterize multiple drug dosing based on the superposition principle.

- *Plasma drug concentration after the first dose (Figure 6-1):*

Based on the equation $C = C_0 \cdot e^{-k_e \cdot t}$, the maximum concentration after the first dose is:

$$C_{max1} = C_0 = \frac{Dose}{V_d} \qquad [6\text{-}1]$$

The minimum concentration after the first dose is the concentration measured right before the second dose is given. The time between two adjacent doses is called *dosing interval*, which is represented by τ. Therefore, the minimum concentration after the first dose is the concentration at time τ.

$$C_{min1} = C_{max1} \cdot e^{-k_e \cdot \tau} \qquad [6\text{-}2]$$

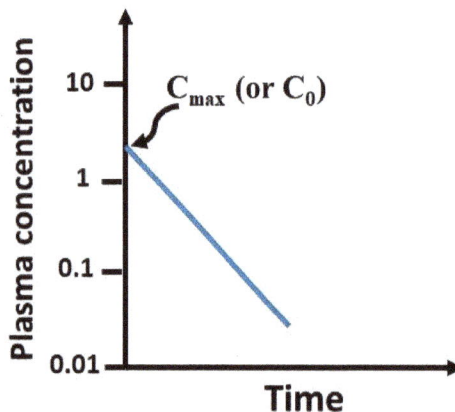

Figure 6-1. Plasma concentration-time profile of a drug after the first I.V. bolus dose.

- *Plasma drug concentration after the second dose (Figure 6-2):*

Based on the superposition principle, the maximum concentration after the second dose can be calculate as:

$$C_{max2} = C_{max1} + C_{min1} \qquad\qquad [6\text{-}3]$$

Where C_{max1} is the concentration from the second dose and C_{min1} is the remaining concentration from the first dose.

Based on Equation 6-2, Equation 6-3 can be further expressed as:

$$C_{max2} = C_{max1} + C_{max1} \cdot e^{-k_e \cdot \tau} \quad \rightarrow \quad C_{max2} = C_{max1}(1 + e^{-k_e \cdot \tau}) \qquad [6\text{-}4]$$

The minimum concentration after the second dose is the concentration measured right before the third dose is given. Therefore, the minimum concentration is the level at time τ since the second dose is given.

$$C_{min2} = C_{max2} \cdot e^{-k_e \cdot \tau} \quad \rightarrow C_{min2} = C_{max1}(1 + e^{-k_e \cdot \tau}) \cdot e^{-k_e \cdot \tau} \qquad [6\text{-}5]$$

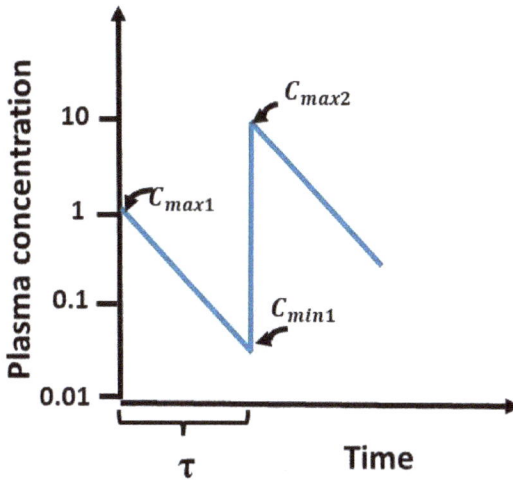

Figure 6-2. Plasma concentration-time profile of a drug after two I.V. bolus doses.

- *Plasma drug concentration after the third dose (Figure 6-3):*

Based on the superposition principle, the maximum concentration after the third dose can be calculate as:

$$C_{max3} = C_{max1} + C_{min2} \qquad\qquad [6\text{-}6]$$

Where C_{max1} is the concentration from the third dose and C_{min2} is the remaining concentration from dose 1 and dose 2.

Based on Equation 6-5, Equation 6-6 can be further expressed as:

$$\begin{aligned} C_{max3} &= C_{max1} + C_{max1}(1 + e^{-k_e \cdot \tau}) \cdot e^{-k_e \cdot \tau} \\ &= C_{max1}(1 + e^{-k_e \cdot \tau} + e^{-2 \cdot k_e \cdot \tau}) \qquad [6\text{-}7] \end{aligned}$$

The minimum concentration after the third dose is the concentration measured at the end of the third dosing interval.

$$C_{min3} = C_{max3} \cdot e^{-k_e \cdot \tau} \rightarrow C_{min3} = C_{max1}(1 + e^{-k_e \cdot \tau} + e^{-2 \cdot k_e \cdot \tau}) \cdot e^{-k_e \cdot \tau} \quad [6\text{-}8]$$

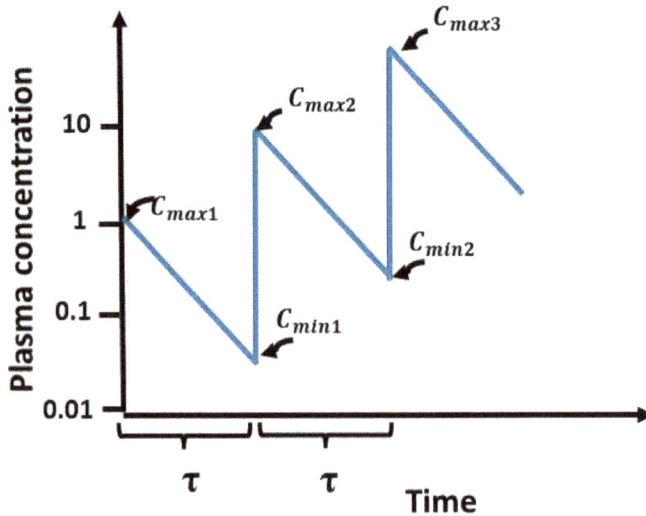

Figure 6-3. Plasma concentration-time profile of a drug after three I.V. bolus doses.

- ***Plasma drug concentration after n doses (Figure 6-4):***

After going through the equations for the first three doses, you probably see a pattern, with which the maximum concentration after any number of doses can be described as:

$$C_{max,n} = C_{max,1}(1 + e^{-k_e \cdot \tau} + e^{-2 \cdot k_e \cdot \tau} + \cdots + e^{-(n-1) \cdot k_e \cdot \tau}) \quad [6\text{-}9]$$

Where n is the number of doses given.

The minimum concentration after n doses is:

$$C_{min,n} = C_{max,n} \cdot e^{-k_e \cdot \tau} \quad [6\text{-}10]$$

Equation 6-9 can be rearranged and simplified to an easier and more useful form:

$$C_{max,n} = C_{max,1} \frac{(1 - e^{-n \cdot k_e \cdot \tau})}{(1 - e^{-k_e \cdot \tau})} \quad [6\text{-}11]$$

Accordingly, the minimum concentration after n doses can be described as:

$$C_{min,n} = C_{max,1} \frac{(1 - e^{-n \cdot k_e \cdot \tau})}{(1 - e^{-k_e \cdot \tau})} \cdot e^{-k_e \cdot \tau} \quad [6\text{-}12]$$

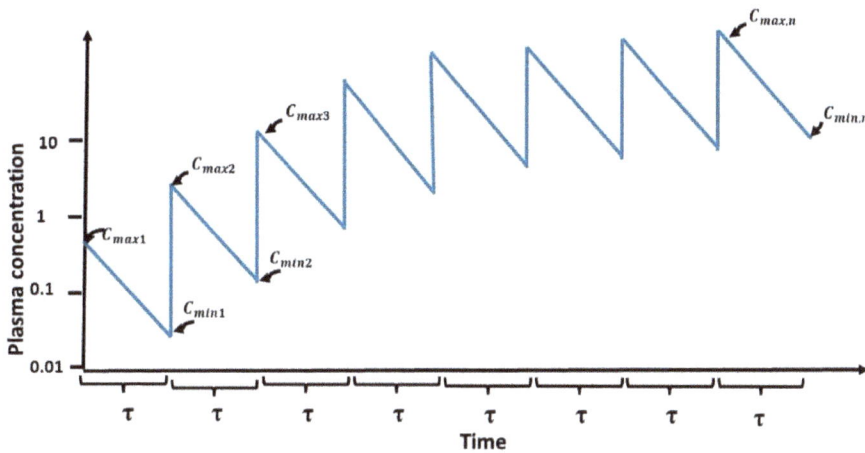

Figure 6-4. Plasma concentration-time profile of a drug after number of n I.V. bolus doses.

Armed with the equations we have learned so far, especially Equation 6-11 and Equation 6-12, we can predict the maximum and minimum concentrations, as well as concentrations at any other time points, after any number of I.V. doses. Let's practice this with the case example below.

Case Example 6-1.

Patient LP received 500 mg of a drug via I.V. bolus every 6 hours for 5 days (i.e., total 20 doses). Two samples were collected at 1 h and 5 h after the first dose, and the concentrations were found to be 12 mg/L and 5 mg/L, respectively. This drug follows first-order kinetics and can be characterized using a one-compartment model. Please calculate:

- k_e, V_d, CL of this drug in this patient.
- $C_{max,1}$, $C_{min,1}$, $C_{max,3}$, $C_{min,3}$, $C_{max,15}$, $C_{min,15}$, $C_{max,20}$, and $C_{min,20}$.
- Drug concentration at 4 h after the 3th dose.

Please work on the above questions yourself before looking at the answers provided below.

~ ~ ~

In this case example, two concentration-time data points were provided. We have learned in Chapter 1 that the pharmacokinetic parameter that can be calculated directly using two data points is k_e.

$$k_e = -slope = -\frac{lnC_2 - lnC_1}{t_2 - t_1} = -\frac{\ln(5) - \ln(12)}{5\,h - 1\,h} \rightarrow k_e = 0.219\,h^{-1}$$

Since $C = C_0\,e^{-ke \cdot t}$, we can get C_0 by plugging in one concentration-time data point and the k_e value we just got:

$12 = C_0\,e^{-0.219\cdot1}$ $\rightarrow C_0 = 14.9\ mg/L$

Why do we calculate C_0? We calculate C_0 because it can be used to estimate V_d based on the following equation:

$$C_0 = \frac{Dose}{V_d} \qquad \rightarrow V_d = \frac{Dose}{C_0} = \frac{500\ mg}{14.9\ mg/L} = 33.6\ L$$

With the information of k_e and V_d, we can obtain CL by the following equation:
CL = $k_e\cdot V_d$ = 0.219 h^{-1}·33.6 L = 7.36 L/h

The drug was given every 6 h, therefore $\tau=6h$. Based on Equations 6-1, 6-11, and 6-12, we can get C_{max} and C_{min} after any number of doses, including the 1st, 3rd, 15th, and 20th doses that are requested:

$C_{max,1} = C_0 = 14.9\ mg/L$

$C_{min,1} = C_{max,1}\cdot e^{-k_e\cdot\tau} = 14.9\cdot e^{-0.219\cdot6} = 4.00\ mg/L$

$C_{max,3} = C_{max,1}\dfrac{(1-e^{-n\cdot k_e\cdot\tau})}{(1-e^{-k_e\cdot\tau})} = 14.9\dfrac{(1-e^{-3\cdot0.219\cdot6})}{(1-e^{-0.219\cdot6})} = 20.0\ mg/L$

$C_{min,3} = C_{max,3}\cdot e^{-k_e\cdot\tau} = 20.0\cdot e^{-0.219\cdot6} = 5.37\ mg/L$

$C_{max,15} = C_{max,1}\dfrac{(1-e^{-n\cdot k_e\cdot\tau})}{(1-e^{-k_e\cdot\tau})} = 14.9\dfrac{(1-e^{-15\cdot0.219\cdot6})}{(1-e^{-0.219\cdot6})} = 20.4\ mg/L$

$C_{min,15} = C_{max,15}\cdot e^{-k_e\cdot\tau} = 20.4\cdot e^{-0.219\cdot6} = 5.48\ mg/L$

$C_{max,20} = C_{max,1}\dfrac{(1-e^{-n\cdot k_e\cdot\tau})}{(1-e^{-k_e\cdot\tau})} = 14.9\dfrac{(1-e^{-20\cdot0.219\cdot6})}{(1-e^{-0.219\cdot6})} = 20.4\ mg/L$

$C_{min,20} = C_{max,20}\cdot e^{-k_e\cdot\tau} = 20.4\cdot e^{-0.219\cdot6} = 5.48\ mg/L$

Drug concentration at 4 h after the 3rd dose can be calculated using the following equation:

$$C_{4h,dose3} = C_{max,3}\cdot e^{-k_e\cdot t} = 20.0\cdot e^{-0.219\cdot4} = 8.33\ mg/L$$

In case example 6-1, we practiced how to use equations to predict drug concentrations at any time points following any number of doses. Based on the maximum and minimum concentrations calculated for the 1st, 3rd, 15th, and 20th doses, we observe the following two phenomena:

- Maximum concentrations at later doses are higher than the maximum concentration after the first dose. The same trend applies to minimum concentrations. This phenomenon is called *accumulation*, which is easily explained by the superposition principle.
- Drug concentration does not increase forever. As demonstrated by $C_{max,15}$ and $C_{max,20}$, the concentration will maintain at the same level after reaching a certain point. The same trend applies to minimum concentrations. This phenomenon is known as *steady state*, which is not very intuitive and will be explained in the next section.

The above two phenomena/terms, along with other terms, are elaborated in Section 6.2.

6.2 Phenomena and Terms Related to Multiple Drug Dosing

6.2.1 Accumulation

Drug accumulation occurs whenever a dose is administered when the drug from a previous dose has not been eliminated completely out of the body. The magnitude of accumulation is reflected by *accumulation ratio*, which is expressed as r and calculated as:

$$r = \frac{C_{max,n}}{C_{max,1}} \hspace{4cm} [6\text{-}13]$$

Based on Equation 6-11, the above equation can be expressed as:

$$r = \frac{C_{max,1}\dfrac{(1-e^{-n \bullet k_e \bullet \tau})}{(1-e^{-k_e \bullet \tau})}}{C_{max,1}} \hspace{0.5cm} \rightarrow \hspace{0.5cm} r = \frac{(1-e^{-n \bullet k_e \bullet \tau})}{(1-e^{-k_e \bullet \tau})} \hspace{1cm} [6\text{-}14]$$

When the number n becomes a large number (e.g., a patient takes a drug regularly for many days, or weeks), $e^{-n \cdot k_e \cdot \tau}$ approaches 0, the accumulation ratio becomes a fixed value ($r = \frac{1}{(1-e^{-k_e \tau})}$) since both k_e and τ are constant values; this means that the drug will not accumulate further no matter how many additional doses are given (i.e., steady state is reached). The accumulation ratio in this situation is expressed as:

$$r_{ss} = \frac{1}{(1-e^{-k_e \bullet \tau})} \hspace{4cm} [6\text{-}15]$$

Accordingly, the maximum concentration at the steady state is:

$$C_{max,ss} = C_{max,1}\frac{1}{(1-e^{-k_e \bullet \tau})} \hspace{0.5cm} \text{or} \hspace{0.5cm} C_{max,ss} = C_{max,1} \bullet r_{ss} \hspace{1cm} [6\text{-}16]$$

It is easy to understand why there is accumulation when multiple doses are administered. However, it is not transparent regarding why a drug eventually will reach steady state; this is elaborated in the next subsection.

6.2.2 Steady State

To reach the steady state, there is one prerequisite - the drug undergoes first-order elimination. The feature of first-order elimination is that the amount of a drug eliminated is proportional to the current amount of drug in the body. In other words, our body eliminates more when there is a higher amount of drug and eliminates less when there is a lower amount in the body. When a patient takes a drug at the same dose regularly for a long period of time, at the beginning, drug concentrations following later doses are higher than those from earlier doses. Because of drug accumulation, the amount of drug in the body increases. Due to first-order elimination, the amount of drug eliminated from the body increases accordingly. Remember the dose (i.e., drug input) remains the same, while the amount of drug eliminated (i.e., drug output) increases with an increase in drug concentration. When the amount of drug eliminated during the dosing interval is identical to the dose (i.e., drug output =drug input), a steady state is reached. After this point, no matter how many more doses a patient takes, the drug will not accumulate further (Figure 6-5).

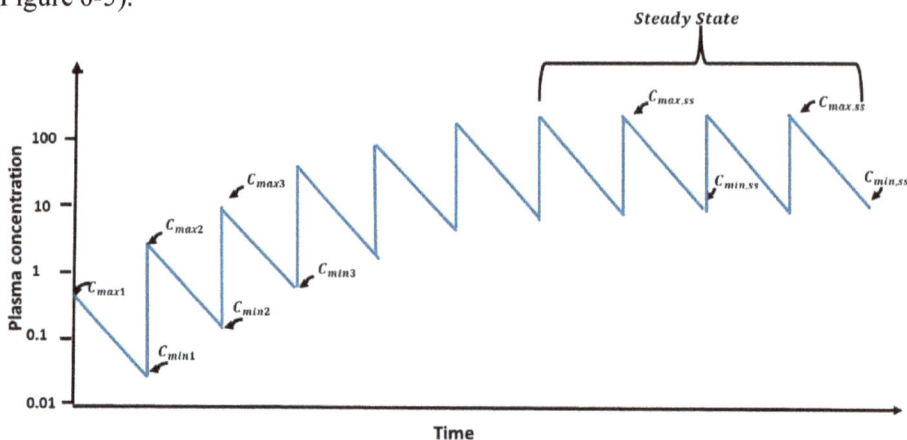

Figure 6-5. The phenomenon of drug accumulation and steady state following multiple drug I.V. bolus dosing.

I hope the above explanation, together with Figure 6-5, could help you comprehend the concept of steady state. In case you are still confused about it, I provide an outside example of Jerry's bank account in Section 6.5. That outside example has helped a lot of PharmD students when I taught the course "Pharmacokinetics and Dose Optimization" over the years. I hope it can help you too.

6.2.3 Time to Reach Steady State

I mentioned earlier that a drug will reach steady state *eventually* following multiple dose regimens. Well, "eventually" is a blurry description. How long does it exactly take for a drug to reach its steady state? It turns out that the time to reach the steady state is dependent only on a drug's half-life. Table 6-1 summarizes the information, and we will learn how we get these numbers in Chapter 7 when I talk about I.V. infusion.

Based on Table 6-1, after one half-life, a drug reaches 50% of the steady state. After two half-lives, 75% of the steady state is achieved. In general, we consider the steady state of a drug is reached after 5 half-lives because that is the time when 97% steady state is achieved.

What does the above information tell us? It means that for a drug with a short half-life, its steady state can be reached quickly. For example, cefazolin, an antibiotic with a half-life around 2 h in a general population, can reach its steady state at 10 h post the first dose. No matter if cefazolin is administered every 4 h, every 12 h, or at any other dosing interval, the time needed to reach its steady state is 10 h (i.e., 5 half-lives). If cefazolin is dosed every 12 h, the steady state can be reached even before the second dose is given.

Table 6-1. The relationship between half-life and percentage of drug steady state achieved.

Number of half-lives	Percentage of steady state
1 $t_{1/2}$	50%
2 $t_{1/2}$	75%
3 $t_{1/2}$	88%
4 $t_{1/2}$	94%
5 $t_{1/2}$	**97%**
6 $t_{1/2}$	98%
7 $t_{1/2}$	99%

For a drug with a long-life, it could take a long time to reach its steady state. For example, the half-life of digoxin in a general population is approximately 2 days, which means that it would take around 10 days to reach its steady state when digoxin is administered under multiple dose regimens. This poses an issue. Imagine digoxin is prescribed to treat a patient with chronic heart failure in ICU, and as the lead pharmacist, you tell the doctor and the patient that it will take 10 days for digoxin to reach its steady state so that the concentrations of digoxin can fall within the desired concentration range. You successfully upset everyone because this treatment plan is not acceptable. In such case, we need to come up with a strategy, with which steady state, along with the desired concentration range, can be achieved right way. This one trick pony is *loading dose*, which is discussed in the next subsection.

6.2.4 Loading Dose and Maintenance Dose

The goal of a loading dose is to achieve steady-state plasma concentrations immediately (Figure 6-6). While this may sound like a mission impossible, it turns out to be a surprisingly easy task. The following is the logic flow and related equations:

As shown in Equation 6-16, the maximum concentration at the steady state is:

$$C_{max,ss} = C_{max,1} \cdot r_{ss}$$

We want to give a dose so that it can reach $C_{max,ss}$ immediately. This dose should be:

$$Loading\ dose = C_{max,ss} \cdot V_d \quad \rightarrow \quad Loading\ dose = C_{max,1} \cdot r_{ss} \cdot V_d$$

Since $C_{max,1} \cdot V_d = Dose$, loading dose can be calculated as:

$$Loading\ dose = Dose \cdot r_{ss} \qquad [6\text{-}17]$$

Where $r_{ss} = \dfrac{1}{(1 - e^{-k_e \cdot \tau})}$ as shown in Equation 6-15.

Therefore, based on the current dose used, the elimination rate constant k_e, and the dosing interval τ, we can calculate the loading dose in a straight-forward manner.

Please note that the loading dose is a one-time deal (that's why I call it "one trick pony"). After the loading dose, the rest doses are back to the one originally administered, which is known as *maintenance dose*.

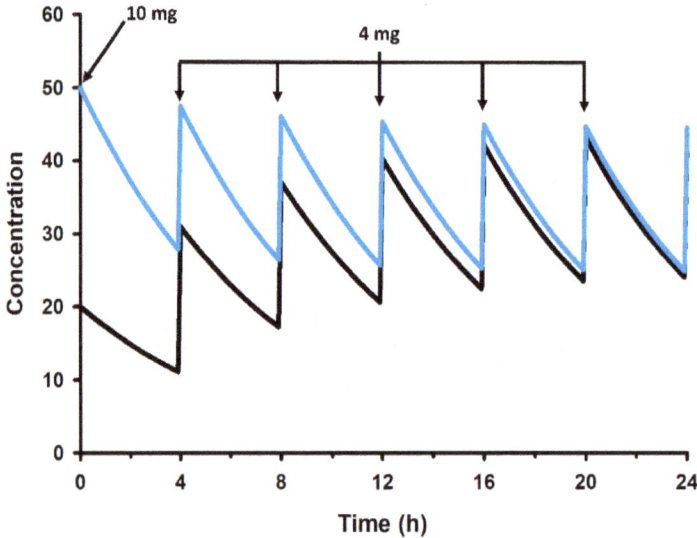

Figure 6-6. The use of loading dose to achieve a drug's steady state immediately.

6.2.5 Steady State Average Concentration

After a drug reaches steady state, sometimes it is useful to calculate the steady state average concentration, expressed as $C_{ave,ss}$, within the dosing interval. If we know the values of $C_{max,ss}$ and $C_{min,ss}$, we can get $C_{ave,ss}$ by using the following equation:

$$C_{ave,ss} = \frac{C_{max,ss} - C_{min,ss}}{lnC_{max,ss} - lnC_{min,ss}} \qquad [6\text{-}18]$$

Steady state average concentration can also be calculated based on the information of AUC using the following equation:

$$C_{ave,ss} = \frac{AUC_{\tau,ss}}{\tau} \qquad [6\text{-}19]$$

Where $AUC_{\tau,ss}$ represents the area under the concentration-time curve within a dosing interval during steady state. τ is the dosing interval.

I would like to provide more information on the calculation of AUC before we revisit $C_{ave,ss}$. The general equation to calculate AUC from time 0 to time t is:

$$AUC_{0-t} = \frac{Amount\ eliminated\ during\ this\ time\ period}{CL} \qquad [6\text{-}20]$$

Following a single I.V. bolus dose, the AUC from time 0 to time infinity is:

$$AUC_\infty = \frac{Amount\ eliminated\ from\ time\ 0\ to\ time\ infinity}{CL}$$

Since the amount eliminated from time 0 to time infinity equates to the amount gets in the body (i.e., dose), therefore, AUC_∞ of a drug after single I.V. dose is:

$$AUC_\infty = \frac{Dose}{CL}$$

Now, let's look at $AUC_{\tau,ss}$. Based on Equation 6-20, it is calculate as:

$$AUC_{\tau,ss} = \frac{Amount\ eliminated\ during\ the\ dosing\ interval\ at\ steady\ state}{CL}$$

What is the amount of drug eliminated during the dosing interval at steady state? If you recall, the amount of drug eliminated out of the body per dosing interval equals the amount of drug that gets in the body (i.e., dose administered) during steady state. Therefore, $AUC_{\tau,ss}$ can be calculated as:

$$AUC_{\tau,ss} = \frac{Dose}{CL} \qquad [6\text{-}21]$$

Therefore, as shown in Figure 6-7, the $AUC_{\tau,ss}$ of a drug following multiple I.V. bolus dose regimens equals to the AUC_∞ of the same drug following a single I.V. bolus dose.

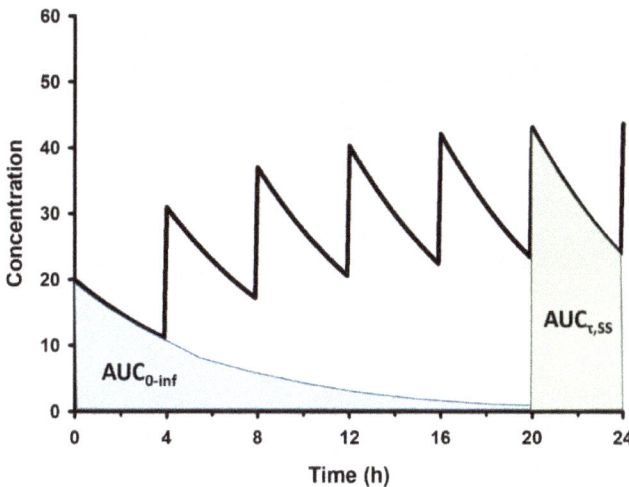

Figure 6-7. $AUC_{\tau,ss}$ of a drug following multiple I.V. bolus dose regimens equals to AUC_∞ of the same drug following a single I.V. bolus dose.

Now let's go back to the topic of $C_{ave,ss}$. Based on Equation 6-19 and Equation 6-21, $C_{ave,ss}$ can be calculated as:

$$C_{ave,ss} = \frac{Dose}{CL \cdot \tau}$$ [6-22]

Equation 6-18 and Equation 6-22 provide two ways of calculating $C_{ave,ss}$. If you know $C_{max,ss}$ and $C_{min,ss}$, you can calculate $C_{ave,ss}$ using Equation 6-18. On the other hand, if you have the information of dose, clearance and dosing interval on hand, you can use Equation 6-22 to calculate $C_{ave,ss}$.

Equation 6-22 is a useful equation because it can be rearranged to calculate the dose:

$$Dose = C_{ave,ss} \bullet CL \bullet \tau$$ [6-23]

Equation 6-23 is important as it allows us to design a dose if we know the desired steady state average concentration, drug clearance, and dosing interval. I highlight this important equation using a different color as we will use it in Section 6.4 when we practice dose regimen design.

Let's revisit $C_{ave,ss}$ again. For example, you give a drug with a dose of 1) 8 mg every 8 h, or 2) 4 mg every 4 h. How does $C_{ave,ss}$ differ? Based on Equation 6-22, $C_{ave,ss}$ remains the same in these two scenarios. But your gut feeling tells you that something is different. What differs? This question is addressed in the next subsection.

6.2.6 Fluctuation

As shown in Figure 6-8, while the dose regimens of 8 mg every 8 h and 4 mg every 4 h yield the same steady state average concentration, the concentration-time curves have different fluctuations. *Fluctuation*, expressed as F', refers to the difference between the maximum and minimum plasma concentrations within a dosing interval.

Fluctuation is calculated as:

$$F' = \frac{C_{max,ss}}{C_{min,ss}}$$ [6-24]

Where $C_{min,ss}$ is calculated as:

$$C_{min,ss} = C_{max,ss} \bullet e^{-k_e \bullet \tau}$$ [6-25]

Based on Equation 6-25, F' can be expressed as:

$$F' = \frac{C_{max,ss}}{C_{min,ss}} = \frac{C_{max,ss}}{C_{max,ss} \bullet e^{-k_e \bullet \tau}} = \frac{1}{e^{-k_e \bullet \tau}} \rightarrow F' = e^{k_e \bullet \tau}$$ [6-26]

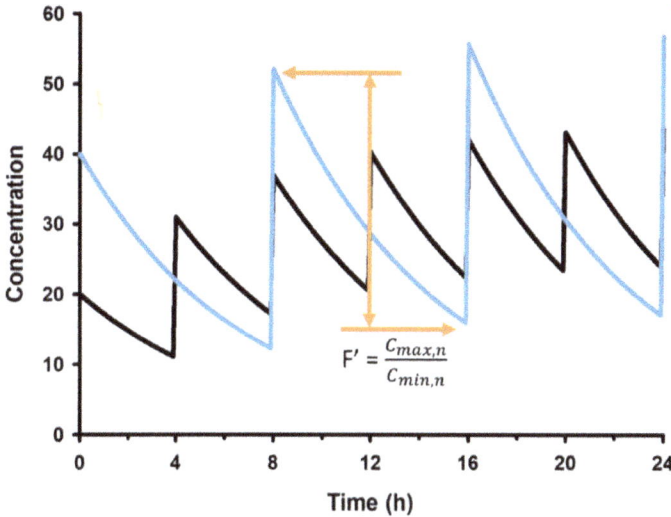

Figure 6-8. An example of two different dosing regimens resulting in the same steady state average concentration but different fluctuation.

Therefore, the fluctuation of a drug concentration-time curve depends on a drug's elimination rate constant k_e and the dosing interval. The larger the value of k_e or τ, the larger the fluctuation of the concentration-time curve. As shown in Figure 6-8, the dose regimen of 8 mg every 8 h has a higher fluctuation than the dose regimen of 4 mg every 4 h because the former has a longer dosing interval.

Equation 6-26 is a useful equation because it can be rearranged to calculate τ:

$$F' = e^{k_e \cdot \tau} \quad \rightarrow \quad lnF' = k_e \cdot \tau \quad \rightarrow \quad \tau = \frac{lnF'}{k_e} \qquad [6\text{-}27]$$

Equation 6-27 is important as it allows us to determine the maximum allowable dosing interval if we know the maximum allowable fluctuation and a drug's elimination rate constant k_e. I highlight this important equation using a different color as we will use it, together with Equation 6-23, in Section 6.4 when we practice dose regimen design.

Up to now, we have learned all new terms related to multiple drug dosing. Let's examine how the changes in drug input (i.e., dose) and primary pharmacokinetic parameters affect drug accumulation, steady-state, and fluctuation in the next section.

6.3 The impact of drug input and primary pharmacokinetic parameters on the accumulation, steady-state, and fluctuation of a drug following multiple dose regimens.

In this section, I provide one case example below, which hopefully could help you gain a good understanding of the impact of changes in drug input and pharmacokinetics parameters on the accumulation, steady-state, and fluctuation of a drug following multiple I.V. dosing regimens.

Case Example 6-2.

Patient AG took drug Iowa-002 4 mg every 4 h for 2 days. The CL and V_d of Iowa-002 in this patient are 30 L/h and 200 L, respectively.

- *Scenario 1.* Recently, patient AG was diagnosed with moderate renal impairment. The CL of Iowa-002 decreased to 10 L/h. V_d stays the same. The doctor recommends the same dose regimen as before (i.e., 4 mg every 4 h).
- *Scenario 2.* The doctor recommends Patient AG to take Iowa-002 every 2 h, instead of the original every 4 h regimen. Dose remains the same. The pharmacokinetics parameters of Iowa-002 remain the same.

Evaluate how the change in CL (scenario 1) or dosing interval (scenario 2) would affect:

a) the accumulation of Iowa-002;
b) time to reach steady state;
c) fluctuation of the concentration-time profile;
d) steady state average concentration;
e) what the old and new plasma concentration-time profiles look like.

As usual, I suggest you work on it yourself before looking at the answers I provide below.

$$\sim \sim \sim$$

- *Scenario 1.*
a) *Based on Equation 6-15, $r_{ss} = \frac{1}{(1-e^{-k_e \cdot \tau})}$, drug accumulation depends on k_e and τ. k_e is a secondary parameter which is dependent on CL and V_d ($k_e = \frac{CL}{V_d}$). Therefore, with a decrease in CL, k_e decreases. Table 6-2 includes the four steps that I usually use to evaluate the direction of change in r_{ss}.*

Therefore, with decrease in CL, k_e decreases. With decrease in k_e, drug accumulation increases in the new condition.

b) *Time to steady state depends on a drug's half-life. With a decrease in CL, Iowa-002's half-life increases based on equation $t_{1/2} = \frac{0.693 \cdot V_d}{CL}$*

Table 6-2. Steps to calculate the direction of change in r_{ss} in scenario 1.

Step	Component	Old condition vs New condition	Notes
1	$k_e = \frac{CL}{V_d}$	k_e (old) > k_e (new)	CL dropped in the new condition
2	$e^{-k_e \cdot \tau}$	old < new	There is a negative sign on the shoulder of e function. The bigger the value of $k_e \cdot \tau$, the smaller the e function
3	$1 - e^{-k_e \cdot \tau}$	old > new	$e^{-k_e \cdot \tau}$ ranges from 0-1. The smaller the value of $e^{-k_e \cdot \tau}$, the larger the value of $(1 - e^{-k_e \cdot \tau})$
4	$\dfrac{1}{(1 - e^{-k_e \cdot \tau})}$	old < new	$(1 - e^{-k_e \cdot \tau})$ is on the denominator; smaller value yields bigger value of $\frac{1}{(1-e^{-k_e \cdot \tau})}$

c) *Based on Equation 6-26, $F' = e^{k_e \cdot \tau}$. In the new condition, k_e decreases due to the decrease in CL. Accordingly, the fluctuation decreases in the new condition.*

d) *Based on Equation 6-22, $C_{ave,ss} = \frac{Dose}{CL \cdot \tau}$. In the new condition, CL drops. Therefore, $C_{ave,ss}$ is higher than that in the old condition.*

e) *Figure 6-9 shows the anticipated concentration time profile of Iowa-002 in the old and new conditions.*

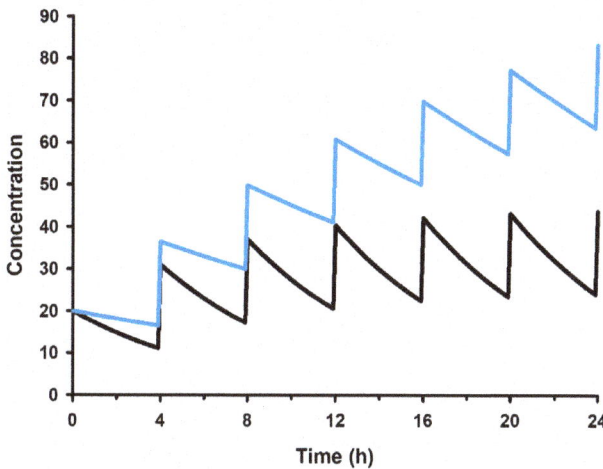

Figure 6-9. Iowa-002 concentration-time profiles following 4 mg every 4 h in the old condition (black curve) and new condition (blue curve). CL of Iowa-002 decreases in the new condition.

- *Scenario 2*.
  a) *Based on Equation 6-15, $r_{ss} = \frac{1}{(1-e^{-k_e \cdot \tau})}$, drug accumulation depends on k_e and τ. In this scenario, τ decreases in the new condition. Table 6-3 lists the four steps that I usually use to evaluate the direction of change in r_{ss}.*

Table 6-3. Steps to calculate the direction of change in r_{ss} in scenario 2.

Step	Component	Old condition vs New condition	Notes
1	$k_e = \frac{CL}{V_d}$	τ (old) > τ (new)	$\tau = 4$ h in the old condition and $\tau = 2$ h in the new condition
2	$e^{-k_e \cdot \tau}$	old < new	There is a negative sign on the shoulder of e function. The bigger the value of $k_e \cdot \tau$, the smaller the e function
3	$1 - e^{-k_e \cdot \tau}$	old > new	$e^{-k_e \cdot \tau}$ ranges from 0-1. The smaller the value of $e^{-k_e \cdot \tau}$, the larger the value of $(1 - e^{-k_e \cdot \tau})$
4	$\dfrac{1}{(1 - e^{-k_e \cdot \tau})}$	old < new	$(1 - e^{-k_e \cdot \tau})$ is on the denominator; a smaller value yields a bigger value of $\frac{1}{(1-e^{-k_e \cdot \tau})}$

Therefore, more drug accumulation occurs in the new condition where Iowa-002 is given more frequently.
  b) *Time to steady state depends on a drug's half-life, not the dosing interval. Therefore, it will take the same amount of time for the drug to reach its steady state in the new condition.*
  c) *Based on Equation 6-26, $F' = e^{k_e \cdot \tau}$. In the new condition, τ decreases from 4 h to 2 h. Accordingly, the fluctuation decreases in the new condition.*
  d) *Based on Equation 6-22, $C_{ave,ss} = \frac{Dose}{CL \cdot \tau}$. In the new condition, τ drops. Therefore, $C_{ave,ss}$ is higher than that in the old condition.*
  e) *Figure 6-10 shows the anticipated concentration time profile of Iowa-002 in the old and new conditions.*

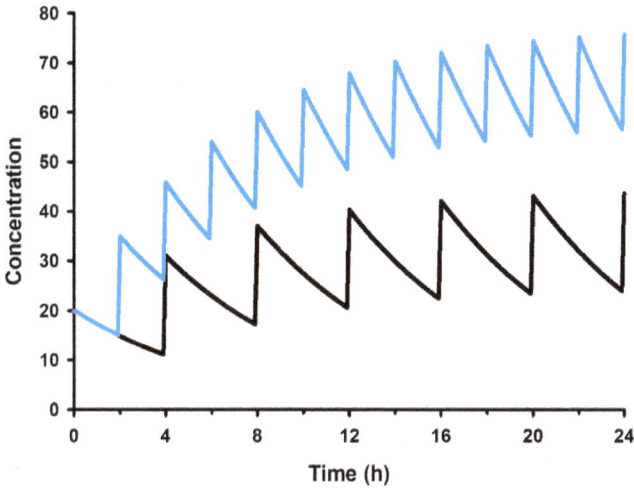

Figure 6-10. Iowa-002 concentration time profiles following 4 mg every 4 h (old condition; black curve) or 4 mg every 2 h (new condition, blue curve).

6.4 Applying the model for dose optimization – a Road Map of Dose Regimen Design.

In this section, I provide one case example below, which will guide you, step by step, on how to perform dose regimen design for drugs following multiple dose regimens.

Case Example 6-3.

A 70 kg male patient MN is diagnosed with meningitis and is about to start amikacin therapy. The elimination half-life of amikacin in this patient is 3 hours with an apparent volume of distribution of 20% of body weight (0.2 L/kg). Amikacin is known to have a narrow therapeutic window. As the lead pharmacist, you aim to keep the drug within 5 mg/L and 15 mg/L after amikacin reaches steady state. Calculate a dosing regimen (multiple IV doses) that will maintain the plasma drug concentrations within the therapeutic window for patient MN.

I strongly recommend you work on it yourself before looking at the answers I provide below.

$$\sim \sim \sim$$

To design a dose regimen, we need to address two questions: what dose to use? What dosing frequency? To answer these questions, we need to find equations related to the calculation of dose and τ. Therefore, Equations 6-23 and 6-27 are the key equations for dose regimen design.

$$Dose = C_{ave,ss} \cdot CL \cdot \tau$$

$$\tau = \frac{lnF'}{k_e}$$

Which equation to start with? Based on Equation 6-23, to calculate the dose, we need to figure out τ. Therefore, we should work on τ first.

To calculate τ, we need to calculate the fluctuation and k_e. Since the goal is to keep the steady state concentrations of amikacin within 5 mg/L and 15 mg/L, this means that $C_{min,ss}$ should not be lower than 5 mg/L and $C_{max,ss}$ should not be higher than 15 mg/L. In this case, the maximum allowable fluctuation is:

$$F' = \frac{C_{max,ss}}{C_{min,ss}} = \frac{15}{5} = 3$$

I would like to emphasize that 3 is the maximum allowable fluctuation. If F' exceeds 3, either $C_{min,ss}$ and/or $C_{max,ss}$ will exceed the predetermined threshold.

$$k_e = \frac{0.693}{t_{1/2}} = \frac{0.693}{3} = 0.231\ h^{-1}$$

Based on the information of F' and k_e, we can get τ based on Equation 6-27:

$$\tau = \frac{lnF'}{k_e} = \frac{ln3}{0.231} = 4.76\ h$$

The above calculated τ is the maximum allowable dosing interval. If you design a dosing interval longer than 4.76 h, the F' will exceed 3, which means that $C_{min,ss}$ and/or $C_{max,ss}$ will exceed the predetermined threshold.

What τ should we choose? While choosing a dosing interval of 4.76 h can keep the concentrations within the desired range, it is impractical in the clinic as the time is difficult to track. You can round it down to an integer, such as 4 h, 3 h, or 2 h. Among these options, 4h is better than 3h and 2h since it reduces the number of injections. To practice, let's propose several dosing intervals, including one that is longer than 4.76, to see what happens.

We have a plan for the dosing interval. Now let's look at the information needed to design a dose.

Based on Equation 6-23, the dose can be determined if we know $C_{ave,ss}$, CL, and τ. With the thresholds of $C_{min,ss}=5$ mg/L and $C_{max,ss}=15$ mg/L, we can calculate $C_{ave,ss}$ using Equation 6-18:

$$C_{ave,ss} = \frac{C_{max,ss} - C_{min,ss}}{lnC_{max,ss} - lnC_{min,ss}} = \frac{15-5}{ln15 - ln5} = 9.1\ mg/L$$

$$CL = k_e \cdot V_d = 0.231 \cdot 0.2 \cdot 70 = 3.23\ L/h$$

If we decide to use a dosing interval of 4 h, the dose will be:

$$Dose = C_{ave,ss} \cdot CL \cdot \tau = 9.1 \left(\frac{mg}{L}\right) \cdot 3.23 \left(\frac{L}{h}\right) \cdot 4\ (h) = 118\ mg$$

If we decide to use a dosing interval of 3 h, the dose will be:

$$Dose = C_{ave,ss} \cdot CL \cdot \tau = 9.1 \left(\frac{mg}{L}\right) \cdot 3.23 \left(\frac{L}{h}\right) \cdot 3\ (h) = 88.2\ mg$$

If we decide to use a dosing interval of 2 h, the dose will be:

$$Dose = C_{ave,ss} \cdot CL \cdot \tau = 9.1 \left(\tfrac{mg}{L}\right) \cdot 3.23 \left(\tfrac{L}{h}\right) \cdot 2 \ (h) = 58.8 \ mg$$

If we decide to use a dosing interval of 6 h (i.e. exceed the threshold of 4.76 h), the dose will be:

$$Dose = C_{ave,ss} \cdot CL \cdot \tau = 9.1 \left(\tfrac{mg}{L}\right) \cdot 3.23 \left(\tfrac{L}{h}\right) \cdot 6 \ (h) = 176 \ mg$$

We can calculate the predicted $C_{max,ss}$ and $C_{min,ss}$ under the dose regimens proposed above using the following two equations:

$$C_{max,ss} = C_{max,1} \frac{1}{(1-e^{-k_e \cdot \tau})} = \frac{Dose}{V_d} \frac{1}{(1-e^{-k_e \cdot \tau})}$$

$$C_{min,ss} = C_{max,ss} \cdot e^{-k_e \cdot \tau}$$

I have summarized all calculated maximum and minimum concentrations under each dosing regimen in Table 6-4 below:

Table 6-4. The predicted $C_{max,ss}$ and $C_{min,ss}$ following different dosing regimens

Dosing regimen		$C_{max,ss}$	$C_{min,ss}$	Note
Dose	T	mg/L	mg/L	
176 mg	6 h	16.8	4.19	Outside of the 5-15 mg/L range
118 mg	4 h	14.0	5.55	Within the 5-15 mg/L range
88.2 mg	3 h	12.6	6.3	Within the 5-15 mg/L range
58.8 mg	2 h	11.4	7.15	Within the 5-15 mg/L range

As shown in Table 6-4, when τ is 6 h, which exceeds the maximum allowable 4.76 h, both $C_{max,ss}$ and $C_{min,ss}$ fall outside of the desired range. In contrast, the other three dosing regimen options are all meet the goal of keeping the steady state concentrations within the 5-15 mg/L range. Since 4 h dosing interval offers the advantage of a smaller number of injections, the best dosing regimen is 118 mg amikacin every 4 h.

Case example 6-3 provides you with a road map regarding how to design a dose regimen to ensure that the steady state concentrations are maintained within a certain range. This calculation is particularly useful for drugs with a narrow therapeutic window. The logic flow and steps used to calculate the dose and dosing interval for amikacin in case example 6-3 can be directly applied to other drugs with a narrow therapeutic index.

6.5 Case Study

In this section, I provide two more case studies. Case example 6-4 aims to help you better understand the concept of steady state. Case example 6-5 is from an interesting case study originally published in the *Journal of Clinical Pharmacology* in 2016.

Case Example 6-4.

Do you remember Jerry, whom I introduced in Chapter 1 (section 1-4)? Jerry and Tom were both freshmen at that time, and I used their bank accounts as examples to explain zero-order kinetics (Tom's bank record) and first-order kinetics (Jerry's bank record). In this case example, I would like to talk about Jerry again. Time flies, Jerry is approaching the end of his senior year. Through 4 years of college study, Jerry has acquired skills, maturity, and experience. Many things have changed, except for one – his habit of spending money. Starting from his senior year, his parents gave him $1,000 on the first day of each month. Same as when he was a freshman, each month Jerry spent half of the money in his bank account. **Figure 6-11** shows the monthly records of Jerry's remaining balance.

Please link Jerry's bank record to what we have learned in this chapter. Work on it yourself before looking at my interpretation.

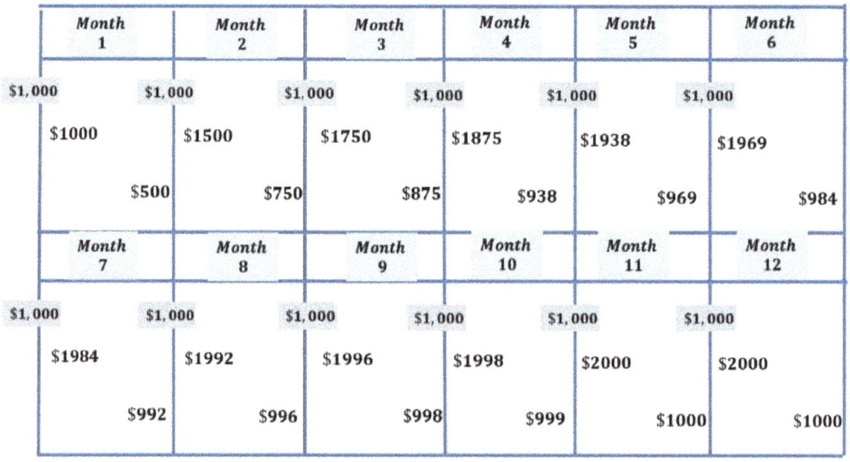

Month 1	Month 2	Month 3	Month 4	Month 5	Month 6
$1,000	$1,000	$1,000	$1,000	$1,000	$1,000
$1000	$1500	$1750	$1875	$1938	$1969
$500	$750	$875	$938	$969	$984

Month 7	Month 8	Month 9	Month 10	Month 11	Month 12
$1,000	$1,000	$1,000	$1,000	$1,000	$1,000
$1984	$1992	$1996	$1998	$2000	$2000
$992	$996	$998	$999	$1000	$1000

Figure 6-11.   Monthly records of Jerry's bank account.

~ ~ ~

Jerry's habit of spending money follows first-order kinetics. He spent more money when he had more in his back account and spent less when he had less money. In contrast, his parents gave him money with zero-order kinetics - $1000 every month (first row of figure 6-11).

As it shows, Jerry's monthly record increased in the first several months (second row), and meanwhile, the money he spent also increased (third row). Once the money he spent every month reached $1000, which is identical to the money he received monthly, his remaining balance stabilized. As shown in month 11 and month 12 records, he had $2000 at the beginning and $1000 at the end.

Now, let's link this case example to what we just learned in this chapter:

- $1000 received from his parent every month = Dose ($1000) and τ (1 month)
- Balance at the beginning of each month = $C_{max,n}$
- Balance at the end of each month = $C_{min,n}$
- Jerry spent half of the money every month = $t_{1/2}$ of 1 month (i.e. k_e=0.693 month^{-1})
- Balance at the beginning of Month 11 and Month 12 = $C_{max,ss}$
- Balance at the end of Month 11 and Month 12 = $C_{min,ss}$

Based on the above information, we can calculate the accumulation ratio of Jerry's record at the steady state:

$$r_{ss} = \frac{1}{(1-e^{-k_e \cdot \tau})} = \frac{1}{(1-e^{-0.693 \cdot 1})} = 2$$

Jerry had $1000 at the beginning of month 1 and had $2000 at the beginning of months 11&12, which verifies that the r_{ss} of 2 calculated above is correct.

If Jerry wants to have a monthly balance stabilized immediately in month 1, what he can do?

Loading dose = dose · rss = $1000 · 2 = $2000

Therefore, if he asks his parents to give him $2000 (loading dose) in month 1, then $1000 (maintenance dose) in each subsequent month, he will have stabilized month records immediately.

Case Example 6-5.

This case study is adapted from *Journal of Clinical Pharmacology 2016, 56(10): 1180-1195*. Credit goes to the original authors of that paper - David J. Greenblatt, MD, and Paul N. Abourjaily, PharmD.

"A 30-year-old man IA has been extensively evaluated for recurrent supraventricular tachycardia (SVT). The treating physician elected to start therapy with digitoxin 0.1 mg daily. One week later the patient reported a reduction in the number of SVT episodes. The plasma digitoxin level was 8 µg/L (usually therapeutic range is 10-20 µg/L). The dose was increased to 0.2 mg per day.

At a follow-up visit 7 days later, the patient claimed that symptoms attributable to SVT had disappeared completely. The plasma digitoxin level was 17.4 µg/L. The patient continued to take 0.2 mg per day of digitoxin. One month later, the patient visited the physician on an urgent basis. He had a diminished appetite and waves of nausea. The electrocardiogram showed T-wave abnormalities, and the plasma digitoxin level was 31.3 µg/L."

Note: digitoxin has a similar structure to digoxin but has a longer half-life; digitoxin $t_{1/2}$=7 days.

Based on what we have learned in this chapter, explain why patient IA had an adverse event in the end. Do you agree with the current dose regimen adjustment? If you were the lead pharmacist or physician, what dose regimen would you give?

Work on this case study yourself before looking at my evaluation provided below.

$$\sim \sim \sim$$

The goal was to give a dose regimen to maintain digitoxin steady state concentrations within the therapeutic range of 10-20 µg/L. The initial dose regimen was 0.1 mg daily (i.e., τ=1 day). after one week, the plasma concentration of digitoxin was 8 µg/L, which is lower than the therapeutic range. Should we increase the dose?

The half-life of digitoxin is 7 days (i.e. 1 week). As shown in Table 6-1, after one half-life, 50% of steady state is reached. If we stick to the dose regimen of 0.1 mg daily, it will take 5 half-lives (i.e., 5 weeks) to reach the steady state; the steady-state concentration would be 16 µg/L based on the data of 8 µg/L at 50% steady state. Therefore, the original dose regimen of 0.1 mg daily can result in steady state concentrations within the therapeutic range of 10-20 µg/L.

However, the physician decided to increase the dose to 0.2 mg every day. Doubling the dose will lead to a 2-fold increase in steady state concentration. We would anticipate that the new steady state concentration is 32 µg/L (i.e., 16 µg/L x 2), which is very close to what was measured (31.3 µg/L). This concentration well exceeds the upper threshold of 20 µg/L, and patient IA experienced side effect, which is not surprising.

Since digitoxin has a long half-life, what should we do if we don't want to wait 5 weeks to reach its steady state?

As $t_{1/2}$= 7 days, k_e of digitoxin is $\frac{0.693}{7}$ = 0.099 day^{-1}

Loading dose = dose · r_{ss} = dose ·$\frac{1}{(1-e^{-k_e \cdot \tau})}$ = 0.1 (mg) ·$\frac{1}{(1-e^{-0.099 \cdot 24})}$ = 1.06 mg ≈ 1 mg

Therefore, we can recommend 1 mg as the loading dose, then 0.1 mg as the maintenance daily dose.

This chapter is an important one. Many important terms are introduced, and several case examples similar to what you may encounter in clinical practice are discussed. I hope you have enjoyed this book so far. We will learn pharmacokinetics and dose regimen optimization following I.V. infusion in the next chapter.

Problem Sets   *(Answers to study problems are in the appendix)*

1. Patient NY is given an I.V. bolus injection of drug A. The followings are the properties of the drug: V_d – 400 L; CL – 100 ml/min; therapeutic range – 2 to 4 mg/L. Recommend a dosing regimen that will maintain the drug concentrations within the therapeutic range.

2. Patient TX received Drug N with the dose of 200 mg every 8 h. After reaching steady state, a peak level of 20 mg/L was measured. And 4 hours after peak, the concentration was 10 mg/L.
    a) Calculate k_e
    b) Calculate the volume of distribution.
    c) Calculate the average steady state concentration.
    d) Find out the trough concentration after the 3rd dose and 10th dose.
    e) How long would it take for Drug N to reach steady state?
    f) If you don't want to wait that long, what loading dose would you recommend?

Chapter 7.
I.V. Infusion (One-Compartment Model)

Learning Objectives

After reading this chapter, the reader shall be able to:

1. Predict drug concentration-time profiles during I.V. infusion and after infusion is stopped.

2. Understand the relationship between pharmacokinetics parameters and concentration time profiles following I.V. infusion.

3. Identify appropriate equations to predict drug pharmacokinetics under different infusion status and steady state conditions.

4. Predict drug concentration-time profiles following multiple intermittent I.V. infusion.

5. Make dosing decisions by applying equations learned in this chapter for patients receiving I.V. infusions.

For drugs given via I.V. administration, there are two different ways: I.V. bolus injection and I.V. infusion. The last two chapters centered on I.V. bolus injection, where a drug is injected into bloodstream in a very short period of time (e.g., within a few minutes). This chapter deals with I.V. infusion, where a drug in an infusion bag is administered at a constant rate as an extended infusion or drip.

In section 7.1, I will go through the equations that can be used to predict concentration-time profiles of a drug following I.V. infusion. Infusion will not go on forever, it will be stopped at a certain point. Infusion may be stopped before or after reaching steady state. When to use what equation? This question is addressed in section 7.2. In addition, several useful topics, such as the determination of clearance, time to reach steady state, and the principle of loading dose, will be discussed in section 7.3. In section 7.4, we will evaluate how changes in drug input and primary pharmacokinetic parameters (i.e., CL and V_d) affect concentration-time profiles of a drug given via I.V. infusion. A patient may receive multiple short-term infusions. Equations related to multiple I.V. infusions are briefly mentioned in section 7.5. A case example showing how to apply I.V. infusion models for dose optimization is provided in section 7.6. Then this chapter ends with additional case studies (section 7.7) and problem sets.

7.1 Pharmacokinetic Equations for a Drug Following I.V. Infusion

For a drug administered through I.V. infusion, the drug is placed in an infusion bag, and there is a tube (i.e., an I.V. line) connects the bag of solution to a patient's vein. Since the drug is delivered to the bloodstream at a constant rate (e.g., 1 mg/min), the drug input follows zero-order kinetics. Once the drug enters bloodstream, the elimination process starts. Most drugs are eliminated via first-order kinetics. Therefore, for a drug administered via I.V. infusion, its pharmacokinetics are determined by a zero-order input and a first-order output.

Figure 7-1 shows the model diagram of a drug administered via I.V. infusion, which includes a one-compartment model with zero-order input (during infusion) and first-order elimination. After the infusion is over, the zero-order input is stopped. Based on this model, the rate of change of drug in body (i.e. amount of drug changes in body per given time) is described as:

During infusion:

$$\frac{dX}{dt} = k_o - k_e \cdot X \qquad\qquad [7\text{-}1]$$

After infusion is stopped:

$$\frac{dX}{dt} = -k_e \cdot X \qquad\qquad [7\text{-}2]$$

$$X_0 = 0$$

Where X represents drug amount in the body; k_o represents infusion rate with unit of amount/time; k_e represents elimination rate constant; and X_0 represents initial amount in the body, which is 0 since the drug is still in the infusion bag at time 0. The rate function of k_o is positive since it represents the amount of drug entering the body per given time. On the other hand, the function of $k_e \cdot X$ is negative since it represents the amount of drug removed from the body per given time.

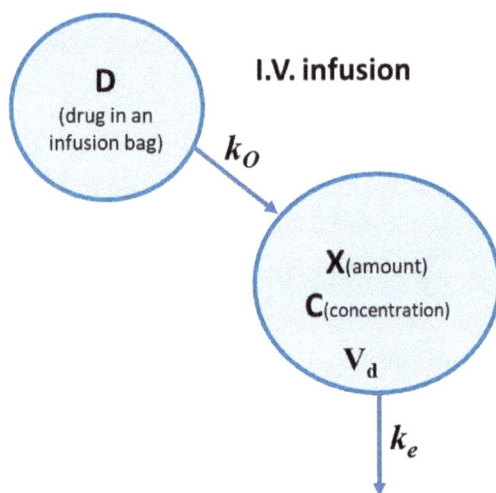

Figure 7-1. Schematic representation of a one-compartment model with zero-order infusion and first-order elimination for a drug administrated via I.V. infusion.

Equations 7-1 and 7-2 can be solved, together with the relationship of $C = \frac{X}{V_d}$, we can get the following general explicit equation for drug concentration C at different time:

$$C = \frac{k_o}{k_e \cdot V_d} (e^{k_e \cdot T} - 1) \cdot e^{-k_e \cdot t}$$ [7-3]

In Equation 7-3, there are two terms for time:

T= time of infusion

t = time after start of infusion

For example, let's assume that an infusion was started at 7:30 AM. Infusion was stopped at 10:00 AM. You were asked to calculate drug concentration at 11:30 AM. What were the T and t?

- *T represents duration of infusion, which was 2.5 h in this case; while t is the time after the start of infusion, which was 4 h.*

What does the concentration-time profile look like for a drug following I.V. infusion? We can get some hints from Equations 7-1 and 7-2. At time 0, plasma drug concentration is 0 since all drug molecules are still in the infusion bag. Then the drug is delivered to the bloodstream at a constant rate (e.g., 1 mg per min). As a result, the drug concentration increases over time. The net amount of drug changes in the body per given time is determined by two rate functions as shown in Equation 7-1: k_o and $k_e \cdot X$. k_o is a zero-order term and it stays constant. $k_e \cdot X$ is a first-order term, and its value gets larger when X is larger. When the amount of drug eliminated per given time (i.e., $k_e \cdot X$) is identical to the amount of drug gets in per given time (i.e., k_o), steady state is reached. As noted earlier, infusion will not go on forever. Once infusion is stopped, there is no input of k_o, while elimination process continues. As a result, the concentration in the body decreases after the infusion is over. Based on the hints from Equations 7-1 and 7-2, for the pharmacokinetics of a drug during and after I.V. infusion, we would expect a concentration-time profile like the one shown in Figure 7-2.

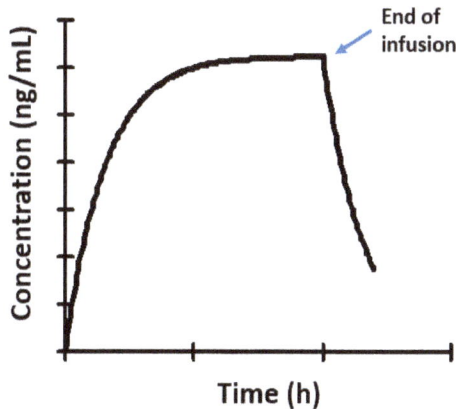

Figure 7-2. Example concentration-time profile of a drug during and after I.V. infusion.

7.2 Identifying Appropriate Equations based on Infusion Status and Steady State Condition

The general equation that can be used to predict drug concentration at different times for a drug following I.V. infusion is shown in Equation 7-3. It is a long equation. In different scenarios, simplified equations can be applied.

Scenario 1. During infusion, the steady state has not been reached.

In this scenario, a sample for concentration measurement is taken during infusion prior to steady state. The condition of "during infusion" means that T (i.e., duration of infusion) equals to t (i.e., time since infusion starts). Since T=t, we can replace T with t in Equation 7-3 and get the following simplified equation:

$$C = \frac{k_o}{k_e \bullet V_d}(e^{k_e \bullet t} - 1) \bullet e^{-k_e \bullet t} \quad \rightarrow \quad C = \frac{k_o}{k_e \bullet V_d}(1 - e^{-k_e \bullet t}) \qquad [7\text{-}4]$$

As shown in Figure 7-3, a sample (represented by a blue circle) is taken during infusion prior to steady state. If we want to calculate the concentration of this sample, Equation 7-4 is the appropriate one to use.

Scenario 2. During infusion, the steady state has been reached.

In this scenario, a sample is taken during infusion after steady state has been achieved. Since it is during infusion, T=t. The drug reaches its steady state when $e^{-k_e \cdot t} \rightarrow 0$. Therefore, Equation 7-4 can be simplified as:

$$C_{ss} = \frac{k_o}{k_e \bullet V_d} \qquad [7\text{-}5]$$

As shown in Figure 7-3, a sample (represented by a red triangle) is taken during infusion after steady state has been achieved. If we want to calculate the concentration of this sample (i.e., concentration at the steady state, C_{ss}), Equation 7-5 is the appropriate one to use.

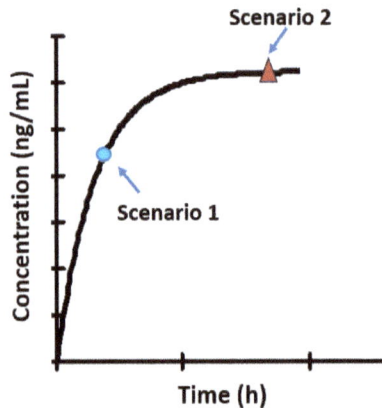

Figure 7-3. Plasma concentration-time profile a drug following I.V. infusion. *Scenario 1.* A sample is taken prior to steady state; *Scenario 2.* A sample is taken after steady state is achieved.

Scenario 3. Infusion is stopped before the steady state has been reached.

In this scenario, infusion is stopped before the steady state has been achieved. A sample, as represented by the blue circle in Figure 7-4, is taken after infusion is stopped. In this scenario, there are three terms that are related to time:

T = infusion time

t= time since infusion starts

t'= time since infusion stops

To calculate the concentration of the sample represented by the blue circle in Figure 7-4, we need to determine the maximum concentration first, then adds an e term to describe the decline of the curve (just like the equation we use for I.V. bolus injection).

$$C = C_{max} \bullet e^{-k_e \bullet t'} \qquad\qquad [7\text{-}6]$$

Where C_{max} is the highest concentration right before infusion is stopped, which means that it is the concentration at T. Therefore, based on Equation 7-4, C_{max} can be expressed as:

$$C_{max} = \frac{k_o}{k_e \bullet V_d}(1 - e^{-k_e \bullet T}) \qquad\qquad [7\text{-}7]$$

Combining Equations 7-6 and 7-7, we get the following equation:

$$C = \frac{k_o}{k_e \bullet V_d}(1 - e^{-k_e \bullet T}) \bullet e^{-k_e \bullet t'} \qquad\qquad [7\text{-}8]$$

Therefore, when infusion is stopped before the steady state is achieved, if we want to calculate the concentration of a sample after infusion is stopped, Equation 7-8 is the appropriate one to use.

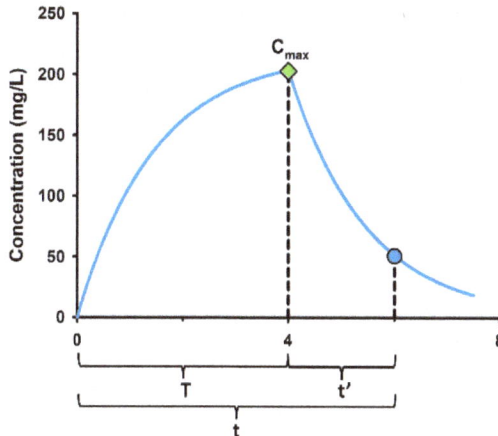

Figure 7-4. Plasma concentration-time profile a drug following I.V. infusion. The infusion is stopped before the steady state is achieved. A sample (blue circle) is taken after infusion is stopped. T, infusion time. t, time since infusion starts; t', time since infusion is stopped.

Scenario 4. Infusion is stopped after the steady state has been reached.

In this scenario, infusion is stopped after the steady state has been achieved. A sample, as represented by the blue circle in Figure 7-5, is taken after infusion is stopped. Since the steady state has been reached, the concentration right before the infusion is stopped is C_{ss}, which can be calculated using equation 7-5 (i.e., scenario 2). Accordingly, the concentration of a sample represented by the blue circle in Figure 7-5 is calculated as:

$$C = C_{ss} \bullet e^{-k_e \bullet t'} \rightarrow \qquad C = \frac{k_o}{k_e \bullet V_d} \bullet e^{-k_e \bullet t'} \qquad\qquad [7\text{-}9]$$

Therefore, when infusion is stopped after the steady state is achieved, if we want to calculate the concentration of a sample after infusion is stopped, Equation 7-9 is the appropriate one to use.

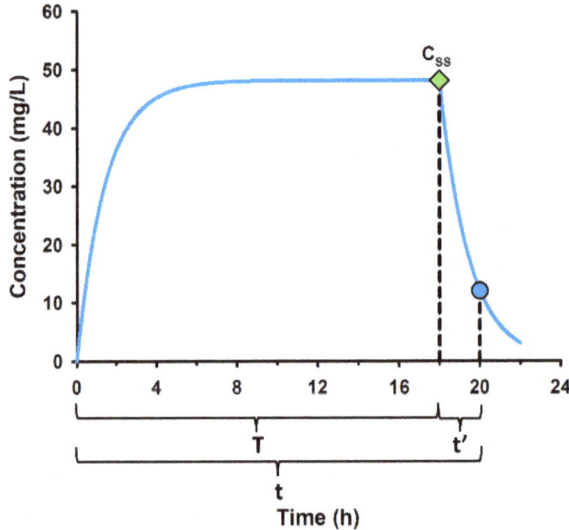

Figure 7-5. Plasma concentration-time profile a drug following I.V. infusion. The infusion is stopped after the steady state is achieved. A sample (blue circle) is taken after infusion is stopped. T, infusion time. t, time since infusion starts; t', time since infusion is stopped.

7.3 Determination of Clearance, Time to Reach Steady State, and Principle of Loading Dose

7.3.1. Determination of clearance

I.V. infusion is a situation highlighting the importance of determining drug clearance. Why? Because steady state concentration C_{ss} is dependent on the infusion rate k_o and CL as shown in Equation 7-5:

$$C_{ss} = \frac{k_o}{k_e \cdot V_d} \quad \rightarrow \quad C_{ss} = \frac{k_o}{CL} \tag{7-10}$$

Equation 7-10 is useful because it can be rearranged to calculate k_o. If we know the desired steady state concentration and the clearance of a drug, we can decide the infusion rate using the following equation:

$$k_o = C_{ss} \cdot CL \tag{7-11}$$

For example, if we know a drug's clearance is 2 L/h, and the targeted steady state concentration is 20 mg/L, then we can design the infusion rate based on Equation 7-11: $k_o = C_{ss} \cdot CL = 20$ mg/L $\cdot 2$ L/h $= 40$ mg/h.

Therefore, there is a clear motive to determine the clearance of a drug in a specific patient so that we can perform individualized therapy. When a patient takes a drug for the first time, we won't know the clearance in this patient. How to estimate the clearance of a drug in this patient? There are two ways:

- The doctor can start an empirical therapy by using an infusion rate based on the drug's clearance in a general population. After infusion starts, wait till the drug reaches the steady state in this patient. Then take a sample, and the concentration measured is C_{ss}. Based on the infusion rate used and the C_{ss} of this specific patient, we can get the drug's clearance in this patient based on the following equation:

$$CL = \frac{k_o}{C_{ss}} \tag{7-12}$$

- Using C_{ss} to estimate CL may not work for drugs with long half-lives as their steady state may take a long time to reach. In order to estimate CL in a timely manner, Chiou equation has been applied for some drugs (e.g., theophylline):

$$CL = \frac{2 \cdot k_o}{C_1 + C_2} + \frac{2 \cdot V_d \cdot (C_1 - C_2)}{(C_1 + C_2)(t_2 - t_1)} \tag{7-13}$$

Where C_1 and C_2 are concentrations of two samples collected at times separated by at least one half-life. For V_d used in the above equation, please note that it is a bodyweight normalized value (i.e., unit is L/kg). Together with the body weight of a specific patient, the volume of distribution of a drug in this patient can be estimated.

7.3.2. Time to reach steady state

In Chapter 6, I said that I will calculate time to reach steady state in Chapter 7. Let's do it. The key equation used for calculation is Equation 7-4.

- After 1 $t_{1/2}$, the concentration is:

$$C = \frac{k_o}{k_e \cdot V_d}(1 - e^{-k_e \cdot t_{1/2}}) \rightarrow C = \frac{k_o}{k_e \cdot V_d}(1 - e^{-k_e \cdot \frac{ln2}{k_e}}) \quad \rightarrow$$

$$C = \frac{k_o}{k_e \cdot V_d}(1 - e^{-\ln2}) \;\rightarrow\; C = \frac{k_o}{k_e \cdot V_d}(1 - \frac{1}{2}) \rightarrow C = 0.5\frac{k_o}{k_e \cdot V_d}$$

$$\rightarrow C = 0.5 \cdot C_{ss}$$

- After 2 $t_{1/2}$, the concentration is:

$$C = \frac{k_o}{k_e \cdot V_d}(1 - e^{-k_e \cdot 2 \cdot t_{1/2}}) \;\rightarrow\; C = \frac{k_o}{k_e \cdot V_d}(1 - e^{-k_e \cdot 2 \cdot \frac{\ln2}{k_e}}) \;\rightarrow$$

$$C = \frac{k_o}{k_e \cdot V_d}(1 - e^{-2 \cdot \ln2}) \;\rightarrow\; C = \frac{k_o}{k_e \cdot V_d}(1 - \frac{1}{4}) \;\rightarrow\; C = 0.75 \cdot C_{ss}$$

- After 3 $t_{1/2}$, the concentration is:

$$C = \frac{k_o}{k_e \cdot V_d}(1 - e^{-k_e \cdot 3 \cdot t_{1/2}}) \rightarrow C = \frac{k_o}{k_e \cdot V_d}(1 - e^{-k_e \cdot 3 \cdot \frac{\ln2}{k_e}}) \rightarrow$$

$$C = \frac{k_o}{k_e \cdot V_d}(1 - e^{-3 \cdot \ln2}) \rightarrow C = \frac{k_o}{k_e \cdot V_d}(1 - \frac{1}{8}) \quad \rightarrow C = 0.875\frac{k_o}{k_e \cdot V_d}$$

$$\rightarrow C = 0.875 \cdot C_{ss}$$

- After 5 $t_{1/2}$, the concentration is:

$$C = \frac{k_o}{k_e \cdot V_d}(1 - e^{-k_e \cdot 5 \cdot t_{1/2}}) \;\rightarrow\; C = \frac{k_o}{k_e \cdot V_d}(1 - e^{-k_e \cdot 5 \cdot \frac{\ln2}{k_e}}) \rightarrow$$

$$C = \frac{k_o}{k_e \cdot V_d}(1 - e^{-5 \cdot \ln2}) \rightarrow C = \frac{k_o}{k_e \cdot V_d}(1 - \frac{1}{32}) \quad \rightarrow C = 0.97\frac{k_o}{k_e \cdot V_d}$$

$$\rightarrow C = 0.97 \cdot C_{ss}$$

In general, we consider that steady state is reached after 5 half-lives since the concentration is approximately 97% of the steady state concentration. For a drug with a long half-life, it may take several days to reach the steady state; this is clearly unideal when the drug is used to treat a life-threatening disease where desired concentrations need to be achieved as soon as possible. That's the situation where loading dose steps in; this is discussed in the next subsection.

7.3.2. Principle of loading dose

The goal of loading dose is to achieve the steady state concentration immediately, instead of waiting for 5 half-lives. Since we know the desired steady state concentration, the loading dose is determined using the following equation:

$$\textit{Loading dose} = C_{ss} \cdot V_d \qquad\qquad\qquad [7\text{-}14]$$

Based on Equation 7-10, the above equation can be expressed as:

$$Loading\ dose = \frac{k_o}{CL} \bullet V_d \ \rightarrow Loading\ dose = \frac{k_o}{k_e} \qquad\qquad [7\text{-}15]$$

Since $k_e = \frac{0.693}{t_{1/2}}$, Equation 7-15 can be expressed as:

$$Loading\ dose = \frac{k_o \bullet t_{1/2}}{0.693} \ \rightarrow Loading\ dose = 1.44 \bullet k_o \bullet t_{1/2} \qquad [7\text{-}16]$$

Please note that the loading dose is given via an I.V. bolus injection, and it is given only once.

7.4 Impact of Change in Drug Input and Pharmacokinetic Parameters in Concentration-Time Profile of a Drug Given via I.V. Infusion

In this section, I use one case example to illustrate how changes in drug input and primary pharmacokinetics parameters affect drug exposure and concentration-time profiles of a drug administered via I.V. infusion.

Case Example 7-1.

Iowa-001 is a new investigational drug with intended indication in alleviating last minute exam panic attacks. It follows the first-order kinetics, and its disposition can be described using a one-compartment model.

Scenario 1. A higher infusion rate of Iowa-001 is administered.

Scenario 2. The clearance of Iowa-001 increases.

Scenario 3. The volume of distribution of Iowa-001 increases.

Please 1) evaluate the impact of each scenario on C_{ss}, AUC, k_e and $t_{1/2}$ of Iowa-001 when it is administered via I.V. infusion; and 2) draw a figure for each scenario to illustrate the old and new pharmacokinetic profiles.

Please work on it yourself before looking at the answer I provide below.

$$\sim\ \sim\ \sim$$

To address this type of question, first we need to list the relevant equations.

- $C_{ss} = \dfrac{k_o}{CL}$
- $AUC = \dfrac{Dose}{CL} \quad\rightarrow\quad AUC = \dfrac{k_o \cdot T}{CL}$
- $k_e = \dfrac{CL}{V_d}$
- $t_{1/2} = \dfrac{0.693}{k_e}$

In scenario 1. The infusion rate (i.e., k_o) of Iowa-001 increases. Based on the above equations, the parameters that are affected by the dose are C_{ss} and AUC. With the increase in the infusion rate, both C_{ss} and AUC of Iowa-001 increase proportionally. k_e and $t_{1/2}$ are not affected by the infusion rate. Accordingly, the time to reach the steady state remains the same.

In scenario 2. Based on the above four equations, with an increase in clearance, C_{ss} decreases; AUC decreases; k_e increases; and $t_{1/2}$ decreases. Since $t_{1/2}$ decreases, it takes a shorter time to reach the steady state.

In scenario 3. With an increase in V_d, both C_{ss} and AUC stay the same; k_e decreases; and $t_{1/2}$ increases. Since $t_{1/2}$ increases, it takes a longer time to reach the steady state.

Below table is provided to facilitate the comparison between your results and the one I provided here:

Table 7-1. Impact of changes in k_o, CL, or V_d on Iowa-001 pharmacokinetics parameters.

	C_{ss}	AUC	k_e	$t_{1/2}$	Time to reach SS
Increase in k_o	↑	↑	↔	↔	↔
Increase in CL	↓	↓	↑	↓	↓
Increase in V_d	↔	↔	↓	↑	↑

Figure 7-6 shows the impact of each scenario in Iowa-001 pharmacokinetics (note: solid black line is the original curve, and solid blue line is the new curve).

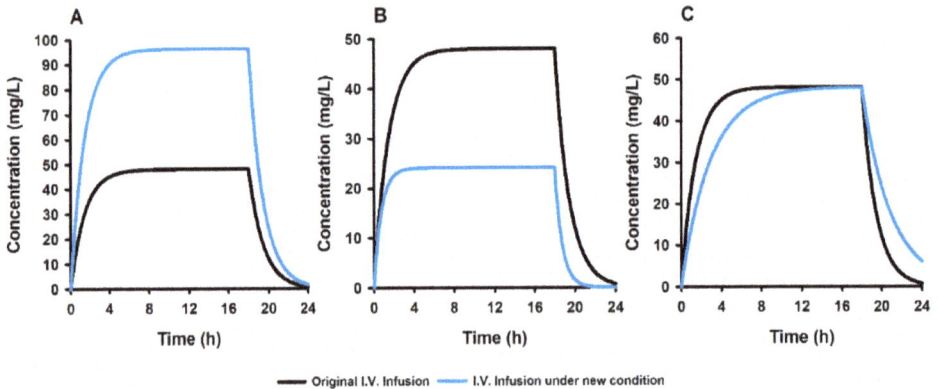

Figure 7-6. The impact of changes in A) infusion, B) CL, or C) V_d on drug pharmacokinetics of Iowa-001 following I.V. infusion.

7.5 Equations Related to Multiple Short-Term I.V. Infusions

In the clinic, there is often a need to give a short-term I.V. infusion of a drug multiple times. For example, you may see a dosing regimen like this in ICU: meropenem 3-h I.V. infusion every 8 h for 5 days. In this example, 3 h is the infusion time (i.e., T), 8 h is the dosing interval (i.e., τ), and 5 days means that the infusion is given for 15 times. How to calculate the concentration of drug following multiple short-term I.V. infusions? The equations are long but are easy to understand after they are broken into pieces. Let's have a brief look.

- During the first dosing interval, the maximum concentration occurs at time T (i.e., right before infusion is stopped), and the minimum concentration is observed just before the next dose (Figure 7-7).

$$C_{max,1} = \frac{k_o}{CL}(1 - e^{-k_e \cdot T})$$ [7-17]

$$C_{min,1} = C_{max,1} \cdot e^{-k_e \cdot t'} \;\rightarrow\; C_{min,1} = \frac{k_o}{CL}(1 - e^{-k_e \cdot T}) \cdot e^{-k_e \cdot t'}$$ [7-18]

where t' = τ – T.

- After n doses of I.V. infusions, the maximum and minimum concentrations are:

$$C_{max,n} = \frac{k_o}{CL}(1 - e^{-k_e \cdot T}) \cdot r$$

Where r is the accumulation ratio, which is same as what we learned in I.V. bolus injection in Chapter 6 (i.e., $r = \frac{(1-e^{-n \cdot k_e \cdot \tau})}{(1-e^{-k_e \cdot \tau})}$).

Therefore $C_{max,n}$ can be expressed as:

$$C_{max,n} = \frac{k_o}{CL}(1 - e^{-k_e \cdot T}) \cdot \frac{(1-e^{-n \cdot k_e \cdot \tau})}{(1-e^{-k_e \cdot \tau})}$$ [7-19]

$$C_{min,n} = C_{max,n} \cdot e^{-k_e \cdot t'}$$

$$\rightarrow C_{min,n} = \frac{k_o}{CL}(1 - e^{-k_e \cdot T}) \cdot \frac{(1-e^{-n \cdot k_e \cdot \tau})}{(1-e^{-k_e \cdot \tau})} \cdot e^{-k_e \cdot t'}$$ [7-20]

- After steady state is reached, the maximum and minimum concentrations during steady state are:

$$C_{max,ss} = \frac{k_o}{CL}(1 - e^{-k_e \cdot T}) \cdot r_{ss}$$

Where r_{ss} is the accumulation ratio at steady state, which is same as what we learned in I.V. bolus injection in Chapter 6 (i.e., $r_{ss} = \frac{1}{(1-e^{-k_e \cdot \tau})}$).

Therefore $C_{max,ss}$ can be expressed as:

$$C_{max,ss} = \frac{k_o}{CL}(1 - e^{-k_e \cdot T}) \cdot \frac{1}{(1-e^{-k_e \cdot \tau})}$$ [7-21]

$$C_{min,ss} = C_{max,ss} \cdot e^{-k_e \cdot t'}$$

$$\rightarrow C_{min,ss} = \frac{k_o}{CL}(1 - e^{-k_e \cdot T}) \cdot \frac{1}{(1-e^{-k_e \cdot \tau})} \cdot e^{-k_e \cdot t'}$$ [7-22]

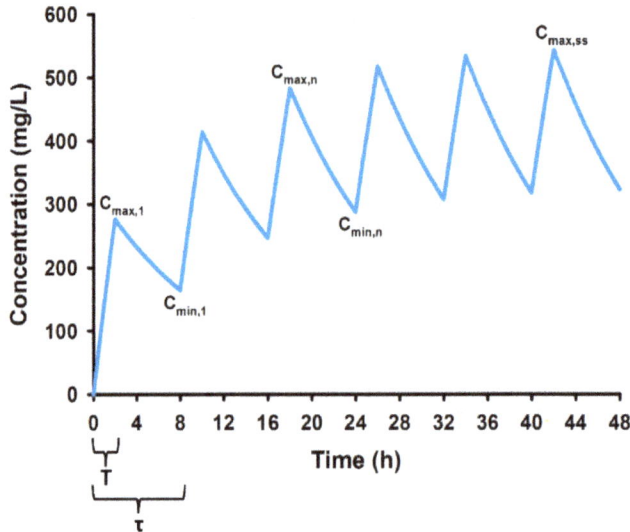

Figure 7-7. Concentration-time profile of a drug following multiple short-term I.V. infusions. T, infusion time; τ, dosing interval.

7.6 Applying I.V. Infusion Models for Dose Optimization

In this section, I provide one case study so that you can apply what you have learned in this chapter for dose optimization.

Case Example 7-2.

Patient MN (60 kg female) started on a continuous I.V. infusion of drug A. This was her first time taking this drug. The desired steady state concentration is 20 mg/L. According to the package insert, the clearance of drug A in the general population is 4 L/h. Based on this information, the doctor prescribed an infusion rate of 80 mg/h (based on equation $k_o = C_{ss} \cdot CL$). However, after the drug reached its steady state, a blood sample was collected, and the steady state concentration was found to be only 10 mg/L. The V_d of drug A is 1 L/kg.

1) propose a treatment plan to keep the steady state concentration at the desired level.
2) estimate how long it would take to reach the steady state.
3) propose a strategy if you want the steady state concentration to be reached immediately.

Please work on it yourself before looking at the answer I provide below.

~ ~ ~

1) *This patient received I.V. infusion with a rate of 80 mg/h and the steady state concentration was 10 mg/L. Based on this information, the clearance of drug A in patient MN is:*

$$CL = \frac{k_o}{C_{ss}} = \frac{80 \; mg/h}{10 \; mg/L} = 8 \; L/h$$

To achieve the desired steady state concentration is 20 mg/L, the infusion rate should be adjusted using the following equation:

$$k_o = C_{ss} \cdot CL = 20 \frac{mg}{L} \cdot 8 \frac{L}{h} = 160 \; mg/h$$

2) *The V_d of drug A in patient MN is 1 L/kg x 60 kg = 60 L. CL of this drug in patient MN is 8 L/h. The half-life of drug A is:*

$$t_{1/2} = \frac{0.693 \cdot V_d}{CL} = \frac{0.693 \cdot 60L}{8 \; L/h} = 5.2 \; h$$

Therefore, it will take 26 h (i.e., 5.2 X 5) to reach the steady state.

3) *In order to immediately achieve the steady state, a loading dose, administered via I.V. bolus injection is needed. The loading dose is:*

$$Loading \; dose = 1.44 \cdot k_o \cdot t_{1/2} = 1.44 \cdot 160 \; mg/h \cdot 5.2 \; h = 1200 \; mg$$

7.7 Case Study

In this section, I provide two additional case studies so that you can further strengthen your dose regimen design skills.

Case Example 7-3.

Patient NY is to be given 100 mg of gentamycin intravenously over 1 h every 8 h. Patient NY is assumed to have an average k_e of 0.2 h^{-1} and a V_d of 15 L.

1) How long will it take to reach steady state.
2) Calculate the peak concentration of gentamycin after the first dose and 20th dose.
3) Calculate the trough concentration of gentamycin after the 20th dose.
4) Calculate average steady state concentration, fluctuation and accumulation ratio.

Please work on it yourself before looking at the answer I provide below.

~ ~ ~

1) *It will take 5 half-lives to reach the steady state. time = $5 \times \frac{0.693}{0.2} = 17.3$ h*

2) $C_{max,1} = \frac{k_o}{CL}\left(1 - e^{-k_e \cdot T}\right) = \frac{100\frac{mg}{h}}{0.2h^{-1} \cdot 15L}\left(1 - e^{-0.2h^{-1} \cdot 8h}\right) = 6.03$ mg/L

$$C_{max,20} = \frac{k_o}{CL}(1 - e^{-k_e \cdot T}) \cdot \frac{(1-e^{-20 \cdot k_e \cdot \tau})}{(1-e^{-k_e \cdot \tau})} = 7.54 \text{ mg/L}$$

3) $C_{min,20} = C_{max,20} \cdot e^{-k_e \cdot t'} = C_{max,20} \cdot e^{-0.2h^{-1} \cdot (8-1)h} = 1.86 \ mg/L$

4) $C_{ave,ss} = \frac{AUC_\tau}{\tau} \rightarrow C_{ave,ss} = \frac{Dose}{CL \cdot \tau} \rightarrow C_{ave,ss} = \frac{k_o \cdot T}{CL \cdot \tau} = \frac{100 \ mg/h \cdot 8h}{0.2h^{-1} \cdot 15L \cdot 8h} = $

$4.17 \ mg/L$

$$F' = \frac{C_{max,ss}}{C_{min,ss}} = e^{k_e \cdot (\tau - T)} = e^{0.2h^{-1} \cdot (8-1)h} = 4.06$$

$$r_{ss} = \frac{1}{(1-e^{-k_e \cdot \tau})} = \frac{1}{(1-e^{-0.2h^{-1} \cdot 8h})} = 1.25$$

Case Example 7-4.

Patient FL (70-kg, male) is admitted to the hospital due to bacterial prostatitis. He is to be given ciprofloxacin multiple I.V. infusion for 5 days. As the lead pharmacist, you are asked to recommend a dosing regimen of ciprofloxacin. You have the following information:

Ciprofloxacin, a broad-spectrum fluoroquinolone antibiotic, exhibits *concentration-dependent killing*, and its antibacterial effect is associated with the ratio of the area under the concentration versus time curve to MIC (i.e., AUC/MIC). MIC represents the lowest concentration of an antibiotic that inhibits the growth of a given strain of bacteria. The treatment goal is to reach AUC_{24}/MIC $\geqslant 125$ for ciprofloxacin.

The volume of distribution of ciprofloxacin is 2 L/kg. The half-life of ciprofloxacin is 4 h. Ciprofloxacin is commonly administered via I.V. infusion (e.g., 1-2 h infusion).

Design a dose regimen to maintain ciprofloxacin AUC_{24}/MIC $\geqslant 125$, with MIC being 2 µg/L.

~ ~ ~

The half-life of ciprofloxacin is 4 h, which means that it will reach steady state within a day (4 x 5 = 20 h). If we plan to give ciprofloxacin once a day (i.e., τ=24 h) and meanwhile reach the goal of AUC_{24}/MIC $\geqslant 125$, AUC_{24} at steady state needs to be at least:

$AUC_{24} \geq 125 \times MIC \rightarrow AUC_{24} \geq 125 \times 2 = 250 \ \mu g/L$

Since $AUC_{24,ss} = \frac{Dose}{CL}$, the dose should be at least:

$Dose = AUC_{24} \times CL = 250 \ \mu g/L \cdot k_e \cdot V_d = 250 \ \mu g/L \cdot \frac{0.693}{4 \ h} \cdot 2L/kg \cdot 70 \ kg = 6064 \ \mu g = 6.1 \ mg$

If we plan to give 1 h infusion (i.e., T=1 h), the minimum infusion rate k_o=dose/T = 6.1 mg/h.

Therefore, one potential dose regimen could be 6.1 mg of ciprofloxacin I.V. infusion over 1 h every 24 h. Please note that 6.1 mg is the minimum dose.

You could also give ciprofloxacin more frequently, as long as the total daily dose is ≥6.1 mg. For example, a dose regimen of 3.1 mg 1-h infusion every 12 h, or 2.1 mg 1-h infusion every 8 h.

Problem Sets   *(Answers to study problems are in the appendix)*

Patient IL (80 kg, male) is to be started on a continuous I.V. infusion of Drug Y. Drug Y has a half-life of 8 h and its volume of distribution is 1L/kg.
1) In order to achieve Css of 25 mg/L, what would be the infusion rate?
2) How long would it take for drug Y to reach steady state?
3) You do not want to wait that long for drug Y to achieve steady state. What would you do?
4) Assume the total infusion time is 8 h. What are the plasma concentrations of Drug Y at 4 h, 8h, and 11 h after the infusion starts?
5) Assume the total infusion time is 50 h. What is the plasma concentration of Drug Y at 53 h after the infusion starts?

Chapter 8.
Oral Administration (One-Compartment Model)

Learning Objectives

After reading this chapter, the reader shall be able to:

1. Understand the concentration-time profile obtained after oral administration.

2. Use feathering to determine absorption rate constant k_a and elimination rate constant k_e from a concentration-time profile of an orally administered drug.

3. Calculate drug concentration at different time points using the Bateman equation.

4. Determine the term "flip flop" and understand the situation where flip flop kinetics may occur.

5. Understand the effect of rate and extent of absorption on the concentration-time profile.

6. Understand the impact of absorption rate on the accumulation, fluctuation, and average steady state level of a drug following multiple oral administrations.

So far, we have learned the pharmacokinetics of drugs following I.V. bolus injections and I.V. infusions. This chapter focuses on a convenient and most commonly used administration route – oral administration. We have learned the fundamentals of absorption process in Chapter 2. I recommend refreshing your understanding of these basic concepts related to oral absorption before diving into this chapter.

In section 8.1, I will go through the equations that can be used to predict the concentration-time profile of a drug following oral administration. When we deal with the pharmacokinetics of an oral drug, it is useful to determine two rate constants: absorption rate constant k_a and elimination rate constant k_e. We will learn about "feathering", a method to determine k_a and k_e, in section 8.2. When the rate of absorption is significantly slower than the rate of elimination, flip-flop kinetics occurs, which may create difficulties in parameter interpretation. We will learn flip-flop pharmacokinetics as well as the situation where flip-flop kinetics may occur in section 8.3. In section 8.4, we will examine how changes in drug absorption and elimination affect concentration-time profiles of a drug following oral administration. A patient may receive an orally administered drug multiple times. Equations related to multiple oral administration are briefly mentioned in section 8.5. Then this chapter ends with a case example (section 8.6).

8.1 Pharmacokinetic Equations for a Drug Following a Single Oral Administration

As noted in Chapter 2, the conventional oral dosage form is the immediate-release dosage form. For immediate-release medications, they are rapidly absorbed from the gastrointestinal tract into the systemic circulation through a first-order absorption process. The pharmacokinetic parameters associated with the rate and extent of drug absorption are *absorption rate constant k_a* and *bioavailability F*, respectively. Once the drug enters the bloodstream, the elimination process starts. Most drugs are eliminated via first-order kinetics. Therefore, for a drug administered via oral administration, its pharmacokinetics is determined by *first-order input* and *first-order output*.

Figure 8-1 shows the model diagram of a drug administered via oral administration, which includes a one-compartment model with first-order absorption and first-order elimination. Based on this model, the rate of change of drug in the gastrointestinal tract (dA/dt) and the rate of change of drug in the body (dX/dt) are described as:

$$\frac{dA}{dt} = -k_a \cdot A \qquad\qquad [8\text{-}1]$$
$$A_0 = Dose \cdot F$$

$$\frac{dX}{dt} = k_a \cdot A - k_e \cdot X \qquad\qquad [8\text{-}2]$$
$$X_0 = 0$$

Where:

A = drug amount in the gastrointestinal tract;

k_a = absorption rate constant (unit is time^{-1});

F = bioavailability;

X = drug amount in the body;

k_e = elimination rate constant (unit is time^{-1});

A_0 =initial amount of drug available to be absorbed, which is Dose·F.

X_0 =initial amount in the body, which is 0 since the drug is still in gastrointestinal tract at time 0.

In Equation 8-2, there are two rate functions. The rate function of $k_a \cdot A$ is positive since it represents the amount of drug that enters the body per given time. On the other hand, the function of $k_e \cdot X$ is negative since it represents the amount of drug eliminated from the body per given time.

Equation 8-2 can be solved to get the explicit equation for drug amount X in the body as a function of time. With the relationship of $C = \frac{X}{V_d}$, we can get the following explicit equation for drug concentration C in the body at different time:

$$C = \frac{F \cdot D \cdot k_a}{V_d \cdot (k_a - k_e)} (e^{-k_e \cdot t} - e^{-k_a \cdot t}) \qquad\qquad [8\text{-}3]$$

Equation 8-3 is known as Bateman equation. With this equation, we can predict drug concentration at any time if we know the information of dose (D), bioavailability (F), absorption rate constant (k_a), volume of distribution (V_d), and elimination rate constant (k_e).

Oral administration

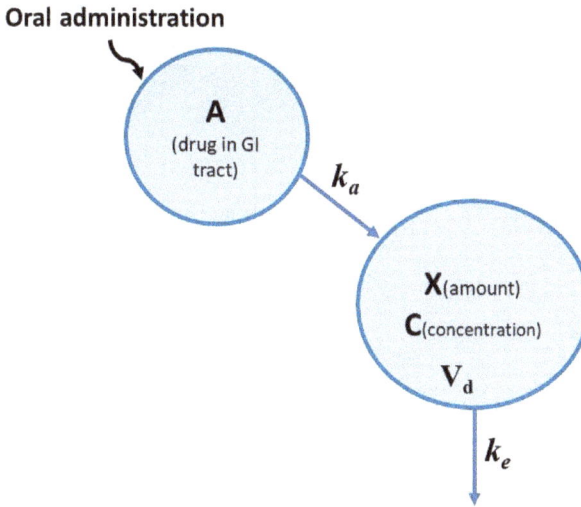

Figure 8-1. Schematic representation of a one-compartment model with first-order absorption and first-order elimination for a drug administrated via oral administration.

What does the concentration-time profile look like for a drug following oral administration? We can get some hints from Equations 8-1 and 8-2. At time 0, plasma drug concentration is 0 since all drug molecules are still in the gastrointestinal tract. The net amount of drug changing in the body per given time is determined by two rate functions, as shown in Equation 8-2: $k_a \cdot A$ and $k_e \cdot X$. $k_a \cdot A$ is a first-order term and how much the drug enters systemic circulation depends on the amount of drug in the gastrointestinal tract. Similarly, $k_e \cdot X$ is also a first-order term, and how much the drug is eliminated from the body depends on the amount of drug in the body.

At the beginning, A, the amount of drug in the gastrointestinal tract, is high, while X, the amount of drug in the body, is minimal. Accordingly, the rate function of $k_a \cdot A$ is a lot larger than $k_e \cdot X$, which means that the net amount of drug changing in the body per given time is a positive value (i.e., $k_a \cdot A - k_e \cdot X > 0$). As a result, drug concentration in the body increases over time. With more drug molecules entering the systemic circulation, A decreases and X increases as time goes by. When the amount of drug eliminated per given time (i.e., $k_e \cdot X$) is identical to the amount of drug entering per given time (i.e., $k_a \cdot A$), the maximum concentration is reached. After that time point, the elimination process dominates since there is not much drug left in the gastrointestinal tract. Accordingly, the concentration in the body decreases in the terminal phase. Based on the hints from Equations 8-1 and 8-2, for the pharmacokinetics of a drug following oral administration, we would expect a concentration-time profile like what is shown in Figure 8-2.

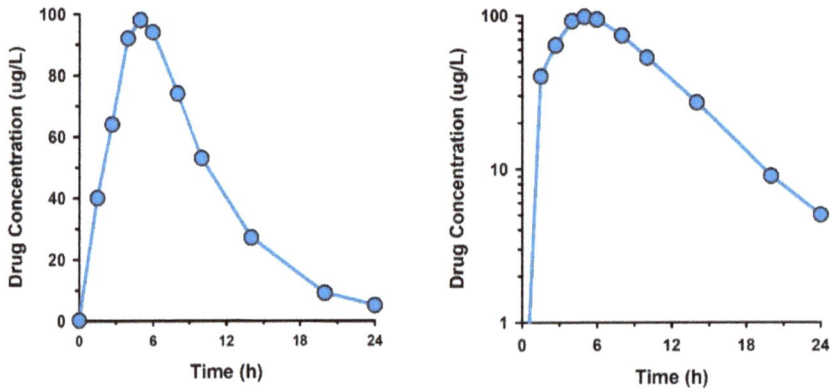

Figure 8-2. An example concentration-time profile after a drug is administered orally. (left) linear scale; (right) semi-logarithm scale.

8.2 Determination of k_a and k_e from a Plasma Concentration-Time Profile Using a Feathering Method

As shown in the Bateman equation, $C = \frac{F \cdot D \cdot k_a}{V_d \cdot (k_a - k_e)} (e^{-k_e \cdot t} - e^{-k_a \cdot t})$, there are two e terms, namely $e^{-k_e \cdot t}$ and $e^{-k_a \cdot t}$. For orally administered drugs, especially those with immediate-release dosage forms, k_a is usually greater than k_e. As a result, at later time points, $e^{-k_a \cdot t}$ approaches zero first. Therefore, in the terminal phase, Equation 8-3 is reduced to:

$$C = \frac{F \cdot D \cdot k_a}{V_d \cdot (k_a - k_e)} (e^{-k_e \cdot t} - 0) \rightarrow C = \frac{F \cdot D \cdot k_a}{V_d \cdot (k_a - k_e)} e^{-k_e \cdot t} \qquad [8\text{-}4]$$

The above equation tells us that k_e can be determined from the terminal slope based on the same equation that we have learned for I.V. bolus administration:

$$k_e = -slope = -\frac{lnC_2 - lnC_1}{t_2 - t_1} \qquad [8\text{-}5]$$

Please note that C_2 and C_1 need to be two concentrations measured at the terminal phase. If you have a concentration-time dataset of an orally administered drug on hand, pick two data points at the later time points when you calculate k_e.

If we connect two data points from the terminal phase, extend the line till it intersects the Y-axis, we will get a dashed line as shown in Figure 8-3. The equation of the dashed line is the reduced equation that I just showed above (i.e., Equation 8-4). For the concentrations on this line, let's call it C'. We will get the following equation:

$$C' = \frac{F \cdot D \cdot k_a}{V_d \cdot (k_a - k_e)} e^{-k_e \cdot t} \qquad [8\text{-}6]$$

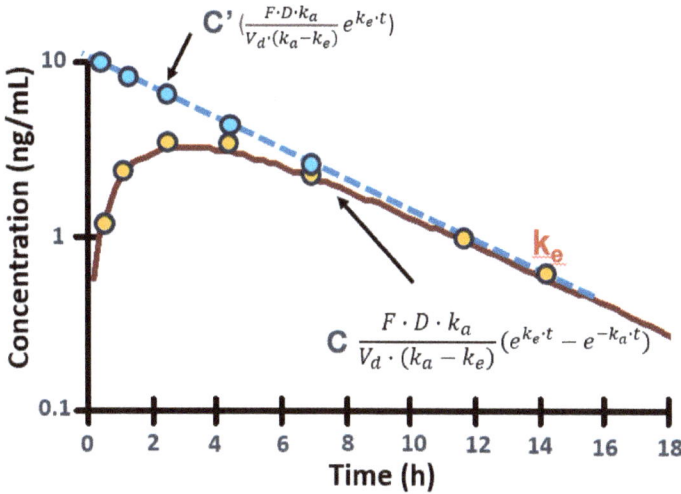

Figure 8-3. Step 1 of feathering – get the profile of C' vs time. k_e can be determined either from the slope of C' vs time profile or from the terminal slope of C vs time profile.

To make the equations easier to be examined, let

$$\text{Constant} = \frac{F \cdot D \cdot k_a}{V_d \cdot (k_a - k_e)} \qquad \text{[8-7]}$$

Based on Equations 8-3 and 8-7, the full equations of C can be expressed as:

$$C = constant \cdot (e^{-k_e \cdot t} - e^{-k_a \cdot t}) \qquad \text{[8-8]}$$

Similarly, based on Equations 8-6 and 8-7, the full equation of C' can be expressed as:

$$C' = constant \cdot e^{-k_e \cdot t} \qquad \text{[8-9]}$$

If we define C'', which is calculated as $C' - C$, we can get the following expression of C'':

$$C'' = C' - C = constant \cdot e^{-k_e \cdot t} - constant \cdot (e^{-k_e \cdot t} - e^{-k_a \cdot t})$$

$$\rightarrow C'' = constant \cdot e^{-k_a \cdot t} \qquad \text{[8-10]}$$

Equation 8-10 tells us that k_a can be determined from the slope of C'' vs time profile, as shown in the green line in Figure 8-4. If you have a concentration-time dataset of an orally administered drug on hand, the following are the steps of feathering:

1. Based on Equation 8-9, calculate C' at the same time points (i.e. blue symbols in Figure 8-4) where you have data for C.
2. After you get C' at each time point, calculate C'' (i.e., C'-C) at each time point (i.e., green symbols in Figure 8-4).

3. Calculate k_a, the negative slope of C'' vs time profile, using the following equation:

$$k_a = -slope = -\frac{\ln C_2'' - \ln C_1''}{t_2 - t_1}$$

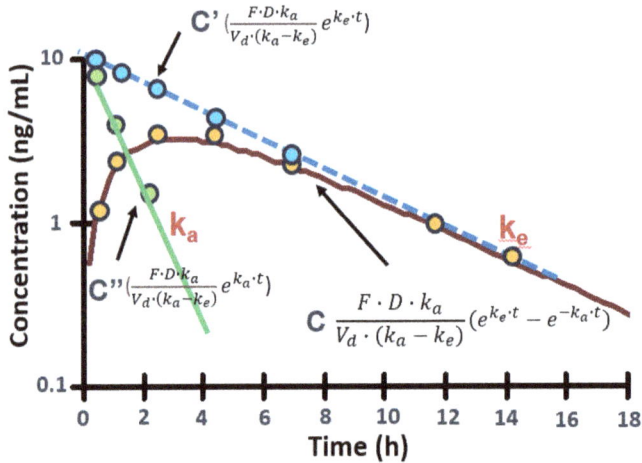

Figure 8-4. Step 2 of feathering – get the profile of C'' vs time. k_a can be determined from the slope of C'' vs time profile.

8.3 Flip-Flop Kinetics

I mentioned in section 8.2 that absorption rate constant k_a usually is much greater than the elimination rate constant k_e for immediate-release drugs. However, this is not the case for all solid dosage forms. For drugs with sustained-release dosage form, the rate of absorption can be much slower than the rate of elimination. Accordingly, k_a is smaller than k_e. This means that for sustained release drugs, $e^{-k_e \cdot t}$ approaches zero first at later time points. As a result, in the terminal phase, Equation 8-3 is reduced to:

$$C = \frac{F \cdot D \cdot k_a}{V_d \cdot (k_a - k_e)}(0 - e^{-k_a \cdot t}) \rightarrow C = \frac{F \cdot D \cdot k_a}{V_d \cdot (k_e - k_a)}e^{-k_a \cdot t} \qquad [8\text{-}11]$$

The above equation tells us that the terminal slope of the concentration-time profile of a sustained-release drug reflects k_a instead of k_e; this phenomenon is known as flip-flop kinetics.

Let's use an example to further elaborate on this. Imagine that we have three choices to administer drug A: 1) I.V. bolus injection; 2) oral administration with immediate-release dosage form; and 3) oral administration with sustained-release dosage form. If a patient tries each choice separately, and pharmacokinetics of drug A are evaluated for each case, we would expect the concentration-time profiles of drug A following different routes/dosage forms to be something like what are shown in Figure 8-5. As it shows, the terminal slopes of I.V. bolus injection and immediate-release dosage form are the same, and they reflect the true elimination rate constant k_e. On the other hand, the terminal slope of the sustained-release drug reflects the absorption rate constant k_a instead, with the real elimination rate constant being masked. When we compare the profiles between the immediate-release and sustained-release dosage forms, we can easily tell that the latter has longer T_{max} and lower C_{max} due to the slower absorption rate.

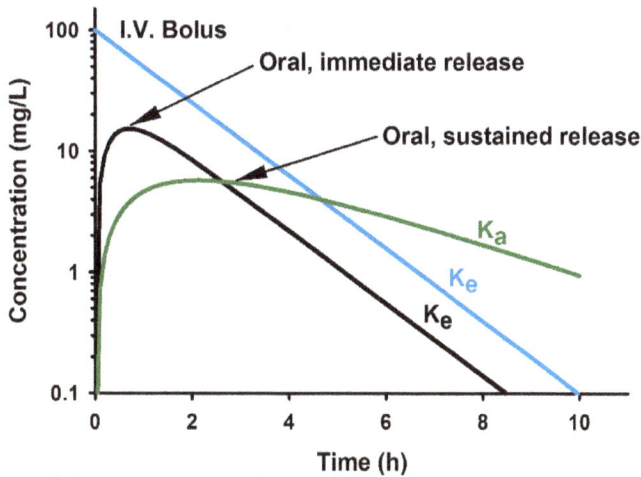

Figure 8-5. Example concentration-time profiles of a drug following I.V. bolus injection (black curve), oral immediate release dosage form (blue curve) and oral sustained release form (green curve). Same dose is given in each scenario. The terminal slope of the sustained release dosage form reflects k_a instead of k_e, a phenomenon known as flip-flop kinetics.

8.4 Impact of Change in Drug Absorption and Elimination in Concentration-Time Profile of an Orally Administered Drug

In Chapter 2, I have used several reports on food/beverage-drug interactions as examples to demonstrate that change in the extent of absorption affects AUC and C_{max}, while change in the rate of absorption affects C_{max} and T_{max}. In this section, I provide one case example below to further elaborate on the impact of changes in the rate and extent of drug absorption on the concentration-time profile of a drug following oral administration.

Case Example 8-1.

Iowa-001 is a new investigational drug with intended indication in alleviating last minute exam panic attacks. It follows the first-order kinetics, and its disposition can be described using a one-compartment model. Iowa-001 is available in two formulations: immediate release dosage form and sustained release dosage form.

Scenario 1. Decrease in the bioavailability of Iowa-001 immediate release dosage form.

Scenario 2. Increase in the absorption rate constant of Iowa-001 immediate release dosage form.

Scenario 3. Decrease in the absorption rate constant of Iowa-001 sustained release dosage form.

Please 1) evaluate the impact of each scenario on T_{max}, C_{max}, AUC, and terminal slope of Iowa-001 when it is oral administered; and 2) draw a figure for each scenario to illustrate the old and new pharmacokinetic profiles.

Please work on it yourself before looking at the answer I provide below.

~ ~ ~

Scenario 1. Bioavailability (i.e., F) of Iowa-001 decreases. The parameters that are affected by F are C_{max} and AUC. With increase in bioavailability, both C_{max} and AUC of Iowa-001 increase proportionally. T_{max} and terminal slope are not affected by the dose.

Scenario 2. k_a of Iowa-001 increases. With increase is absorption rate, more drug molecules are absorbed into systemic circulation per given time, and maximum concentration can be reached sooner. Therefore, T_{max} decreased and C_{max} increased. AUC and terminal slope are not affected by k_a.

Scenario 3. Please note that this is a sustained release form, which means that the terminal slope reflects k_a due to flip-flop kinetics. When k_a of Iowa-001 decreases, the terminal slope is shallower, T_{max} is prolonged and C_{max} decreases.

Table 8-1 is provided to facilitate the comparison between your results and the one I provided here:

Table 8-1. Impact of changes in F and k_a on Iowa-001 pharmacokinetics parameters following oral administration of an immediate release form (scenarios 1 and 2) or a sustained release form (scenario 3).

Scenario	T_{max}	C_{max}	AUC	Terminal slope
1. Decrease in F	↔	↓	↓	↔
2. Increase in k_a	↓	↑	↔	↔
3. Decrease in k_a	↑	↓	↔	↓

Figure 8-6 shows the impact of each scenario on Iowa-001 pharmacokinetics (note: solid black line is the original curve, and blue dashed line is the new curve).

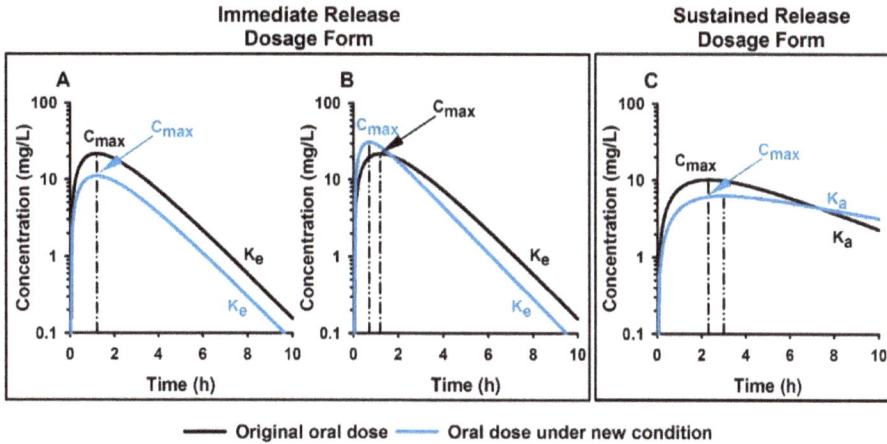

Figure 8-6. The effect of F and k_a on the pharmacokinetics of Iowa-001 following oral administration of an immediate release form (scenarios 1 and 2) or a sustained release form (scenario 3). *Solid black line represents the original condition, and blue dashed line represents the new condition.*

8.5 Equations Related to Multiple Oral Administrations

For orally administered drugs, they are often given multiple times. Therefore, it is useful to learn the equations that can be used to characterize drug pharmacokinetics following multiple oral administrations. The good news is that the principles of accumulation, steady state, and fluctuation learned in the context of multiple I.V. bolus injection and multiple short-term I.V. infusions can be applied directly to the oral dosage forms.

As we learned in section 8.1, following a single oral dose, plasma concentrations over time can be calculated based on the Bateman equation listed below:

$$C = \frac{F \cdot D \cdot k_a}{V_d \cdot (k_a - k_e)} \left(e^{-k_e \cdot t} - e^{-k_a \cdot t} \right)$$

Following multiple oral doses, the steady state concentration can be calculated by below equation, with each exponential function being multiplied by its own accumulation ratio:

$$C_{ss} = \frac{F \cdot D \cdot k_a}{V_d \cdot (k_a - k_e)} \left(\frac{e^{-k_e \cdot t}}{1 - e^{-k_e \cdot \tau}} - \frac{e^{-k_a \cdot t}}{1 - e^{-k_a \cdot \tau}} \right) \qquad [8\text{-}12]$$

Following a single oral dose, the AUC, which is the area under the concentration-time curve from time 0 to time infinity, can be calculated as:

$$AUC_\infty = \frac{Dose \cdot F}{CL} \tag{8-13}$$

Following multiple oral doses, the AUC within each dosing interval at the steady state is calculated as:

$$AUC_{ss} = \frac{Dose \cdot F}{CL} \tag{8-14}$$

Therefore, similar to what we have learned in Chapter 6, the $AUC_{\tau,ss}$ of a drug following multiple oral dose regimens equals to the AUC_∞ of the same drug following a single oral dose. Please review Chapter 6, section 6.2.5 for more detailed information regarding how AUC is calculated.

The average concentration of an orally administered drug during the steady state is:

$$C_{ave,ss} = \frac{Dose \cdot F}{CL \cdot \tau} \tag{8-15}$$

$C_{ave,ss}$ is independent of k_a. While ka does not impact the average steady state concentration, it affects the fluctuation as shown in Figure 8-7. In general, the slower the absorption (i.e., the smaller the k_a), the less the fluctuation. Based on this information, you may recognize the advantage of sustained-release drug as it has smaller k_a compared to immediate-release drug and accordingly has less fluctuation in concentrations at steady state.

8.6 Case Study

In this section, I provide one case example for you to practice calculating drug concentrations at different time points for an orally administered drug.

Case Example 8-2.

500 mg of Drug A was given through I.V. bolus and the half-life and AUC_{inf} were found to be 8 h and 50 mg.hr/L, respectively. When drug A was given orally with the dose of 100 mg, its half-life and AUC_{inf} were found to be 20 h and 8 mg.hr/L, respectively. What is the concentration of Drug A 6 h and 24 h after oral dose administration (dose is 100 mg)?

Please work on it yourself before looking at the answer I provided below.

~ ~ ~

The equation needed to estimate Drug A concentrations at different time points, including 6 h and 24 h post dose, is the Bateman equation:

$$C = \frac{F \cdot D \cdot k_a}{V_d \cdot (k_a - k_e)} (e^{-k_e \cdot t} - e^{-k_a \cdot t})$$

To calculate C_{6h} and C_{24h}, we need to obtain the values of the following parameters: F, k_a, V_d, and k_e.

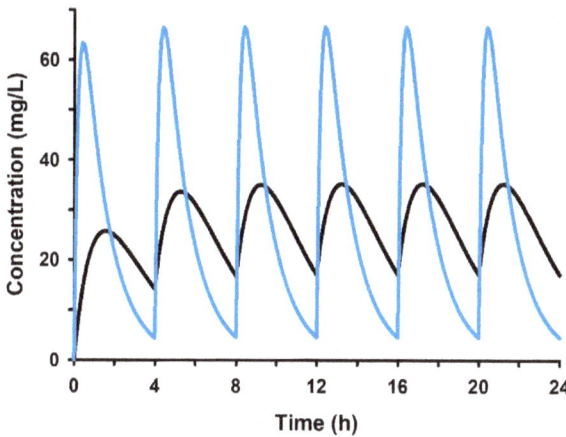

Figure 8-7. The effect of k_a on fluctuation of the concentration-time profile of a drug following multiple oral doses.

As we have learned in Chapter 2, F can be calculated using the following formula:

$$F = \frac{AUC_{oral} \times Dose_{iv}}{AUC_{iv} \times Dose_{oral}} = \frac{8 \times 500}{50 \times 100} = 0.8$$

Based on the information, the half-life of Drug A administered via oral route is much longer than the one obtained after I.V. administration (20 h vs 8 h). This indicates that Drug A has flip-flop kinetics following oral administration, which means that its terminal slope reflects k_a, instead of k_e. Therefore, ke can be calculated based on the half-life of Drug A when it was given via I.V. route, and ka can be estimated using the half-life of Drug A following oral administration.

$$k_e = \frac{0.693}{8} = 0.0866 \ h^{-1}$$

$$k_a = \frac{0.693}{20} = 0.0347 \ h^{-1}$$

CL can be calculated based on the dose and AUC information obtained following I.V. administration:

$$CL = \frac{Dose}{AUC} = \frac{500}{50} = 10 \ ^L/_h$$

With k_e and CL on hand, we can calculate V_d:

$$V_d = \frac{CL}{k_e} = \frac{10}{0.0866} = 115 \ L$$

Now we can calculate C_{6h} and C_{24h} using the Bateman equation:

$$C_{6h} = \frac{0.8 \cdot 100 \cdot 0.0347}{115 \cdot (0.0347 - 0.0866)} (e^{-0.0866 \cdot 6} - e^{-0.0347 \cdot 6}) = 0.101 \; mg/L$$

$$C_{24h} = \frac{0.8 \cdot 100 \cdot 0.0347}{115 \cdot (0.0347 - 0.0866)} (e^{-0.0866 \cdot 24} - e^{-0.0347 \cdot 24}) = 0.144 \; mg/L$$

Chapter 9.
Two-Compartment Model

Learning Objectives

After reading this chapter, the reader shall be able to:

1. Understand the concentration-time profile of a drug following biexponential decline.

2. Use feathering to determine slopes related to α phase and β phase, as well as intercepts A and B for a drug demonstrating biexponential decline following a single I.V. bolus injection.

3. Understand the relationship between macro and micro rate constants.

4. Understand the difference among initial volume of distribution (V_c), volume of distribution at the steady state (V_{ss}), and volume of distribution at the elimination phase (V_β).

5. Understand the physiological basis for the two-compartment model and apply the knowledge in clinical practice by choosing appropriate sampling times for half-life determination, making right decision in loading dose calculation, and linking drug exposure to drug effect appropriately.

So far, we have been focusing on the one-compartment model, in which our body is viewed as a single and uniform compartment and the drug distributes instantaneously to all body areas once it gets in the body. As noted in Chapter 1, the assumption of immediate distribution works well for many drugs, but not for all. For some drugs, after entering systemic circulation, they first reach highly perfused organs (e.g., heart, lung, liver, kidneys), then distribute to poorly perfused organs (e.g., fat, skin, bone) at a slower rate. To characterize this distribution pattern, a *two-compartment model* is needed, which is the topic of this chapter.

In section 9.1, I will walk you through the equations used to characterize the concentration-time profile of a drug using a two-compartment model, and I will explain why the concentration-time profile displays a biexponential decline. The parameters related to the distribution phase and elimination phase, as well as the relationship between macro and micro rate constants will be covered in section 9.2. When characterizing drug pharmacokinetics using a two-compartment model, it is useful to determine two rate constants: α, the hybrid rate constant for distribution, and β, the hybrid rate constant for elimination. We will learn "feathering", a method to determine α and β, in section 9.3. In a two-compartment model, the values of the volume of distribution determined at different times differ. I will explain the difference among three volume of distribution terms, namely initial volume of distribution (V_c), volume of distribution at the steady state (V_{ss}), and volume of distribution at the elimination phase (V_β), in section 9.4. Understanding the physiological basis for the two-compartment model is important as it will help us to choose appropriate sampling times for half-life determination, make right decision in loading dose calculation, and link drug exposure to drug effect appropriately; we will learn these clinical applications of the two-compartment model in section 9.5. Then this chapter ends with a case example based on a real story (section 9.6).

9.1 Pharmacokinetic Equations Related to a Two-Compartment Model and the Corresponding Concentration-Time Profile

For drugs that have rapid distribution to some tissues and slower distribution to the other tissues in the body, their pharmacokinetics can be characterized using a two-compartment model, which consists of a *central compartment* representing plasma and highly perfused organs and a *peripheral compartment* representing poorly perfused organs. Once the drug enters bloodstream, both the distribution and elimination processes start. Drug distribution between the central and the peripheral compartments is a two-way traffic – the drug can be transferred from the central to the peripheral compartments, and vice versa. Drug elimination occurs in the central compartment since both liver and kidney are highly perfused organs and belong to the central compartment. Distribution is a first-order process. Most drugs are eliminated via first-order kinetics. Therefore, for a drug characterized by a two-compartment model, its pharmacokinetics is determined by *first-order distribution* and *first-order elimination*.

Figure 9-1 shows the two-compartment model diagram of a drug following an I.V. bolus injection. Based on this model, the rate of change of the drug in the central compartment (dX_1/dt) and the rate of change of the drug in the peripheral compartment (dX_2/dt) are described as:

$$\frac{dX_1}{dt} = -k_{12} \cdot X_1 + k_{21} \cdot X_2 - k_e \cdot X_1 \qquad [9\text{-}1]$$
$$X_1(0) = Dose$$

$$\frac{dX_2}{dt} = k_{12} \cdot X_1 - k_{21} \cdot X_2 \qquad [9\text{-}2]$$
$$X_2(0) = 0$$

Where:

X_1= drug amount in the central compartment;

X_2= drug amount in the peripheral compartment;

k_{12} = rate constant from the central to the peripheral compartment (unit is time^{-1});

k_{21} = rate constant from the peripheral to the central compartment (unit is time^{-1});

k_e = elimination rate constant (unit is time^{-1});

$X_1(0)$ = initial amount of drug in the central compartment, which is dose;

$X_2(0)$ = initial amount of drug in the peripheral compartment, which is 0 since the drug is still in the central compartment.

In addition, as shown in Figure 9-1, volumes of distribution of the drug in the central and peripheral compartments are denoted as V_1 and V_2, respectively. The drug concentrations in the central and peripheral compartments are denoted as C_p and C_t, respectively, and they are calculated as:

$$C_p = \frac{X_1}{V_1}$$ [9-3]

$$C_t = \frac{X_2}{V_2}$$ [9-4]

I.V. bolus injection

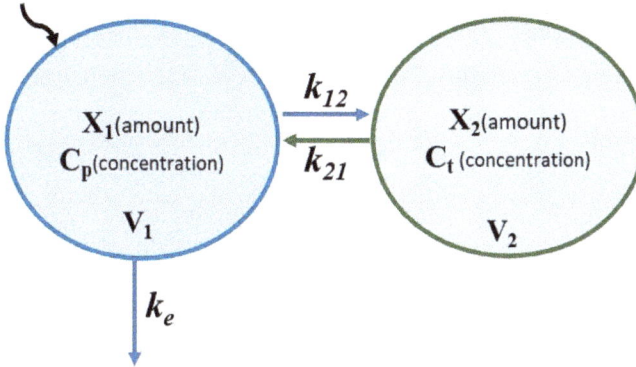

Figure 9-1. Schematic representation of a two-compartment model for a drug administrated via I.V. bolus injection.

The above equations can be integrated and solved to get the explicit equation for drug concentration in the central compartment (i.e., C_p), which is our primary interest. As the equation is long, the equation for C_p is often represented using a simplified form:

$$C_p = A \bullet e^{-\alpha \bullet t} + B \bullet e^{-\beta \bullet t}$$ [9-5]

Where:

α = hybrid rate constant for distribution.

β = hybrid rate constant for elimination.

A = intercept of the first exponential function.

B = intercept of the second exponential function.

For drugs that need to be characterized using a two-compartment model, their pharmacokinetics following an I.V. bolus dose typically look like what is presented in Figure 9-2. The hallmark is a biphasic curve when concentrations are presented on the logarithmic scale (i.e., biexponential decline). This is fundamentally different from drugs characterized by a one-compartment model, where a straight line is observed when concentrations are presented on the logarithmic scale (i.e., mono-exponential decline).

The biexponential decline in drug concentrations is the result of intertwined processes of drug distribution and elimination. Initially, upon I.V. bolus injection, all the drug is in systemic circulation, entering the central compartment. On the other hand, there is no drug in the peripheral compartment at time 0. Due to the concentration gradient, there is a driving force to move drug molecules from the central to the peripheral compartment. Meanwhile, drug molecules in the central compartment start to be eliminated by eliminating organs (i.e., the liver and/or kidney). Therefore, drug plasma concentrations decrease rapidly because there are two processes, occurring at the same time, to move drug molecules out of the central compartment. That's why we see a steep decline in the concentration-time profile at the beginning (Figure 9-2). This phase of rapid decline is called *α phase*.

With decrease in drug concentration in the central compartment and increase in drug concentration in the peripheral compartment, the difference in drug levels between these two compartments gets smaller and smaller. At a certain point, the free drug levels in these two compartments are equal. Beyond this point, drug concentration in the central compartment falls below that in the peripheral compartment because drug continues to be eliminated from the central compartment. As a result, the drug molecules in the peripheral compartment start to be redistributed back to the central compartment. At this stage, drug plasma concentrations decrease slower because some drug molecules return to the central compartment while others continue to be eliminated from it. That's why we see a shallower decline of the concentration-time profile at the later time points (Figure 9-2). This phase of slower decline is called *β phase*. During the β phase, the drug concentration in the peripheral compartment is always higher than in plasma, although they run in parallel. Drug is drained by elimination from the central compartment.

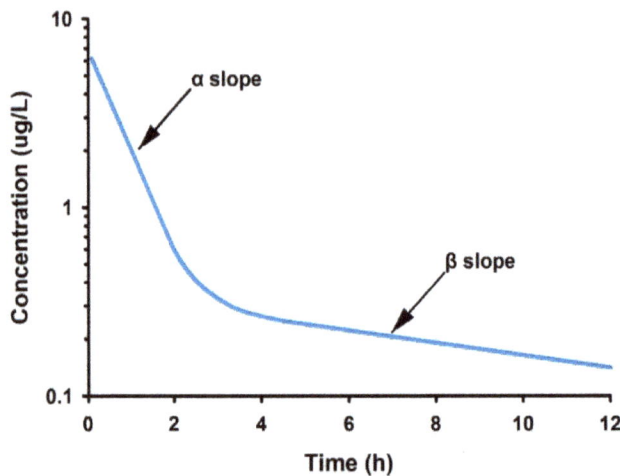

Figure 9-2. Example concentration time profile of a drug administrated via I.V. bolus injection with biexponential decline.

9.2 Key Parameters and Relationship between Macro and Micro Rate Constants

Equation 9-5 (i.e., $C_p = A \cdot e^{-\alpha \cdot t} + B \cdot e^{-\beta \cdot t}$) contains two exponential terms. $A \cdot e^{-\alpha \cdot t}$ describes the characteristics of the plasma concentration-time profile during the distribution phase, while $B \cdot e^{-\beta \cdot t}$ capture the kinetics of the drug during the elimination phase. The half-life determined during the α phase is referred to as the *distribution half-life ($t_{1/2,\alpha}$)*:

$$t_{1/2,\alpha} = \frac{0.693}{\alpha} \qquad\qquad [9\text{-}6]$$

On the other hand, the half-life determined during the β phase is known as the *elimination half-life ($t_{1/2,\beta}$)*:

$$t_{1/2,\beta} = \frac{0.693}{\beta} \qquad\qquad [9\text{-}7]$$

As noted earlier, both distribution and elimination are first-order processes. Therefore, it takes one $t_{1/2,\alpha}$ to finish 50% of the distribution process, and it takes 5 $t_{1/2,\alpha}$ for the distribution phase to complete. Similarly, it takes one $t_{1/2,\beta}$ to eliminate 50% of the dose, and it takes 5 $t_{1/2,\beta}$ eliminate almost all the drug from the body.

Equation 9-5 contains 4 terms, namely α, β, A, and B. α and β are hybrid rate constants, and they are considered as *macro rate constants* because they are complex functions of the first-order *micro rate constants* k_e, k_{12} and k_{21}. A and B are intercepts, and they are dependent on the dose and the pharmacokinetics parameters of a drug. Followings are the relationship between macro and micro rate constants:

$$\alpha + \beta = k_{12} + k_{21} + k_e \qquad\qquad [9\text{-}8]$$

$$\alpha \bullet \beta = k_{21} \bullet k_e \qquad\qquad [9\text{-}9]$$

$$A = \frac{D_{iv} \bullet (\alpha - k_{21})}{V_1 \bullet (\alpha - \beta)} \qquad\qquad [9\text{-}10]$$

$$B = \frac{D_{iv} \bullet (k_{21} - \beta)}{V_1 \bullet (\alpha - \beta)} \qquad\qquad [9\text{-}11]$$

Where D_{iv} is the intravenous dose.

$$k_{21} = \frac{A \bullet \beta + B \bullet \alpha}{A + B} \qquad\qquad [9\text{-}12]$$

$$k_e = \frac{\alpha \bullet \beta}{k_{21}}$$ [9-13]

$$k_{12} = \alpha + \beta - k_{10} - k_{21}$$ [9-14]

9.3 Determination of α, β, A, and B from a Plasma Concentration-Time Profile Using a Feathering Method

For a drug whose concentration-time profile is similar to Figure 9-2, it is useful to find a way to determine the values of α, β, A, and B so that we can use Equation 9-5 to predict concentrations at different time points. Although nowadays several commercial software options are available for parameter determination, it is still valuable to use simple curve stripping, also called feathering, to determine α, β, A, and B, without the need of software. If you have a concentration-time dataset on hand, all you need is a calculator. Following is the procedure for feathering (or curve stripping):

- Step 1. Choose two data points at the terminal phase of C_p vs time profile, calculate β using the following equation:

$$\beta = - slope = - \frac{lnC_2 - lnC_1}{t_2 - t_1}$$ [9-15]

- Step 2. If we connect these two data points, extend the line till it hits the Y-axis, we will get a green dashed line as shown in Figure 9-3, which can be expressed as:

$$C' = B \cdot e^{-\beta \bullet t}$$ [9-16]

  Since β is calculated from the previous step, we can plug in any of these two data points in Equation 9-16 to get the intercept B.

- Step 3. Now we get the values of B and β. Based on Equation 9-16, calculate the value of C' at 2-3 early time points (note: need to be the same time points as the C vs time curve) represented by the green circles in Figure 9-3.

- Step 4. If we define C'', which is calculated as $C - C'$, we can get the values of C'' at the same two to three time points, and get the following expression of C'':

$$C'' = C - C' = A \cdot e^{-\alpha \cdot t} + B \cdot e^{-\beta \cdot t} - B \cdot e^{-\beta \cdot t} \rightarrow C'' = A \cdot e^{-\alpha \cdot t}$$ [9-17]

- Step 5. Based on the calculated C'' at two to three time points (orange triangles in Figure 9-3), determine α using the following equation:

$$\alpha = -\ slope = -\ \frac{lnC_2 - lnC_1}{t_2 - t_1} \qquad [9\text{-}18]$$

- Step 6. Since α is calculated from the previous step, we can plug in any of two data points calculated in Step 4 to get the intercept A.

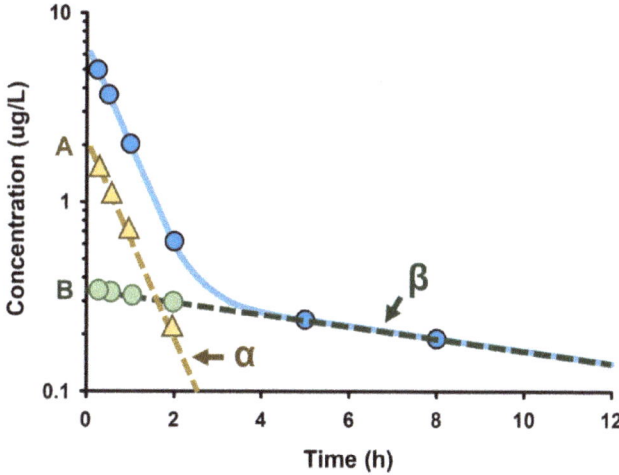

Figure 9-3. Determination of α, β, A, and B from a plasma concentration-time profile using a feathering method.

9.4 Different Terms of Volume of Distribution

As shown in Figure 9-1, a two-compartment model involves two volume terms, namely V_1 and V_2. You may wonder how these volumes are related to the volume of distribution. If you recall, volume of distribution, V_d, is calculated as the amount of drug *in the body* at any time over the concentration of drug *in the plasma* at that time. For a two-compartment model, the general equation for V_d calculation is:

$$V_d = \frac{Amount\ of\ drug\ in\ the\ body}{Plasma\ concentration} \quad \rightarrow \quad V_d = \frac{X_1 + X_2}{C_p}$$

$$\rightarrow V_d = \frac{C_p \bullet V_1 + C_t \bullet V_2}{C_p} \qquad [9\text{-}19]$$

In a two-compartment model, V_d determined at different times differs, with three different terms, namely initial volume of distribution (V_c), volume of distribution at the steady state (V_{ss}), and volume of distribution at the elimination phase (V_β). The relationship between these volume of distribution terms and V_1 and V_2 is elaborated in the subsections below.

9.4.1. Initial volume of distribution (V_c)

As its name indicates, the initial volume of distribution V_c represents the volume of distribution determined immediately after I.V. bolus administration of a drug (i.e., at time 0). At this time, the entire dose is in the central compartment (i.e., $X_1 = dose$), which means that the concentration in the peripheral compartment (i.e., C_t) is 0. Based on Equation 9-19, V_c is calculated as:

$$V_c = \frac{C_p \cdot V_1 + C_t \cdot V_2}{C_p} = \frac{C_p \cdot V_1 + 0 \cdot V_2}{C_p} = \frac{C_p \cdot V_1}{C_p}$$

$$\rightarrow V_c = V_1 \qquad\qquad [9\text{-}20]$$

Therefore, the initial volume of distribution reflects the volume of the central compartment. V_c may be determined:

$$V_c = \frac{Dose}{C_0} = \frac{Dose}{A + B} \qquad\qquad [9\text{-}21]$$

Please note that the dose needs to be an I.V. bolus dose. Equation 9-21 does not apply to the oral dose.

9.4.2. Volume of distribution at the steady state (V_{ss})

As its name indicates, V_{ss} represents the volume of distribution determined at the steady state. At the steady state, $C_t = C_p$ since there is no concentration gradient at that moment. Therefore, V_{ss} is calculated as:

$$V_{ss} = \frac{C_p \cdot V_1 + C_t \cdot V_2}{C_p} = \frac{C_p \cdot V_1 + C_p \cdot V_2}{C_p} \quad \rightarrow \quad V_{ss} = V_1 + V_2 \qquad [9\text{-}22]$$

9.4.3. Volume of distribution at the elimination phase (V_β)

V_β represents the volume of distribution determined in β phase, also known as elimination phase or terminal phase. In β phase, the drug concentration in the peripheral compartment is higher than that in the central compartment, which means that $C_p < C_t$. Based on this relationship, we can have a good guess that $V_\beta > V_1 + V_2$. V_β is usually calculated using the following equation:

$$V_\beta = \frac{Dose}{\beta \cdot AUC} \qquad\qquad [9\text{-}23]$$

Therefore, based on the above information, we can conclude that $V_c < V_{ss} < V_\beta$.

9.5 Clinical Applications of the Two-Compartment Model

As noted in Chapter 1 (sections 1.7 and 1.8), drug concentrations measured with a rich sampling schedule in humans mainly occur in two scenarios: 1) when a drug is still in the development phase; the pharmacokinetics of the drug needs to be thoroughly evaluated prior to its approval; 2) in a research study where there is a need to rigorously evaluate the pharmacokinetics of the drug to address a specific research question.

However, in clinical practice, we rarely see pharmacokinetic samples being collected at a rich sampling schedule. What we commonly see is that plasma concentrations are measured only at 2-3 time points. That's all the pharmacokinetics data we have on hand to make dosing decisions. What does that mean? It means that we won't see the distribution phase of a drug even if it has one. That's also why the one-compartment model is extensively discussed in this book because it is the most frequently used model in clinical practice.

If you are a PharmD student (or a clinical pharmacist already), you may feel that there is no strong rationale for you to learn the two-compartment model since you rarely encounter it in clinical practice anyway. Actually, this is not true. While you may not need to spend time studying all equations mentioned in this chapter, it is important to understand the concept of the two-compartment model. In this section, I share several important clinical applications of the two-compartment model.

9.5.1 Estimation of the elimination half-life in the post-distribution phase.

For many drugs, the time needed to distribute the drug from systemic circulation to the rest of body is very short (in minutes). This situation indicates that the concentration-time profiles of these drugs can be handled using a one compartment model since the distribution phase (i.e., α phase) is short. However, do not make the mistake of taking blood samples for therapeutic drug monitoring (TDM) during the α phase. In clinical practice, to perform TDM, usually a drug's half-life in an individual patient is determined from only two blood samples. If one or both samples is/are collected during the α phase, the calculated slope, which is supposed to indicate the elimination rate constant, will be steeper than the one from the real elimination phase. As a result, the half-life determined is shorter than the real elimination half-life $t_{1/2,\beta}$. Accordingly, if we make dosing decision based on the calculated half-life, we may recommend a higher dose or more frequent dosing interval, which may increase the risk of side effects of the drug.

To avoid the underprediction of a drug's half-life, we need to wait till the α phase is over to draw the first blood sample. How long would it take for the distribution phase to be done? As mentioned in section 9.2, it takes 5 $t_{1/2,\alpha}$ for the distribution phase to complete. With this information in mind, we can decide what the appropriate time is to collect samples. For example, for a drug that have a $t_{1/2,\alpha}$ of 5-6 minutes (e.g. aminoglycosides), wait at least 30 minutes to draw the first sample.

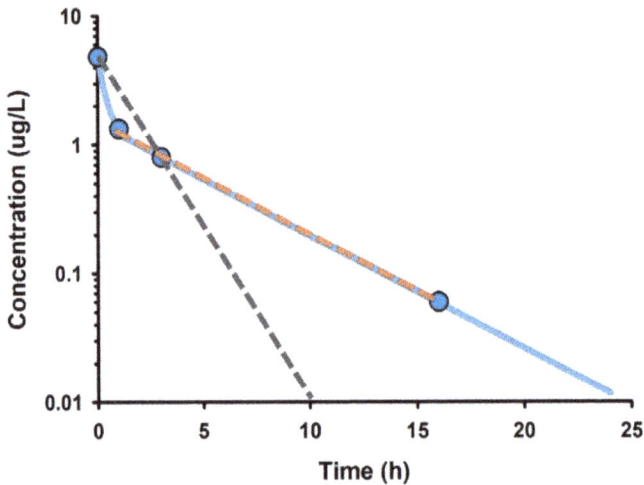

Figure 9-4. Data points used to determine the elimination half-life. Inaccurate estimation of half-life happens when plasma samples in the distribution phase are used to determine $t_{1/2,\beta}$.

9.5.2 Evaluation of a dose based on the compartment containing the site of action.

9.5.2.1 Site of action is in the central compartment.

I would like to use a case example to elaborate how to evaluate a dose when the site of action is in the central compartment.

Case Example 9-1.

This case study is adapted from *Journal of Clinical Pharmacology 2016, 56(10): 1180-1195*. Credit goes to the original authors of that paper - David J. Greenblatt, MD, and Paul N. Abourjaily, PharmD.

"A fourth-year dental student is doing a clerkship in a dental surgeon's practice. A healthy 34-year-old woman scheduled to undergo procedures estimated to last approximately 2 h. Following instillation of local anesthesia, the patient is still extremely agitated and fearful. The surgeon administers an I.V. bolus dose of 0.5 mg/kg of propofol. The patient becomes calm, relaxed, and falls into a light sleep. The surgical procedure is initiated and proceeds without incident for about 45 min. At this time, the patient becomes alert, and again is fearful and agitated. The surgeon administers another 0.5 mg/kg of propofol intravenously, the patient again becomes calm, and the surgical procedure proceeds to completion without incident.

The student is confused. He/she asks the surgeon, "Why did the patient wake up after only 45 min? The half-life of propofol usually is at least 8 h."."

I encourage you to think about this case study and propose a response yourself before looking at the answer provided below.

~ ~ ~

Propofol is a small lipophilic psychotropic drug, and its site of action is in the brain, a highly perfused organ. Following an I.V. bolus injection of propofol, it enters the brain rapidly; that's why the onset of action is fast. However, the pharmacodynamic effect won't last long because once propofol is distributed to organs belonging to the peripheral compartment, such as adipose, it can accumulate there. Adipose tissue creates a large reservoir for accumulated propofol, and the drug is slowly redistributed from the peripheral compartment to the central compartment, eventually being eliminated. Therefore, for propofol, its duration of the pharmacodynamic effect is dependent more on duration of the distribution phase rather than the elimination phase. The pharmacokinetics of propofol can be described by a two-compartment model or even a three-compartment model. Although propofol has not been eliminated from the body, its distribution from systemic circulation into peripheral tissue results in lower concentrations in plasma and brain. As a result, the patient becomes more alert, and a second dose is required.

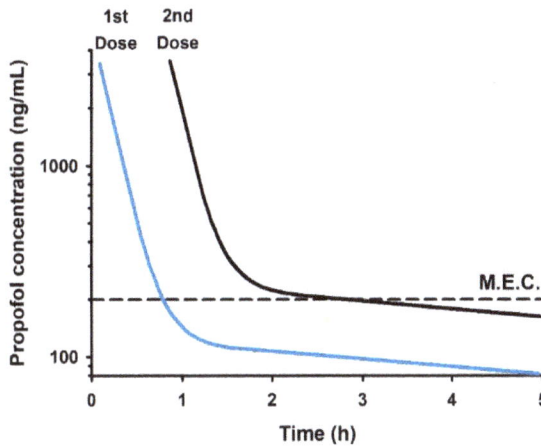

Figure 9-5. Anticipated plasma concentration-time profiles of propofol. A 0.5 mg/kg intravenous dose of propofol is initially given at time 0. The plasma propofol concentrations rapidly fall below the hypothetical minimum effective concentration (MEC) of 200 ng/mL at 0.75 hours, at which time the patient emerges from the sedated condition. An additional 0.5 mg/kg dose of propofol is required at the 0.75-hour time to maintain plasma concentrations above the MEC and maintain the patient in a sedated condition for the remainder of the procedure. This figure is adapted from *Greenblatt DJ & Abourjaily PN. Journal of Clinical Pharmacology 2016, 56(10): 1180-1195.*

9.5.2.2 Site of action is in the peripheral compartment.

I would like to use a case example to elaborate how to evaluate a dose when the site of action is in the peripheral compartment.

Case Example 9-2.

This case study is adapted from *Basic Pharmacokinetics and Pharmacodynamics (2017) Second edition, John Wiley & Sons*. Credit goes to the original author Sara E Rosenbaum, PhD.

"Patient NY has congestive heart failure and has been taking digoxin 250 µg for several years. On a routine visit to the community health center, she discusses her medication with her health team. She says she finds it easy to remember to take digoxin as it is a once-daily regimen, and she always takes it with her breakfast at 8:00 AM. Her physician would like to maintain her plasma digoxin in the range of 0.5- 1.5 µg/L. A blood sample is taken just before she leaves at 9:30 AM. The following day, the result comes back form the laboratory and reveal a plasma level of 2.6 µg/L. Is this patient at risk for digoxin toxicity?"

I encourage you to think about this case study and propose a response yourself before looking at the answer provided below.

~ ~ ~

In the two-compartment model, the highly perfused organs (i.e., tissues in the central compartment) are always in equilibrium with the plasma. However, this is not the situation for the poorly perfused organs (i.e., tissues in the peripheral compartment). At the beginning, plasma concentration is highest at time 0 following an I.V. bolus dose, and drug concentration in the peripheral compartment is 0. During the α phase, drug concentration in the peripheral compartment increases and approaches equilibrium with the plasma at the end of distribution phase. This means that if a drug's site of action is in the peripheral compartment, the plasma concentration will mirror the concentration at the site of action only during the post-distribution phase (i.e., after β phase begins).

Digoxin's site of action and toxicity is in the peripheral compartment. Different from aminoglycosides whose distribution phase is very short, digoxin has an exceptionally long distribution phase, with an α phase of over 4 h for an I.V. dose and over 6 h for an oral dose. To ensure that the plasma levels monitored reflect the concentration at the site of action, it is important to collect samples at least 6 h after an I.V. dose and 8 h after an oral dose. Patient NY's plasma level of 2.6 µg/L is obtained from a sample collected at 1.5 h post dose, which is still in the distribution phase. The plasma level of 2.6 µg/L overpredicts digoxin exposure at the site of action. Therefore, this patient has minimal risk of digoxin toxicity.

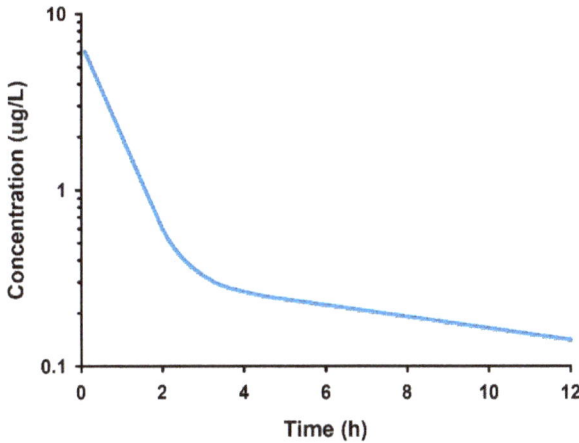

Figure 9-6. The concentration-time profile of digoxin follows a clear biphasic decline on a semi-log plot. The α phase of digoxin last about 4-6 h.

9.6 Case Study

This case study is based on a real story that happened in August 2023. A former Mayo Clinic doctor poisoned his wife, who was a pharmacist, using liquid colchicine. If you google "mayo physician poisons wife", you can easily find the news yourself and learn the whole story.

Case Example 9-3.

Let's call this former Mayo Clinic doctor CB, and his wife BB. CB and BB were having marital problems and were talking about a divorce. On the night of August 15, 2023, BB texted a friend that she was drinking at home with CB and, upon falling ill, thought the cause was something mixed into a large smoothie she had been given. She was admitted to the hospital on August 16 with severe gastrointestinal distress and dehydration. The standard treatment for food poisoning did not work and she rapidly deteriorated with multi-organ dysfunction. BB died on August 20, 2023. The toxicology report revealed a high colchicine concentration (29 ng/mL) in her blood from a sample drawn on August 16, the day she was admitted to the hospital and a day after drinking the suspicious smoothie.

All information in this case study is based on the real story, including the result of the toxicology report.

Imagine that an expert team is assembled to investigate this case. You are invited to join the team as a pharmacokinetics expert. You are asked to:

- provide the rest of the team with key background information of colchicine;
- estimate the initial colchicine concentration as well as the dose of colchicine based on the concentration of 29 ng/mL measured approximately 24 h after BB took it via smoothie. You were provided a concentration-time profile of colchicine following a 0.5 mg oral dose (see Figure 9-7). Assuming that the oral absorption of colchicine is so fast that you can use I.V. model to capture its pharmacokinetics.

Please work on this case example yourself before reading my response provided below.

Colchicine 0.5 mg oral dose

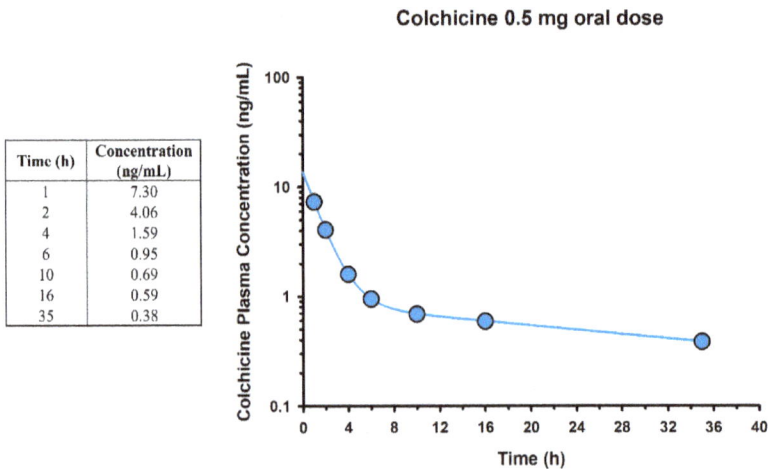

Time (h)	Concentration (ng/mL)
1	7.30
2	4.06
4	1.59
6	0.95
10	0.69
16	0.59
35	0.38

Figure 9-7. The concentration-time profile of colchicine in a subject following an oral dose of 0.5 mg colchicine. *This profile was simulated based on the data from a real study published by Ferron GM et al. Journal of Clinical Pharmacology 1996;36:874-883.*

~

Colchicine is a centuries-old treatment for gout, an inflammatory arthritis that causes pain in joints. Colchicine binds to the protein tubulin in cells, preventing the generation of microtubules. Colchicine has a narrow therapeutic index and is usually given 0.5 mg daily. With sufficiently high dose, the drug can demolish microtubular function and halt cell division, leading to multi-organ failure. While the lethal dose is suggested to be ≥0.8 mg/kg, there is a report showing that two patients died after ingestion of approximately 12 mg colchicine (i.e. about 0.2 mg/kg for a 60-kg patient). Therefore, there is no clear separation between nontoxic, toxic, and lethal dosages of colchicine.

The clinical presentation of acute colchicine toxicity can be divided into three stages:

- 1st *stage: Early stage develops within a day - gastrointestinal symptoms, including nausea, vomiting, diarrhea, abdominal pain. Autopsy may show profound mucosal damage.*
- 2nd *stage: Intermediate stage usually develops 1-3 days after colchicine ingestion – multi-organ dysfunction, including pulmonary, neurologic, renal, hematologic, and cardiovascular problems.*
- 3rd *stage: Recovery stage which can last from 7- 21 days.*

BB's symptoms were in close agreement with the first two stages of acute colchicine toxicity. Unfortunately, BB did not make it to the third stage. She died 5 days after she was poisoned.

To estimate the initial colchicine concentration as well as the amount of colchicine that BB ingested, we need to learn more about the pharmacokinetics of colchicine. As shown in Figure 9-7, the colchicine concentration-time profile on a semi-logarithm scale is biphasic, indicating that a two-compartment model is required to characterize its pharmacokinetics.

Based on the dataset shown in Figure 9-7, we can pick the last two data points to calculate β:

$$\beta = -slope = -\frac{lnC_2-lnC_1}{t_2-t_1} = \frac{ln0.38-ln0.59}{35-16} = 0.0232\ h^{-1}$$

Based on Equation 9-16, we can plug in one of the data points and the value of β that we just calculated:

$$C' = B \cdot e^{-\beta \cdot t} \rightarrow 0.59 = B \cdot e^{-0.0232 \cdot 16} \rightarrow B=0.855\ ng/mL$$

Therefore, following a dose of 0.5 mg, the concentration at 24 h post dose, namely C_{24h} is:

$$C_{24h} = 0.855 \cdot e^{-0.0232 \cdot 24} = 0.49\ ng/mL$$

Following a dose of 0.5 mg, the concentration of colchicine 24 h post dose is 0.49 ng/mL. The colchicine concentration in BB's blood 24 h post dose is 29 ng/mL. Assuming colchicine has linear pharmacokinetics, the amount of colchicine that BB ingested was:

$$Amount\ of\ colchicine\ that\ BB\ took = \frac{29\frac{ng}{mL} \cdot 0.5\ mg}{0.49\frac{ng}{ml}} = 29.6\ mg$$

Therefore, the amount of colchicine that BB ingested via the smoothie is estimated to be 29.6 mg, which was 59-fold higher than the recommended daily dose (i.e., 0.5 mg).

To calculate the initial concentration, we need to get both A and B since $C_0=A+B$. We got the value of B earlier, which is 0.855 ng/mL for the 0.5 mg dose. To calculate A, based on the curve stripping method that we learned in section 9.3, we need to first calculate C' at two early time points:

$$C'_{1h} = 0.855 \cdot e^{-0.0232 \cdot 1} = 0.836\ ng/mL$$
$$C'_{2h} = 0.855 \cdot e^{-0.0232 \cdot 2} = 0.816\ ng/mL$$

With the information of C_{1h} and C_{2h} in the dataset, and C'_{1h} and C'_{2h} that we just calculated, we can calculate C''_{1h} and C''_{2h} using the equation of $C''=C - C'$:

$$C''_{1h} = 7.30 - 0.836 = 6.46 \, ng/mL$$

$$C''_{2h} = 4.06 - 0.816 = 3.24 \, ng/mL$$

$$\alpha = -slope = -\frac{lnC''_{2h} - lnC''_{1h}}{t_2 - t_1} = \frac{ln3.24 - ln6.46}{2-1} = 0.69 \, h^{-1}$$

$$C'' = A \cdot e^{-\alpha \cdot t} \rightarrow 6.46 = A \cdot e^{-0.69 \cdot 1} \rightarrow A = 12.9 \, ng/mL$$

Therefore, following 0.5 mg dose, the concentration-time profile is:

$$C = A \cdot e^{-\alpha \cdot t} + B \cdot e^{-\beta \cdot t} = 12.9 \cdot e^{-0.69 \cdot t} + 0.855 \cdot e^{-0.0233 \cdot t}$$

$$C_0 = A + B = 13.7 \, ng/mL$$

BB took 29.6 mg of colchicine, the C_0 in her blood was: $\frac{29.6 \, mg \cdot 13.7 \, ng/mL}{0.5 \, mg} =$ **811 ng/mL, which was 59-fold higher than the initial concentration of 13.7 ng/mL obtained following the dose of 0.5 mg.**

Chapter 10.
Nonlinear Pharmacokinetics

Learning Objectives

After reading this chapter, the reader shall be able to:

1. Differentiate the features of linear and nonlinear pharmacokinetics.

2. Explain the potential biopharmaceutic processes that can lead to nonlinear pharmacokinetics.

3. Use the Michaelis-Menten model to characterize nonlinear pharmacokinetics.

4. Perform individualized therapy based on estimation of V_{max} and K_m obtained from one or two concentrations for a drug following nonlinear pharmacokinetics.

5. Understand how the nonlinear pharmacokinetics of phenytoin is handled clinically.

The motivation for me to write this book is to provide a useful reference book for PharmD students in my class. This pharmacokinetics book aims to provide essentials, *only essentials*, in clinical pharmacokinetics, as it is supposed to be an introductory level book for beginners. Nonlinear pharmacokinetics is more complicated than linear pharmacokinetics. Should I include this topic in this book? I asked myself. It didn't take much time for me to make up my mind – I should. Why? Because clinical pharmacists and other healthcare professionals encounter nonlinear pharmacokinetics in clinical practice. Therefore, if you are a PharmD student, you need to learn, sooner or later, how to deal with nonlinear pharmacokinetics.

So far, we have been focusing on *linear pharmacokinetics* because most drugs used clinically demonstrate linear pharmacokinetics when they are administered within therapeutic dose ranges. However, for a number of drugs, they follow *nonlinear pharmacokinetics*. What is the difference between linear pharmacokinetics and nonlinear pharmacokinetics? What are the "symptoms" of nonlinear pharmacokinetics? The above questions are addressed in section 10.1. Nonlinear pharmacokinetics can arise from different sources. The various biopharmaceutic processes that can lead to nonlinear pharmacokinetics is discussed in section 10.2. Once we see the "symptoms" of nonlinear pharmacokinetics and understand the causes of nonlinear pharmacokinetics, there is a natural desire (and meanwhile a clinical need) to build a mathematical model to quantitatively characterize nonlinear pharmacokinetics. The model that has been extensively used for describing nonlinear pharmacokinetics is the Michaelis-Menten model, which is elaborated in section 10.3. As noted earlier, nonlinear pharmacokinetics is more complicated than linear pharmacokinetics. Accordingly, dose regimen selection for a drug following nonlinear pharmacokinetics is more challenging than a drug with linear pharmacokinetics. How is nonlinear pharmacokinetics handled in clinical practice? This question is addressed in section 10.4 using phenytoin as a case example.

10.1 "Symptoms" of Nonlinear Pharmacokinetics

For someone who just stepped into the field of pharmacokinetics, the terms "linear pharmacokinetics" and "nonlinear pharmacokinetics" can be misleading. You have seen a lot of pharmacokinetics plots in the previous 9 chapters, most of which present the time-course of drug concentrations. At the first glance of the name "linear pharmacokinetics", intuitively you may think that it indicates the relationship between concentration and time. Actually, this is not what this term meant to indicate. Many pharmacokinetics profiles show straight lines because the concentrations are plotted on a logarithm scale, not on a linear scale. Therefore, the term *linear* does not indicate the concentration-time relationship. Instead, what the term *linear* really refers to is the dose-concentration relationship - the plasma concentration at any time after a dose is proportional to the dose for a drug following linear pharmacokinetics.

For example, following a 10 mg dose, the plasma concentration of drug A is 50 ng/mL at 2 h post dose. When a dose of 20 mg is administered, what would be the concentration at 2 h post dose? If drug A has linear pharmacokinetics, doubling the dose will double the drug concentration. As a result, drug A's plasma concentration at 2 h following a 20 mg dose will be 100 ng/mL. Some pharmacokinetic scientists do not like the term *linear pharmacokinetics* and prefer to use the term *dose proportional*; these two terms are interchangeable, and both are commonly used in literature.

Once we have a good understanding of the term *linear pharmacokinetics*, the term *nonlinear pharmacokinetics* is self-evident – it means that the dose-concentration relationship is nonlinear. For example, for a drug following nonlinear pharmacokinetics, doubling the dose will not double the drug concentration. The concentration could be more than doubled (e.g., 3-times higher), which is known as a *more than dose-proportional* increase, or less than doubled (e.g., only 50% higher), which is usually called *less than dose-proportional* increase.

How to differentiate linear and nonlinear pharmacokinetics? The following are a few tips and some useful ways to diagnose if a drug's pharmacokinetics is nonlinear.

- To evaluate if a drug has linear or nonlinear pharmacokinetics, the bottom line is that you need to have concentration-time data from at least two doses. Pharmacokinetics linearity is difficult to assess with just one dose level. To make a robust evaluation, data from ≥ three doses covering a wide therapeutic dose range are ideal.

- Let's assume that you have concentration-time data from three doses of a drug. A simple way to evaluate pharmacokinetic linearity is to plot the dose-normalized concentration-time profiles. For example, there are 3 doses: 2 mg, 5 mg, and 10 mg. For the concentrations obtained from the 2 mg dose group, divide each concentration by 2. Similarly, for the concentrations from the 5 mg dose group, divide each concentration by 5.

Do the same calculation with data from the 10 mg dose. Then you plot the dose-normalized concentration vs time curve. If all the curves overlay (Figure 10-1, upper panel), the drug has linear pharmacokinetics. If the curves are not overlapping with each other (Figure 10-1, lower panel), the drug has nonlinear pharmacokinetics.

- In addition to dose-normalized concentration-time profiles, another common way to evaluate pharmacokinetic linearity is to plot AUC vs dose. If the AUC values are proportional to the doses (Figure 10-2, left), the drug has linear pharmacokinetics.   Otherwise, the drug has nonlinear pharmacokinetics, either with a more-than dose proportional increase in AUC (Figure 10-2, middle) or a less-than dose proportional increase in AUC (Figure 10-2, right).

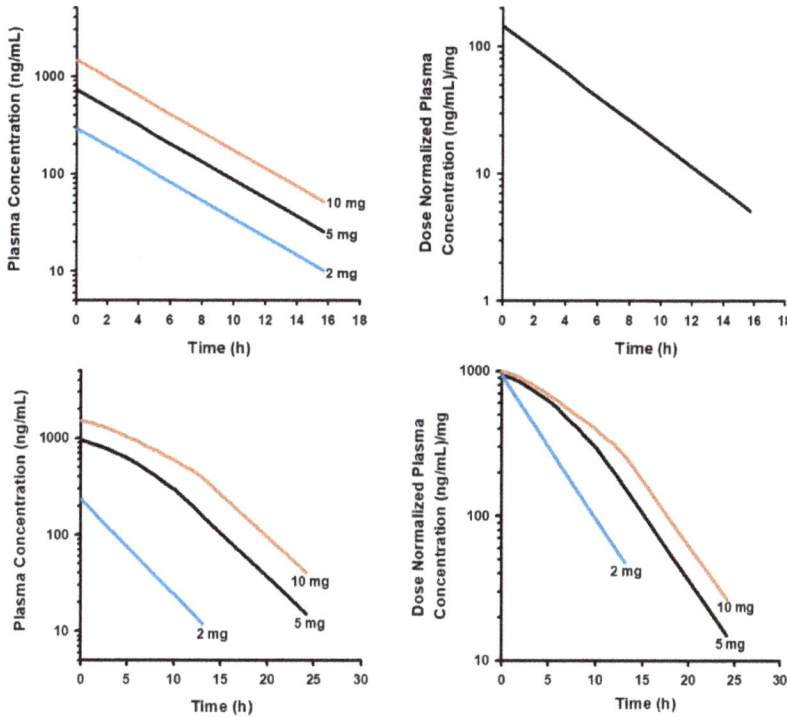

Figure 10-1. Original concentration-time profiles (left column) and dose-normalized concentration-time profiles (right column) for a drug with linear pharmacokinetics (upper panel) or nonlinear pharmacokinetics (lower panel).

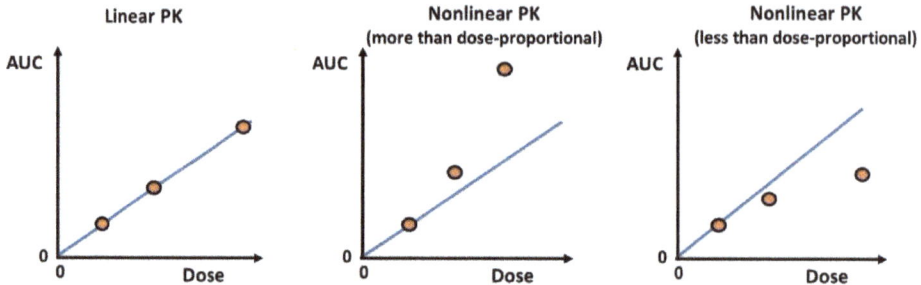

Figure 10-2. Relationship between AUC vs dose for a drug with linear pharmacokinetics (left), nonlinear pharmacokinetic with more than dose-proportional increase in AUC (middle), and nonlinear pharmacokinetic with less than dose-proportional increase in AUC (right). The blue line serves as a reference line which links the data point [0,0] and AUC-dose pair from the lowest dose. If all AUC-dose pairs fall on the blue line, the drug has linear pharmacokinetics. Otherwise, the drug has nonlinear pharmacokinetics.

10.2 Causes of Nonlinear Pharmacokinetics

You have seen what nonlinear pharmacokinetics look like in the last section, and you may wonder what the causes are. One common mechanism is the saturation of an enzyme or transporter involved in ADME, which happens when drug concentrations/doses are high enough. Nonlinear pharmacokinetics can arise from different sources. The following are some examples of the biopharmaceutic processes that can lead to nonlinear pharmacokinetics:

- *Saturation of the absorption process.* For example, for an orally administered drug undergoing first-pass metabolism, the enzyme responsible for the first-pass loss may be saturated at high doses. As a result, the bioavailability of the drug increases with dose escalation, leading to a more than dose proportional increase in drug exposure. In addition to enzymes, saturation could also happen to drug transporters, including both the uptake transporters and efflux transporters.

- *Saturation of the distribution process.* For example, if a drug binds to a high-affinity low-capacity plasma protein, the fraction of unbound drug will increase when the plasma protein gets saturated at high doses, resulting in an increase in volume of distribution and decrease in plasma concentrations.

- *Saturation of the metabolism process.* A typical example is the saturation of a drug metabolizing enzyme expressed in the liver. The result of this saturation is the decreased hepatic clearance, which causes a more than dose-proportional increase in drug exposure with dose escalation. Saturable metabolism (also called capacity-limited metabolism) is the most common source of nonlinearity and *is the focus of the remaining sections of this chapter.*

- *Saturation of the excretion process.*   For example, if a drug is a substrate of a transporter that is responsible for the tubular secretion of the drug, saturation of the transporter at high doses could lead to decrease in renal excretion. Accordingly, with an increase in doses, drug exposure increases more than dose proportionally. Conversely, if a drug is a substrate of a transporter involved in its tubular reabsorption, saturation of the transporter would lead to increase in renal excretion, resulting in a less than dose proportional increase in drug exposure with an increase in doses.

- *Other sources of nonlinear kinetics* In addition to saturation of the ADME processes, nonlinear kinetics can arise from the saturation of the pharmacological target, a phenomenon known as target-mediated drug disposition (TMDD). TMDD is viewed as the consequence of pharmacodynamics affecting pharmacokinetics, which is counter intuitive and considered as a special source of nonlinear pharmacokinetic. TMDD is beyond the scope of this book; it will be elaborated upon in great detail in another book of mine ("*Advanced Pharmacokinetics and Pharmacodynamics*"), which is anticipated to be published by the end of 2025.

10.3   The   Michaelis-Menten   Model   for   Describing   Nonlinear Pharmacokinetics

Saturable metabolism, also referred to as capacity-limited metabolism, represents the most important type of nonlinear pharmacokinetics from clinical practice perspective. The mathematical equation that has been used extensively to describe nonlinear pharmacokinetics is the Michaelis-Menten equation. Michaelis-Menten kinetics was named after Leonor Michaelis and Maud Menten based on their famous paper published in 1913, a paper that has had an enormous influence on the progress of biochemistry. Following is the Michaelis-Menten equation used in the nonlinear pharmacokinetics arena:

$$\text{Drug elimination rate} = -\frac{dX}{dt} = \frac{V_{max} \cdot C_P}{K_m + C_P} \qquad\qquad [10\text{-}1]$$

Where:

$-\frac{dX}{dt}$ = drug elimination rate. X represents drug amount in the body. The unit of drug elimination rate is amount/time. In some articles, it is also expressed as V, which stands for velocity of drug metabolism.

V_{max} = maximum amount of drug that can be eliminated in the given time period. The unit of V_{max} is amount/time.

K_m = Michaelis-Menton constant which is the drug concentration at which the rate of elimination is half of V_{max}. The unit is amount/volume, which is same as the unit of drug concentrations.

C_P = drug plasma concentration.

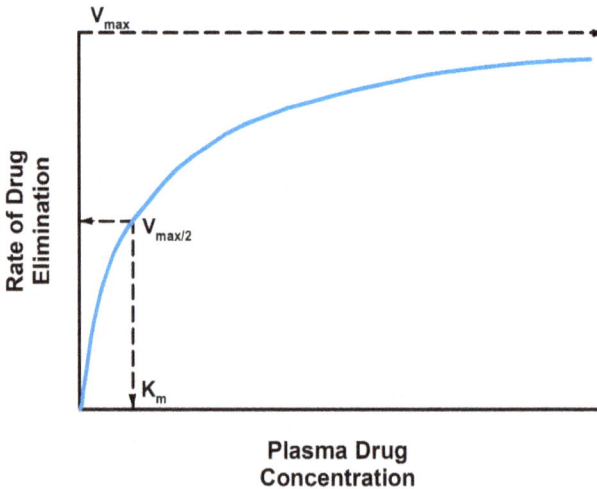

Figure 10-3. Michaelis-Menton kinetics to characterize the relationship between drug elimination rate and plasma drug concentration with saturable metabolism. At low concentration, $C_P \ll K_m$, the rate of drug elimination is first order. With increase in concentration, some saturation is seen, and the rate of drug metabolism can not keep up with increases in the drug concentration. At sufficiently high concentrations, $C_P \gg K_m$, the enzyme is fully occupied, and the maximum rate of metabolism is reached. As a result, the rate of drug elimination is zero order.

Equation 10-1 provides the following valuable insights on the pattern of drug concentration decline over time:

- At low drug concentrations, $C_P \ll K_m$. Therefore, $K_m + C_P \approx K_m$. Equation 10-1 can be simplified as:

$$\text{Drug elimination rate} = \frac{V_{max} \cdot C_P}{K_m} \rightarrow \text{Drug elimination rate} = \text{constant} \cdot C_P \quad [10\text{-}2]$$

Equation 10-2 indicates that drug elimination rate is proportional to the plasma concentration, which is a key feature of a first-order process. This represents a situation where there is an excess amount of drug metabolizing enzyme. Most drugs are given at mg dose range, and their therapeutic concentrations are typically less than K_m. As a result, drug elimination, as indicated in Equation 10-2, is a first-order process (i.e., behaves like Jerry as mentioned in Chapter 1). This explains why most drugs follow linear pharmacokinetics.

- At very high drug concentrations, $C_P >> K_m$. Therefore, $K_m + C_P \approx C_P$. Equation 10-1 can be simplified as:

Drug elimination rate = $\dfrac{V_{max} \cdot C_P}{C_P}$ → Drug elimination rate = V_{max} [10-3]

Equation 10-3 indicates that drug elimination rate no longer depends on current drug concentration/amount in the body. It becomes a constant at its maximum value (i.e. V_{max}) because the enzyme is fully saturated. This is a zero-order process (i.e., behaves like Tom as mentioned in Chapter 1).

Equations 10-2 and 10-3 describe two extreme situations. When the drug is high (e.g. $C_P > K_m$) but not high enough to fully saturate the enzyme, drug elimination rate could be mixed-order and nonlinear.

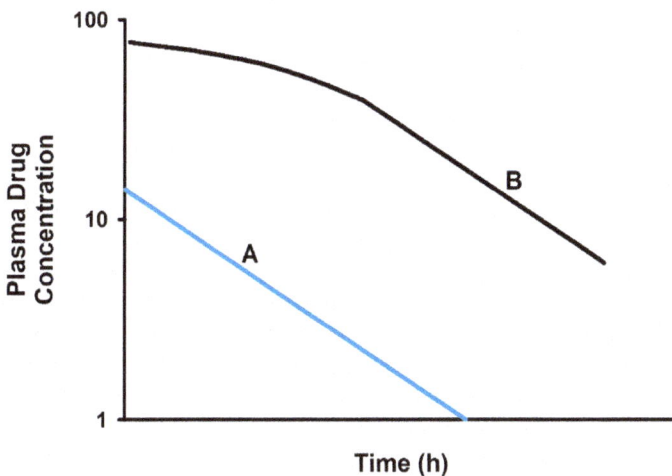

Figure 10-4. Concentration-time profiles of a drug following a low dose and a high dose. At the low dose (curve A), the drug undergoes first-order elimination and demonstrates linear pharmacokinetics. At the high dose, the drug undergoes zero-order elimination at high concentrations due to enzyme saturation, then transitioned to first-order elimination after concentrations decline to a certain threshold. Curve B is the result of mixed order elimination and displays a clear nonlinear pharmacokinetics behavior.

Figure 10-4 demonstrates the concentration-time profiles that we would anticipate for a drug with saturable metabolism. At the low dose (curve A), the drug undergoes first-order elimination and demonstrates linear pharmacokinetic behavior. This is in line with what Equation 10-2 indicates. At the high dose, the drug undergoes zero-order elimination at high concentrations due to enzyme saturation, then transitions to first-order elimination after concentrations decline to a certain threshold. Curve B is the result of mixed-order elimination and displays a clear nonlinear pharmacokinetics behavior.

For a drug following nonlinear pharmacokinetics, dose regimen optimization can be challenging as the dose-concentration relationship is no longer straightforward. Determining the values of V_{max} and K_m is important because these values are critical in estimating the dose necessary to achieve desired plasma concentrations. How to determine V_{max} and K_m? How long would it take to eliminate a drug with nonlinear pharmacokinetics? How long would it take for a drug with nonlinear pharmacokinetics to reach steady state? How to make dose adjustment for a drug following nonlinear pharmacokinetics? All these important questions are addressed in the next section using phenytoin as a case example.

10.4 Handling Nonlinear Pharmacokinetics in Clinical Practice – Case Example of Phenytoin

When discussing how nonlinear pharmacokinetics is handled in clinical practice, one drug that cannot be overlooked is phenytoin, an anticonvulsant agent that is commonly used to treat and prevent seizure disorders. Phenytoin undergoes saturable hepatic metabolism, and nonlinear pharmacokinetics occurs at concentrations within the therapeutic range. Phenytoin is commonly prescribed, and many patients take phenytoin for years. Meanwhile, phenytoin has a very narrow therapeutic window (10-20 mg/L) - plasma concentrations lower than the minimum effective concentration are associated with risk of breakthrough seizures, while concentrations above the upper threshold place patients at risk of many side effects, including nystagmus, ataxia, slurred speech, lethargy, confusion, and coma. Therefore, it is important to keep plasma concentrations of phenytoin within the therapeutic range.

The features of nonlinear pharmacokinetics, widespread use for decades, and narrow therapeutic window have made phenytoin a classic example for discussing the therapeutic implications of nonlinearity. Therapeutic drug monitoring (TDM) has been routinely performed for phenytoin. Plasma concentrations usually are collected at steady state, and the Michaelis-Menten model is then applied to obtain V_{max} and/or K_m of phenytoin in each individual patient to initiate personalized therapy aiming to maintain its plasma concentrations within the therapeutic range.

Over the years, extensive experience has been gathered for phenytoin. The average value of V_{max} for phenytoin is 7 mg/kg/day, which is equivalent to around 500 mg/day for a typical 70-kg adult. The average K_m is around 4 mg/L. Please note that these are just average values in a population. It is well known that there is large interindividual variability of V_{max} and/or K_m among patients. Therefore, it is important to estimate these two parameters in each individual patient. The following subsections discuss how mathematical equations have been used to deal with the nonlinear pharmacokinetics of phenytoin.

10.4.1 Equations for Steady State Condition

Phenytoin has good oral bioavailability, and F is generally assumed to be 1. The salt factors (S) are 0.92 for capsules and the injectable preparations and 1 for the suspension and chewable tablets. An S of 0.92 means that, for phenytoin sodium, 92% (by weight) is phenytoin. For 100 mg of phenytoin sodium administered, 92 mg of phenytoin reaches the systemic circulation. Since the salt factor of phenytoin is high, to simplify the situation, S is assumed to be 1 even for capsules and injectables. Accordingly, both F and S are not included in the equations.

Phenytoin is known to have a very slow oral absorption process. It has been assumed that phenytoin is absorbed at a constant rate over a large portion of the dosing interval. This assumption enables the use of an infusion model to characterize the drug input, which is represented as $\frac{Dose}{\tau}$ (Figure 10-5). Meanwhile, the drug output, expressed as the drug elimination rate, is characterized by the Michaelis-Menten kinetics as shown in Equation 10-1. Taken together, the change in the amount of drug in the body per given time is:

$$\frac{dX}{dt} = drug\ input - drug\ output \quad \rightarrow \quad \frac{dX}{dt} = \frac{D}{\tau} - \frac{V_{max} \bullet C_P}{K_m + C_P} \qquad [10\text{-}4]$$

Where D is dose, τ is dosing interval, C_P is the plasma concentration, V_{max} and K_m have been defined earlier.

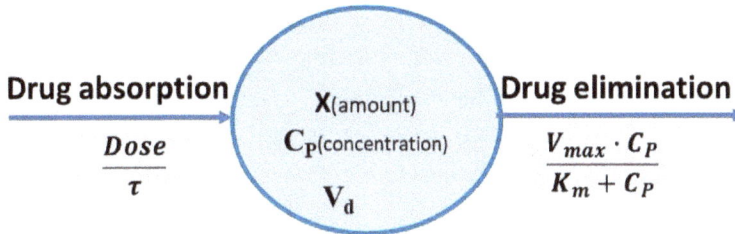

Figure 10-5. One compartment model of phenytoin with zero-order absorption and saturable elimination.

At steady state, drug input equals drug output. As a result, $\frac{dX}{dt} = 0$. accordingly

$$\frac{D}{\tau} = \frac{V_{max} \cdot C_{p,SS}}{K_m + C_{p,SS}} \qquad [10\text{-}5]$$

I boxed the above equation because it is used extensively for phenytoin and other drugs with saturable elimination. Equation 10-5 tells us that if we know the V_{max} and K_m values of phenytoin, together with the desired steady-state concentration, we can determine the dose.

Case Example 10-1.

Estimation of initial phenytoin dose

Patient WI (60 kg Female) has focal seizure and is about to begin phenytoin therapy. WI has never taken phenytoin before. The desired steady state plasma concentration of phenytoin is 15 mg/L. You, as the lead pharmacist, are asked to recommend a dose regimen.

Please work on it yourself first before checking my response below.

~ ~ ~

Patient WI has no history of phenytoin usage. As a starting point, we can use the population mean values of V_{max} and K_m, which are 7 mg/kg/day and 4 mg/L, respectively. Using Equation 10-5:

$$\frac{D}{\tau} = \frac{7 \cdot 60 \cdot 15}{4 + 15} \qquad \rightarrow \frac{D}{\tau} = 332 \, mg/day$$

Therefore, a dose of 332 mg of phenytoin per day would be used as the first-time therapy.

In addition to dose calculation, Equation 10-5 can be rearranged to the following equation to estimate steady state plasma concentration of phenytoin:

$$C_{P,ss} = \frac{K_m \cdot \frac{D}{\tau}}{V_{max} - \frac{D}{\tau}} \qquad [10\text{-}6]$$

Equation 10-6 tells us that if we know the V_{max} and K_m values of phenytoin, together with the daily dose prescribed to the patient, we can predict the steady state plasma concentration of phenytoin in this patient.

Case Example 10-2.

Estimation of steady-state plasma concentration of phenytoin

Patient IL (60 kg Female) has focal seizure and starts phenytoin therapy. IL's individual V_{max} and K_m are found to be 8 mg/kg/day and 4.5 mg/L, respectively. You, as the lead pharmacist, proposed three options: 1) 300 mg/day; 2) 350 mg/day; and 3) 400 mg/day. What is the estimated steady state plasma concentration of phenytoin from each dose regimen?

Please work on it yourself first before looking at my response below.

~ ~ ~

The steady state plasma concentration of phenytoin can be predicted based on Equation 10-6:

- *For a dose regimen of 300 mg/day:*

$$C_{P,ss} = \frac{4.5 \cdot 300}{8 \cdot 60 - 300} = 7.5 \; mg/L$$

- *For a dose regimen of 350 mg/day:*

$$C_{P,ss} = \frac{4.5 \cdot 350}{8 \cdot 60 - 350} = 12.1 \; mg/L$$

- *For a dose regimen of 400 mg/day:*

$$C_{P,ss} = \frac{4.5 \cdot 400}{8 \cdot 60 - 400} = 22.5 \; mg/L$$

Since the therapeutic range of phenytoin is 10-20 mg/L, among the three dosing regimens, the one that is appropriate is 350 mg per day. A modest decrease in dose (i.e. 300 mg/day) leads to subtherapeutic steady state concentration (i.e., 7.5 mg/L), while a modest increase in dose (i.e., 400 mg/day) results in toxic steady state level (i.e. 22.5 mg/L).

This example clearly shows how plasma concentrations of phenytoin increase disproportionally with increase is doses. A _33.3%_ increase in dose from 300 mg/day to 400 mg/day leads to _3-fold_ increase in the steady state plasma concentration of phenytoin from 7.5 mg/L to 22.5 mg/L.

10.4.2 Time to Eliminate the Drug

For drugs with nonlinear pharmacokinetics, the concept of half-life is meaningless since the time needed to decrease half of the concentration is no longer constant. Following is the equation to estimate the time needed to for the plasma concentration to drop from the one value ($C_{P,t1}$) to another ($C_{P,t2}$):

$$t = \frac{V_d}{V_{max}} \left(C_{P,t1} - C_{P,t2} + K_m \cdot \ln \frac{C_{P,t1}}{C_{P,t2}} \right) \qquad [10\text{-}7]$$

Case Example 10-3.

Estimation of time to eliminate phenytoin

Patient IL (60 kg Female) has focal seizure and has been taking phenytoin 425 mg/day for 2 weeks. Her individual V_{max} and K_m are 8 mg/kg/day and 4.5 mg/L, respectively. V_d of phenytoin in this patient is 50 L. A blood sample was drawn, and the steady state plasma concentration was found to be 35 mg/L. If patient IL stops taking phenytoin, how long would it take to drop to the therapeutic concentration of 17.5 mg/L (i.e., half of the current value)? How long would it take to drop to the subtherapeutic concentration of 8.75 mg/L (i.e., another 50% decrease)?

Please work on it yourself first before looking at my response below.

~ ~ ~

Equation 10-7 is used to address these questions.

- *Time for the plasma concentration to fall from 35 mg/L to 17.5 mg/L:*

$$t = \frac{50}{480}\left(35 - 17.5 + 4.5 \cdot \ln\frac{35}{17.5}\right) = 2.4 \ days$$

- *Time for the plasma concentration to fall from 17.5 mg/L to 8.75 mg/L:*

$$t = \frac{50}{480}\left(17.5 - 8.75 + 4.5 \cdot \ln\frac{17.5}{8.75}\right) = 1.5 \ days$$

10.4.3 Time to Reach Steady State

For drugs with nonlinear pharmacokinetics, the time needed to reach the steady state is no longer as simple as the 5 half-lives seen in drugs with linear pharmacokinetics. If we consider that steady state is reached when the concentration is about 90% of the steady state concentration, following is the equation to estimate the time:

$$t_{90\%} = \frac{K_m \cdot V_d}{\left(V_{max} - \frac{D}{\tau}\right)^2}\left(2.3 \cdot V_{max} - 0.9 \cdot \frac{D}{\tau}\right) \qquad [10\text{-}8]$$

As indicated in the above equation, the time to steady state (i.e. $t_{90\%}$) is dependent on V_{max}, K_m, as well as the daily dose administered. For a higher dose, it takes longer time to reach steady state than for a lower dose. When the daily dose approaches V_{max}, the denominator $\left(V_{max} - \frac{D}{\tau}\right)$ tends towards zero, indicating that steady state may never be reached.

Case Example 10-4.

Estimation of time to reach phenytoin steady state

Patient IL (60 kg Female) has focal seizure and will start phenytoin therapy soon. Her individual V_{max} and K_m are 8 mg/kg/day and 4.5 mg/L, respectively. V_d of phenytoin in this patient is 50 L. How long would it take to reach steady state if IL takes 1) 350 mg daily dose; or 2) 450 mg daily dose?

Please work on it yourself first before looking at my response below.

~ ~ ~

Equation 10-8 is used to address the above questions.

- *Time to reach steady state when patient IL takes 350 mg daily dose:*

$$t_{90\%} = \frac{4.5 \cdot 50}{(8 \cdot 60 - 350)^2}(2.3 \cdot 8 \cdot 60 - 0.9 \cdot 350) = 10.5 \ days$$

- *Time to reach steady state when patient IL takes 450 mg daily dose:*

$$t_{90\%} = \frac{4.5 \cdot 50}{(8 \cdot 60 - 350)^2} (2.3 \cdot 8 \cdot 60 - 0.9 \cdot 350) = 175 \; days$$

10.4.4 Individualized therapy - dose adjustment based on the Steady-State Levels

When phenytoin is administered for the first time to a patient, as elaborated in Case example 10-1, we can use the population average values of V_{max} and K_m to estimate the initial dose. However, these are just population mean values. Considering the large interindividual variability of V_{max} and K_m among patients, the chance that the individual patient you are treating has the same V_{max} and K_m as those population mean values is low. Therefore, you need to figure out the V_{max} and K_m values in each individual patient and adjust the dose accordingly. The following is the typical procedure of V_{max} and K_m determination and dose adjustment:

1) Calculate initial dose based on population mean values of V_{max} and K_m as well as the desired steady state plasma concentration of phenytoin using Equation 10-5.

2) Patient takes the daily dose calculated from step 1. Two weeks after the start of therapy, collect one blood sample, and measure the steady state plasma concentration of phenytoin.

3) If the measured concentration is satisfactory, lucky you. No dose adjustment is needed. However, if the concentration is not ideal, and you need to adjust dose, here are the next steps: Now you have the information of a) the actual daily dose used; b) the actual steady state plasma concentration in this specific patient, and c) the population mean of K_m. With this information, you can calculate the V_{max} of phenytoin in this specific patient using the following equation, which is rearranged based on Equation 10-5:

$$V_{max} = \frac{\frac{D}{\tau} \cdot (K_m + C_{P,ss})}{C_{P,ss}} \qquad [10\text{-}9]$$

4) With the value of V_{max} calculate in step 3 for this specific patient, together with the population mean K_m value and the desired steady state plasma concentration of phenytoin, calculate the dose again based on Equation 10-5.

5) The patient takes the adjusted dose. Then one blood sample is collected two weeks later, and the steady state plasma concentration of phenytoin following the adjusted dose is measured.

6) If the concentration from step 5 is satisfactory, no further dose adjustment is needed. However, if the concentration is still not satisfactory, a new daily dose needs to be determined. In that case, you have two daily dose-$C_{p,ss}$ data pairs on hand, which can be used to estimate the K_m value in this specific patient. K_m can be estimated from the slope of the daily dose (i.e. $\frac{D}{\tau}$) vs daily dose/$C_{p,ss}$ plot:

$$\frac{D}{\tau} = V_{max} - K_m \frac{\frac{D}{\tau}}{C_{P,ss}}$$

[10-10]

7) Now you have the values of V_{max} (from step 3) and K_m (from step 6) of phenytoin in this specific patient. Together with the desired steady state plasma concentration, you can adjust the dose based on Equation 10-5.

I provide two case examples below so that you can practice the individuation of phenytoin doses.

Case Example 10-5.

Adjusting phenytoin dose based on one steady-state level

Patient ND (70 kg Male) has tonic-clonic seizure and has been taking 400 mg phenytoin per day for 2 weeks. During a doctor's visit, a blood sample was collected, and the plasma concentration was found to be 30 mg/L. Recommend a new dose to achieve the desired steady state plasma concentration of phenytoin, which is 15 mg/L.

Please work on it yourself first before checking my calculations below.

~ ~ ~

The population average K_m= 4 mg/L is assumed. The dose used is 400 mg daily, and the concentration is 30 mg/L. Vmax of phenytoin in patient ND can be calculate using Equation 10-9:

$$V_{max} = \frac{\frac{D}{\tau} \cdot (K_m + C_{P,ss})}{C_{P,ss}} = \frac{400 \cdot (4+30)}{30} = 453 \, mg/day$$

Based on the Vmax calculated above, together with the Km of 4 mg/L and the desired concentration of 15 mg/L, the new dose should be:

$$\frac{D}{\tau} = \frac{453 \cdot 15}{4+15} \qquad \rightarrow \qquad \frac{D}{\tau} = 358 \, mg/day$$

Therefore, a new dose regimen of 358 mg of phenytoin per day should be used.

Case Example 10-6.

Adjusting phenytoin dose based on two steady-state levels

Continuing with Case example 10-5, patient ND (70 kg Male) has been taking the adjust daily dose of 358 mg/day. He visited the doctor 2 weeks later for the blood draw and the concentration was found to be 21 mg/L, which is still unideal. Recommend a new dose to achieve the desired steady state plasma concentration of phenytoin, which is 15 mg/L.

Please work on it yourself first before checking my response below.

$$\sim \sim \sim$$

Now you have two data pairs on hand:

When $\dfrac{D}{\tau} = 400\ mg/day$, Cp,ss = 30 mg/L

When $\dfrac{D}{\tau} = 358\ mg/day$, Cp,ss = 21 mg/L

Also you know the Vmax of phenytoin in patient ND is 453 mg/day

As shown in Figure 10-6, a plot of $\dfrac{D}{\tau}$ against $\dfrac{\frac{D}{\tau}}{C_{P,ss}}$ yields a straight line and the negative slope of the line is K_m.

Therefore, K_m is:

$$K_m = -\,slope = -\,\dfrac{\dfrac{D_1}{\tau} - \dfrac{D_2}{\tau}}{\dfrac{\frac{D_1}{\tau}}{C_{P,ss,1}} - \dfrac{\frac{D_2}{\tau}}{C_{P,ss,2}}} = -\,\dfrac{400 - 358}{\dfrac{400}{30} - \dfrac{358}{21}} = 11.3\ mg/L$$

The new dose is calculate using Equtation 10-5:

$$\dfrac{D}{\tau} = \dfrac{453 \bullet 15}{11.3 + 15} \qquad \rightarrow \qquad \dfrac{D}{\tau} = 258\ mg/day$$

Therefore, to reach the desired steady state concentration of 15 mg/L, a new dose regimen of 258 mg of phenytoin per day should be used.

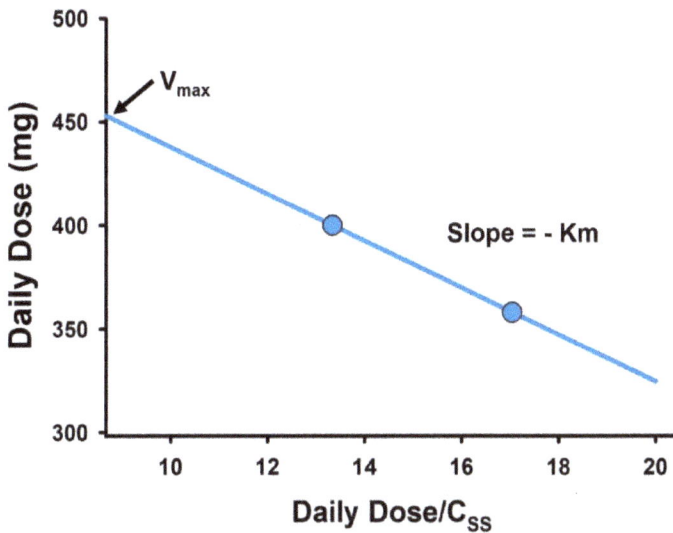

Figure 10-6. Linear plot of the Michaelis-Menten equation.

References

- Basic Pharmacokinetics and Pharmacodynamics (2017). 2nd edition. John Wiley & Sons, Inc.
- Concepts in Clinical Pharmacokinetics (2014). 6th edition. American Society of Health-System Pharmacists, Inc.

Chapter 11.
Pharmacokinetics and Dose Optimization in Special Population

Learning Objectives

After reading this chapter, the reader shall be able to:

1. Understand the variability in pharmacokinetics and list the sources of variability.

2. Describe physiological/ pathophysiological processes that are altered in special populations, including children, the elderly, people with obesity, patients with renal disease, and pregnant women.

3. Explain how the changes in physiological/ pathophysiological processes affect pharmacokinetics

4. Perform dose adjustment for a patient in a special population.

As noted in Chapter 1, there is variability in pharmacokinetics. Following the same dose, drug concentrations may vary substantially among different patients. Drug variability can arise from various sources. One source is enzyme- and transporter-mediated drug-drug interactions, which have been discussed with examples in Chapter 4 (sections 4.1.1 and 4.1.2). Another source is pharmacogenetics, which has been briefly mentioned in Chapter 4 (section 4.1.3). In addition to the above two, other common sources of variability include age, difference in body weight and body fat composition, diseases, as well as special condition (e.g., pregnancy). This chapter focuses on pharmacokinetics and dose optimization in special populations, including children (section 11.1), the elderly (section 11.2), people with obesity (section 11.3), patients with renal disease (section 11.4), and pregnant women (section 11.5). Patients falling into the category of special population are no longer the "typical patients" due to altered physiological/pathophysiological processes. The altered physiological/ pathophysiological conditions subsequently lead to changes in drug pharmacokinetics. As a result, the "usual dosage regimen" derived from the standard/typical population often does not apply to the special population. The goal of this chapter is to learn how changes in physiological/pathophysiological processes affect pharmacokinetics and how to adjust dose regimen accordingly in these special populations.

11.1 Pediatric Population

The life of a human is often divided into several stages. Society's view of which age belongs to which stage is changing. There is no universal agreement on the cut off values. In this book, adulthood and the different stages of "pre-adulthood" are defined as follows:

- *Neonate*: The first month of a child's life. A neonate is also called *newborn*. Babies born before 36 weeks of pregnancy is considered as premature (or preterm) neonates, while those with > 36 weeks gestational age are called full-term (or term) neonates.

- *Infant*: Between the ages of 1 month and 2 years.
- *Child*: Between 2-12 years of age
- *Adolescent*: Between 12 and 18 years of age
- *Adult*: > 18 years

Results from numerous pharmacokinetics studies have consistently conveyed one message – a child is not a small adult; this is not surprising as the above groups differ in terms of physical size, body composition, biochemistry, and physiology. Figure 11-1 provides an overall picture of the developmental changes in physiologic factors that influence drug ADME in children.

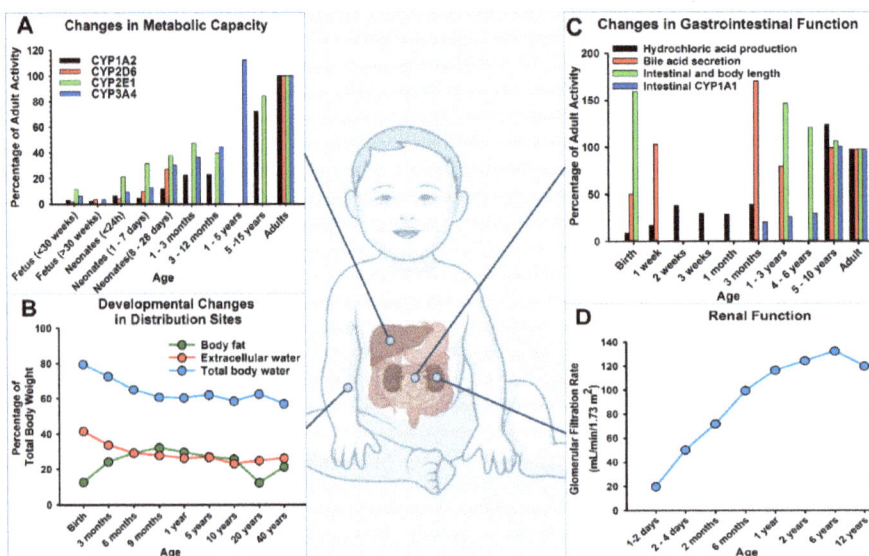

Figure 11-1. Developmental changes in physiologic factors that influence drug ADME in children. This figure is made based on data from two papers: 1) Kearns GL, et al. N Engl J Med 2003;349:1157-67. 2)van Groen BD, et al. Pharmacol Rev 2021;73:597–678.

11.1.1. Absorption:

Gastric pH is neutral at birth due to the presence of amniotic fluid and drops to 1-3 within 1-2 days after birth. The pH gradually returns to neutral again after a week, then declines and slowly reaches adult values after 2 years of age. Frequent feedings with milk may also influence gastric pH. Changes in gastric pH affect drug stability, dissolution rate, and degree of ionization, which subsequently influence the extent and rate of drug absorption. Gastric emptying in neonates and infants is slower than in adults, resulting in delayed drug absorption. In addition, neonates and infants have diminished biliary function, which compromises the body's ability to solubilize and subsequently absorb some lipophilic drugs. Additionally, developmental changes in the expression and activity of intestinal drug-metabolizing enzymes and drug transporters could potentially influence the bioavailability of drugs.

11.1.2 Distribution:

Figure 11-1 B shows developmental changes in total body water, extracellular water, and body fat. As it shows, total body water, expressed as a percentage of body weight, is highest in newborns (80%) and reaches adult value (60%) after 1 year of age. Body fat demonstrates the opposite trend – it increases from 10-15% in a term neonate to 20-25% in a 1-year-old. The body fat in a premature neonate is only 1-2%. The primary pharmacokinetic parameter that is affected by the changes in body water and body fat is the volume of distribution (V_d). How much impact these developmental changes have on V_d is dependent on the physiochemical properties of the drug.

The "water-loving" hydrophilic drugs face difficulty passing through the membrane, and they usually are confined within the extracellular space. As a result, the V_d of a hydrophilic drug in infants and children is usually higher than the value in adults. A typical example is aminoglycosides, such as gentamicin, amikacin, tobramycin, and streptomycin. The V_d of aminoglycosides is 0.5-1.2 L/kg in infants and children, which is higher than the value of 0.2-0.3 L/kg observed in adults. Conversely, lipophilic drugs have a higher volume of distribution in adults compared with neonates and infants because the former has a higher percentage of body fat. For example, diazepam, a highly lipophilic drug, has a V_d of 1.3-2.6 L/kg in neonates/infants, which is lower than the values of 1.6-3.2 L/kg in adults.

Another factor that affects the volume of distribution is plasma protein binding, which tends to be reduced in neonates and infants. For example, the protein binding of ampicillin is 10% in newborns, which is lower than the 18% reported in adults. The protein binding of phenytoin is 80% in newborns and 90% in adults, which means that the fraction of unbound in newborns is 2-fold higher than in adults. The reduced protein binding seen in neonates and infants could be due to not only the lower expression of plasma proteins but also the diminished binding affinity caused by high concentrations of endogenous substances competing with drugs.

Dose adjustment strategy: Clinically, V_d is an important parameter because it is used to calculate the loading dose. In addition, the differences in V_d will affect the half-life values. Using aminoglycosides as an example, the higher value of V_d in infants and children compared to adults highlights the need of prescribing a higher loading dose and a longer dosing interval.

11.1.3 Metabolism:

As shown in Figure 11-1 A, several important CYP450 enzymes have either no or very low expression in neonates. Then, their expression levels increase during the first several months of life, and often reach adult level after 1 year (e.g.,

CYP3A4) or 5 years of age (e.g., CYP1A2). Figure 11-2 shows the concentration-time profiles of caffeine, a sensitive CYP1A2 substrate, in the same baby at 6 and 10 weeks of age. The half-life of caffeine decreased from 41 h (at 6 weeks of age) to 16 h (at 10 weeks of age), which is well explained by the developmental change in CYP1A2.

Another classic example is chloramphenicol's "grey baby syndrome". Chloramphenicol is eliminated exclusively through glucuronidation by the phase II enzyme glucuronyl transferase (UGT), which is depressed at birth and reaches adult levels in children by three years of age. When chloramphenicol is linearly scaled according to body weight, the resulting exposure in newborns is five-fold higher than that reached in adults, causing the well-known grey baby syndrome. Therefore, the dose recommendation for neonates and infants up to 1 month age is to give half of the dose recommended to other groups (25 mg/kg/day).

Dose adjustment strategy: As many clinically important Phase 1 and Phase 2 enzymes have lower expression in neonates and infants than in adults, the clearance of the substrates of these enzymes is reduced, leading to higher plasma exposures and longer drug half-lives in neonates and infants. Therefore, lower doses and longer dosing intervals may be needed for drugs with relatively narrow therapeutic windows.

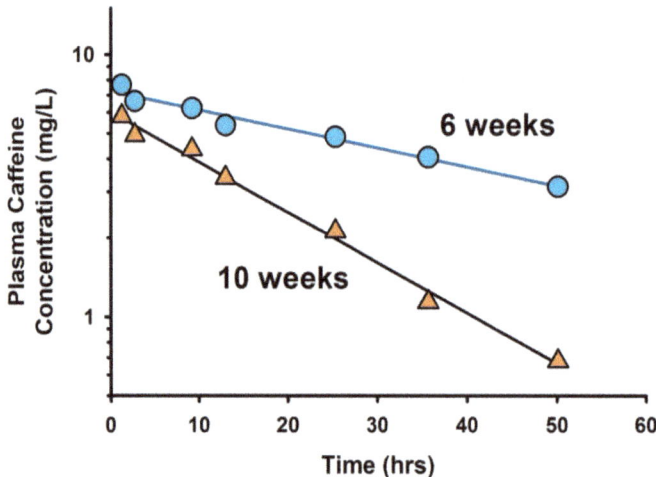

Figure 11-2. The concentration-time profiles of caffeine in the same baby at 6 and 10 weeks of age. Caffeine is metabolized in liver through CYP1A2. The half-life decreased from 41 h (at 6 weeks of age) to 16 h (at 10 weeks of age). *This figure is adapted from Aranda et al., Archives of Disease in Childhood 1979;54:946-949.*

11.1.4 Excretion:

Figure 11-1 D shows the changes in glomerular filtration rate (GFR) across different age groups. GFR is around 15-45 ml/min within the first week of life and increases to 30-60 ml/min at 1 month of age, 50-100 ml/min at 6 months of age, and typically reaches adult levels by 1 year of age. We learned in Chapter 4 that Cock-croft Gault equation is the most common method to calculate creatinine clearance for renal function estimation in adult. In children, different methods are used, among which the most frequently used creatinine-based eGFR equation is the revised bedside Schwartz formula:

eGFR= [(0.413 × Height (cm)) / Scr (mg/dL)]   [11-1]

This formula is recommended by the National Kidney Disease Education Program for creatinine methods with calibration traceable to isotope dilution mass spectrometry.

Dose adjustment strategy: Neonates and infants have immature renal clearance processes, leading to reduced renal excretion and prolongation of the half-lives of drugs that are primarily eliminated by the kidney. For such drugs (e.g., aminoglycosides), initial dose adjustment can be performed by either reducing the dose or increasing the dosing interval.

11.2 Elderly Population

Same as the situation of defining pediatric population, society's view of who is elderly is changing as well, and there is no universal agreement on the cut off value. In this book, individuals aged ≥ 65 years are considered elderly.

11.2.1. Absorption:

Gastric emptying time is prolonged in the elderly. As a result, the rate of absorption of an orally administered drug can be reduced. In general, the extent of absorption is usually unaltered. However, the bioavailability of certain drugs may increase due to the reduced first-pass effect. A typical example is propranolol, a beta blocker subject to extensive hepatic first-pass metabolism following oral administration. As shown in Figure 11-3, following the same oral dose, the plasma concentrations of propranolol in the elderly were significantly higher than those in the young adults, a result of the reduced first-pass effect.

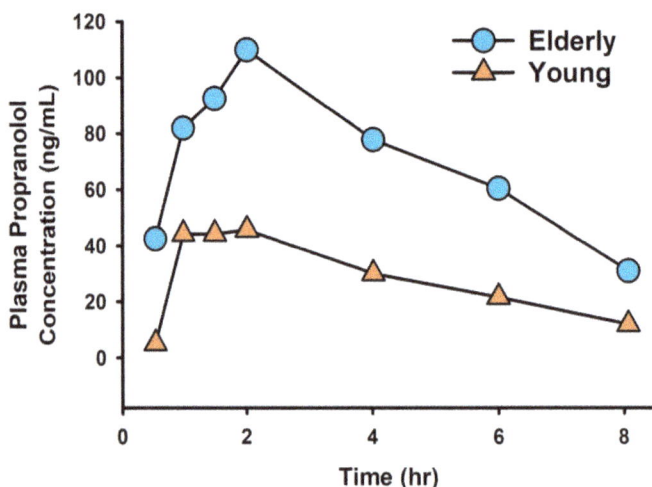

Figure 11-3. The plasma concentration-time profiles of propranolol in elderly (average 78 years, N=8) and young adults (average 29 years, N=7) following a single oral dose of 40 mg propranolol. *This figure is adapted from Castleden CM and George CF. Br J Clin Pharmac 1979;7:49-54.*

11.2.2. Distribution

Compared to young adults, elderly people have decreased total body water, deceased intracellular water, and little change in extracellular water. Plasma albumin was found to decrease with increase in age during adulthood, while α-acid glycoprotein showed no age-dependent change. In addition, the elderly have a higher percentage of fat tissue and less lean body mass (i.e., muscle). The influence of these changes in body composition on drug distribution depends on the physicochemical characteristics of the drug.

For drugs that distribute primarily into lean tissue (many hydrophilic drugs), a age-related decrease in volume of distribution is expected (e.g., ethanol). On the other hand, for drugs that distribute primarily into fatty tissue (many lipophilic drugs), a age-related increase in volume of distribution is anticipated (e.g., thiopental, diazepam). Figure 11-4 shows the representative thiopental serum concentration-time profiles for a young (29 years) and an elderly (77 years) patient after I.V. administration of a single dose of thiopental, a highly lipophilic drug. Further investigation indicated that the increase in thiopental half-life in the elderly was primarily a function of volume of distribution, but not clearance.

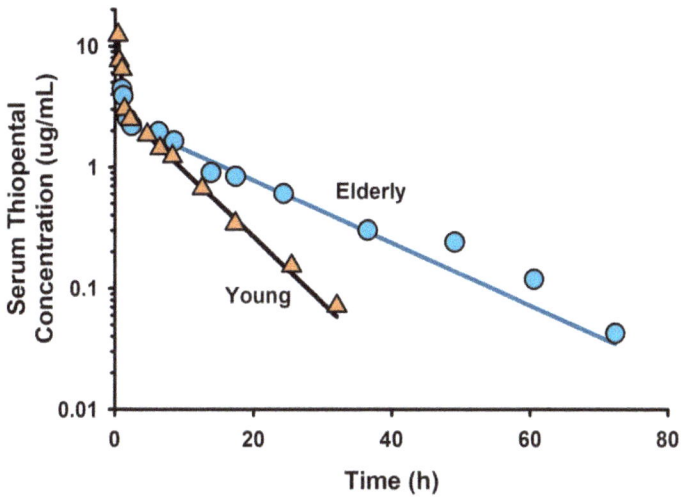

Figure 11-4. Representative thiopental serum concentration-time profiles for a young (29 years) and an elderly (77 years) patient after I.V. administration of a single dose of thiopental. *This figure is adapted from Jung D et al. Anesthesiology 1982; 56:263-268.*

11.2.3. Metabolism

Regarding drug metabolism, in general the hepatic clearance in the elderly is reduced due to the decreased liver blood flow and decreased liver mass. Deceased hepatic clearance has been reported for several drugs such as antipyrine and pethidine. In a report evaluating 10 different drugs that are substrates of CYP3A, the result showed that clearance in the elderly decreased, on average, about 30% to 40% compared to the younger adult group.

11.2.4. Excretion:

It has been reported that many physiologic functions diminish by approximately 1% per year with increasing age during adulthood. Renal function is no exception. As shown in Figure 11-5, GFR, tubular excretory capacity and renal blood flow all decrease with age.

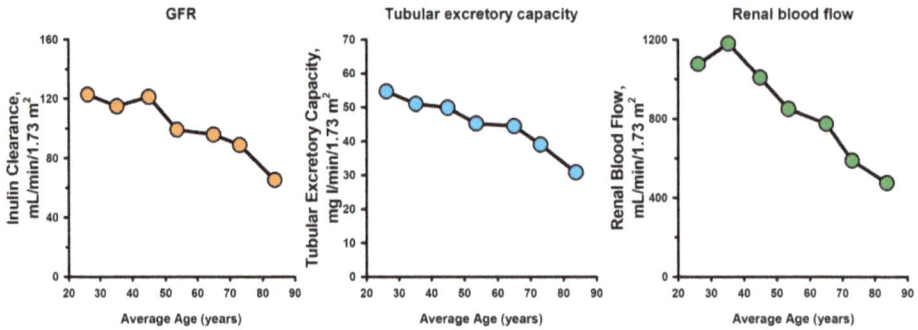

Figure 11-5. Effect of age on different parameters of renal function in adult males. *This figure is adapted from Davies DF and Shock NW. J Clin Invest 1950:29:496-507.*

For drugs primarily eliminated through the kidney, their renal clearance is usually decreased, and the half-lives are often prolonged (if V_d remains the same or changes in a less magnitude). As shown in Figure 11-6, kanamycin, a renally excreted antibiotic, demonstrated a clear age-dependent decrease in renal clearance and increase in the half-life.

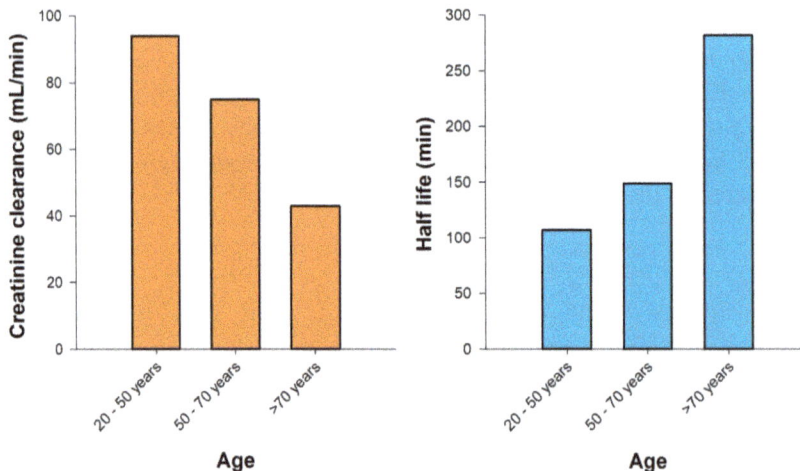

Figure 11-6. Effect on age on kanamycin pharmacokinetics. *This figure is adapted from Applied Pharmacokinetics (Third Edition).*

11.2.5. Dose adjustment

In summary, the pharmacokinetic changes in the elderly include reduced first-pass effect, decreased protein binding (for drugs bound to albumin), altered volume of distribution (Vd↑ for lipophilic drugs and Vd↓ for hydrophilic drugs), decreased renal clearance, decreased hepatic clearance, usually longer half-lives. Dose adjustment, either reducing the dose or increasing the dosing interval, may be needed for elderly people.

11.3 People with Obesity

Obesity, characterized by an abnormally high percentage of body fat, frequently refers to body fat content greater than 25% and 30% of total body weight for men and women, respectively. Obesity is defined as a body mass index (BMI) of 30 or higher; BMI is calculated as a person's weight in kilograms divided by the square of height in meters. It is projected that 49% of the US adult population will have obesity by 2030.

As obese people have a higher percentage of body fat, the primary pharmacokinetic parameter that is affected by obesity is the volume of distribution (V_d). The magnitude of the effect of obesity on V_d depends on the lipophilicity of the drug. For hydrophilic drugs, there could be little change or a slightly increase in V_d, and the body weight normalized V_d (i.e., V_d/kg) is reduced in obese people. For lipophilic drugs, increase in both V_d and V_d/kg is expected. Figure 11-7 describes the impact of obesity on the volume of distribution of a drug characterized by a two-compartment model. In this figure, two cases are presented, with Case A indicating hydrophilic drugs and Case B resembling lipophilic drugs. To further elaborate the impact of obesity on V_d, examples are provided in each case in the subsections 11.3.1 -11.3.3.

Case A: Example of a drug that does not readily distribute into excess adipose tissue, such that the Vd is similar in lean and obese individuals

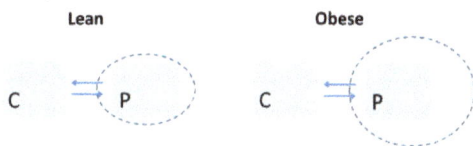

Lean   Obese

C ⇄ P   C ⇄ P

Case B: Example of a drug with extensive distribution into excess adipose tissue, such that the Vd is markedly increased in obese individuals

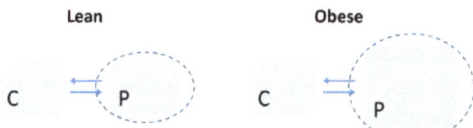

Lean   Obese

C ⇄ P   C ⇄ P

Figure 11-7. Impact of obesity on the volume of distribution of a drug characterized by a two-compartment model. Two scenarios are presented. The dashed circle represents the degree of adiposity. *This figure is adapted from Hanley MJ et al. Clinical Pharmacokinetics 2010; 49(2):71-87.*

11.3.1. Case A, example 1- Cefotaxime

Cefotaxime is a third-generation cephalosporin antibiotic. Figure 11-8 shows the mean concentration-time profiles of cefotaxime in 12 normal (90-110% ideal body weight) and 11 obese (190-210% ideal body weight) individuals following a single dose of 1g cefotaxime. Despite the extreme case of 100% difference in body weight investigated in this study, the concentration-time profiles, and pharmacokinetic parameters between these two groups are comparable. This can be explained by the hydrophilic nature of cefotaxime. The result indicated that very little dose adjustment is needed to treat obese patients with cefotaxime. Obese patients may receive an overdose if using total body weight based dosing approach.

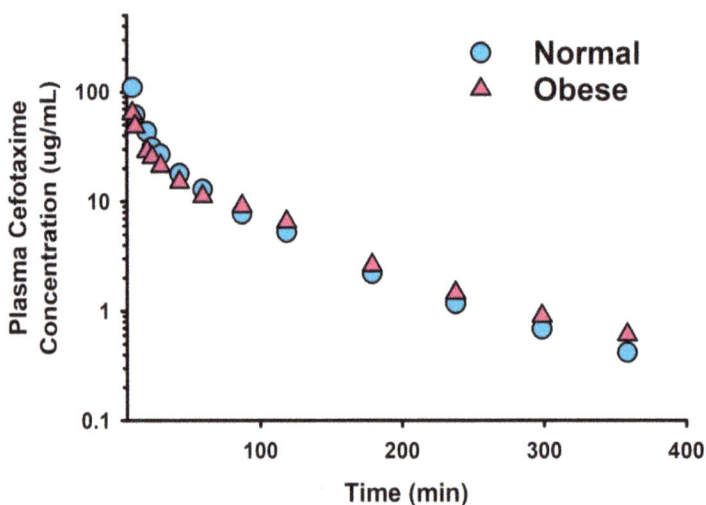

Figure 11-8. Mean concentration-time profiles of cefotaxime in normal (90-110% ideal body weight) and obese (190-210% ideal body weight) following a single dose of 1g cefotaxime. *This figure is adapted from Yost RL and Derendorf H. Therapeutic Drug Monitoring. 1986;8:189-194.*

11.3.2. Case A, example 2- Aminoglycosides

The aminoglycosides, such as gentamicin, tobramycin, amikacin, and kanamycin, are hydrophilic antibiotics commonly used for serious gram-negative infections. Aminoglycosides are very toxic. They are known to cause nephrotoxicity and ototoxicity due to accumulation in the kidney and middle ear, respectively. Aminoglycosides are hydrophilic and they distribute primarily into intravascular space and only moderately into interstitial space (V_d=0.25 L/kg). The clearance, volume of distribution, and half-life of all aminoglycosides are similar.

Aminoglycosides typically display a slightly larger volume of distribution in obese patients than in lean patients. The need for dosing adjustment in obesity has been established in gentamicin, tobramycin, and amikacin. It was found that the uptake of aminoglycosides into excess body mass is about 40% of uptake into lean body mass. Therefore, for obese patients, dosing aminoglycosides using *actual body weight* (or total body weight, TBW) may result in increased drug exposure, leading to an elevated risk for nephrotoxicity and ototoxicity in obese individuals. On the other hand, dosing aminoglycosides for obese patients using *ideal body weight* (IBW) may result in decreased drug concentrations, which may decrease its therapeutic efficacy. To address this issue, *adjusted body weight* (ABW) is usually used when dosing aminoglycosides in obese patients. Adjusted body weight is calculated as below:

$$ABW = IBW + 0.4 \cdot (TBW - IBW) \tag{11-2}$$

11.3.3. Case B, example - Diazepam

Diazepam is used to treat anxiety disorders, alcohol withdrawal, and seizures. It is a lipophilic drug. A study comparing the pharmacokinetics of diazepam between normal weight (mean weight 60 kg) and obese people (mean weight 92 kg) showed that diazepam elimination half-life was significantly prolonged in the obese subjects. Figure 11-9 shows the results from two representative participants, with a $t_{1/2}$ of 99 h in the obese woman and 39 h in the matched control with normal weight. Further data analysis revealed that there was no change in clearance. Instead, a large increase in volume of distribution (228 L in obese participants vs. 70 L in normal weight participants) was the reason for the prolonged terminal half-life in obese participants. This result indicated that during chronic dosing with diazepam, obese patients may experience a much slower onset of maximal drug effect compared to normal weight patients due to the delayed accumulation of diazepam. On the other hand, residual drug effects may persist for a prolonged period in obese patients after discontinuation of the drug.

11.3.4. Dose adjustment

In terms of bodyweight-based dose adjustment, the general rule is that if total body weight (TBW) is less than 20% above ideal body weight (IBW), use TBW. If TBW is more than 20% above IBW, use IBW, adjusted body weight (ABW), lean body weight (LBW) or TBW, depending on the physicochemical properties and individual drug recommendations.

Due to the high prevalence of obesity in the US and worldwide, there is an increased appreciation of the importance of rational drug use in patients with obesity. However, although more studies have been conducted in recent years than

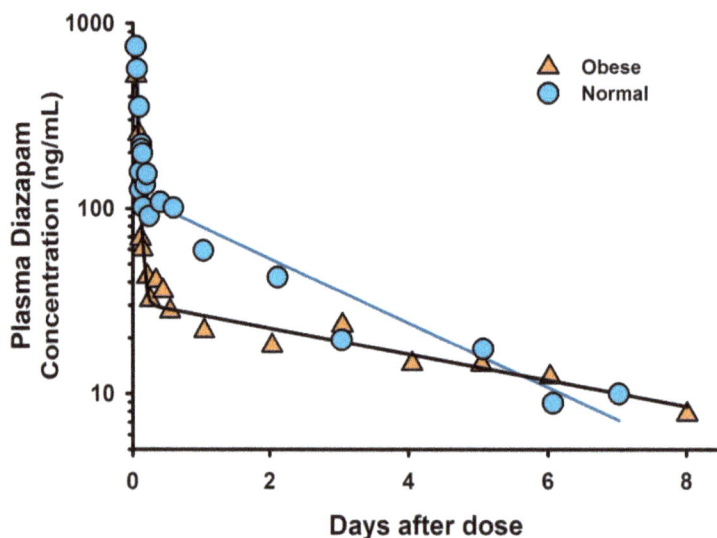

Figure 11-9. Plasma concentration-time profiles of diazepam in an obese woman (triangle) and a matched control female (circle) of normal weight. Both participants received 10 mg diazepam via I.V. injection. *This figure is adapted from Abernethy DR, et al. Journal of Clinical Pharmacology 1983;23:369-376.*

in the past, there is still a lot more to learn and a lot of "holes" to fill. As discussed in a recent review (Apovian CM et al. Current Obesity Reports. 2023), many drugs are difficult to properly administer in people with obesity, and dosing changes for these drugs performed in practice may not be in line with the product labeling. Table 11-1 shows the comparison of dosing recommendations between a critical care textbook and package inserts. It's clear that there is a discrepancy between these recommendations. More research is needed to fill in the gap between what is known about the effects of obesity on drug disposition and the current use of drugs according to drug prescribing information and clinical practice.

Table 11-1. Difference between practical and package insert dosing recommendations. *This table is adapted from Apovian CM et al. Current Obesity Reports. 2023;12:429–438.*

Drug	Recommendation from evidence-based critical care		Package insert dosing recommendation
	Induction	**Maintenance**	
Aminoglycosides	ABW	ABW	Dose calculated on mg/kg of TBW
Aminophylline	IBW	IBW	Loading dose based on IBW, then flat infusion rate based on age
Atracurium	TBW	TBW	Dose calculated based on mg/kg of TBW
B-blockers	IBW	IBW	Fixed dose not based on weight; titrate to effect
Corticosteroids	IBW	IBW	Variable based on disease state
Cyclosporine	IBW	IBW	Dose calculated based on mg/kg of TBW
Digoxin	IBW	IBW	Loading dose calculated using TBW; maintenance dose based on LBW and renal function
Lidocaine	TBW	IBW	Dose calculated based on mg/kg of TBW
Phenytoin	TBW	IBW	Fixed dose not based on weight; titrate to effect
Vancomycin	ABW	ABW	Dose calculated based on mg/kg of TBW and renal function
Vecuronium	IBW	IBW	Dose calculated based on mg/kg of TBW

TBW: total body weight; IBW: ideal body weight; ABW: adjusted body weight

11.4 Patients with Renal Disease

For drugs primarily eliminated by the kidney, when administered to patients with renal impairments, one pharmacokinetic parameter that is affected directly is renal clearance, which is often reduced due to decreased renal excretion. Besides renal excretion, the pathophysiological conditions of renal diseases may affect other pharmacokinetics processes. For example, albumin level often decreases under renal impairment condition, while α-acid glycoprotein may increase when the kidney is injured. Changes in plasma protein levels can affect the fraction of unbound (f_u), subsequently influencing the volume of distribution, clearance, and free drug concentrations. Renal dysfunction may even alter non-renal elimination due to the accumulation of active metabolites and/or endogenous substances.

In Chapter 4, I have discussed the measurement of renal function using the unit nephron hypothesis, the markers for GFR estimation, the advantages and limitations of using creatinine as the marker, the Cockcroft-Gault equation for creatinine clearance (CL_{cr}) estimation, as well as considerations regarding which body weight should be used for CL_{cr} calculation. To avoid redundancy, this information will not be elaborated again in this chapter.

For drugs primarily eliminated through the renal pathway, there is often a good correlation between creatinine clearance and the total clearance of the drug. Cefepime serves as a good example. Figure 11-10 shows the mean plasma concentration-time profiles of cefepime in patients with normal renal function and various degrees of renal insufficiency following 1g dose of cefepime intravenously. As it shows, the more severe the renal impairment, the higher the plasma exposure of cefepime. Further analysis demonstrated a linear correlation between creatinine clearance and cefepime total clearance.

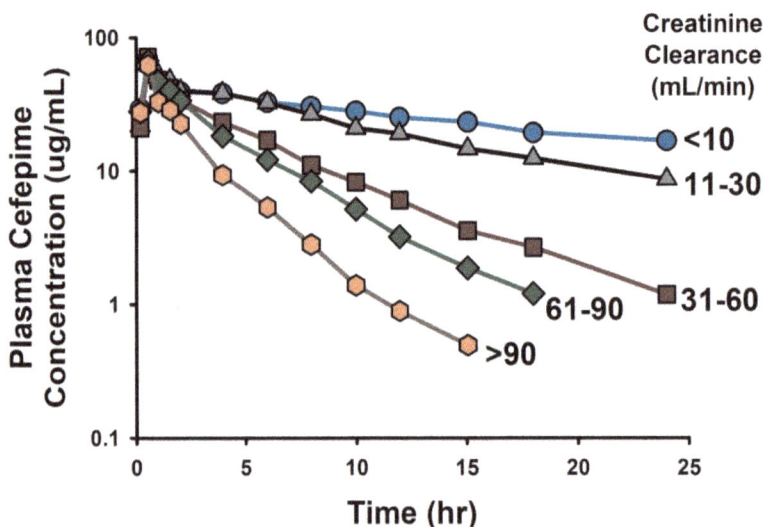

Figure 11-10. Mean plasma concentration-time profiles of cefepime in patients with normal renal function and various degrees of renal impairment. All participants received 1 g I.V. dose of cefepime. *This figure is adapted from Barbhaiya RH, et al. Clin Pharmacol Ther 1990;48:268-276.*

Creatinine serves as a reflection of renal function. The robust correlation between CL_{cr} and total clearance of renally eliminated drugs provide a foundation for CL$_{cr}$-based dose adjustment. The following equation provides an option for dose adjustment in renal impairment:

$$D_{pat} = D_{norm} \cdot [1 - f_e \cdot (1 - RF)$$ [11-3]

Where:

D$_{pat}$ = Dose for patient with renal impairment;

D$_{norm}$ = Dose in patient with normal renal function;

f$_e$ = Fraction of drug excreted into urine;

RF = Renal function, which is expressed as fraction of normal. For example, CLcr of 25 ml/min (20 % of normal) means RF = 0.2.

Another way of adjusting dose in renal impairment is provided below:

Dosing adjustment factor = (Fraction eliminated hepatically) + [(Fraction eliminated renally) · (Fraction of normal renal function)]   [11-4]

For example, drug A is 30% metabolized and 70% renally eliminated. The standard dose regimen is 200 mg every 12 h. Drug A will be administered to a patient who has only 30% of normal renal function. Based on Equation 11-4, the dosing adjustment factor is:

Dosing adjustment factor = 0.3+(0.7·0.3) = 0.51

The dosing adjustment factor of 0.51 indicates that the dose should be reduced to half of standard dose, which could be achieved by using 100 mg every 12 h or 200 mg every 24 h, or by a combination of dose and dosing interval.

Please note that, for the above dose adjustment approaches to be applicable, following conditions have to be met:

- Renal function does not affect the non-renal elimination of the drug;
- Drug metabolites are pharmacologically inactive and do not accumulate in renal insufficiency;
- The pharmacodynamic response to the drug is not altered in renal disease.

11.5 Pregnant Women

Pregnancy is a complex state where changes in maternal physiology may result in changes in ADME processes. Accordingly, dose adjustment may be needed. Many physiological parameters, such as cardiac output, heart rate, plasma volume, hepatic blood flow, renal blood flow, and GFR are significantly increased during pregnancy (Figure 11-11). In addition, the activities of drug metabolizing enzymes have been found to be altered. For example, CYP3A4, CYP2D6, CYP2C9, and UGT1A have demonstrated increased activity, while CYP2C19, CYP1A2, and NAT2 have shown decreased activity.

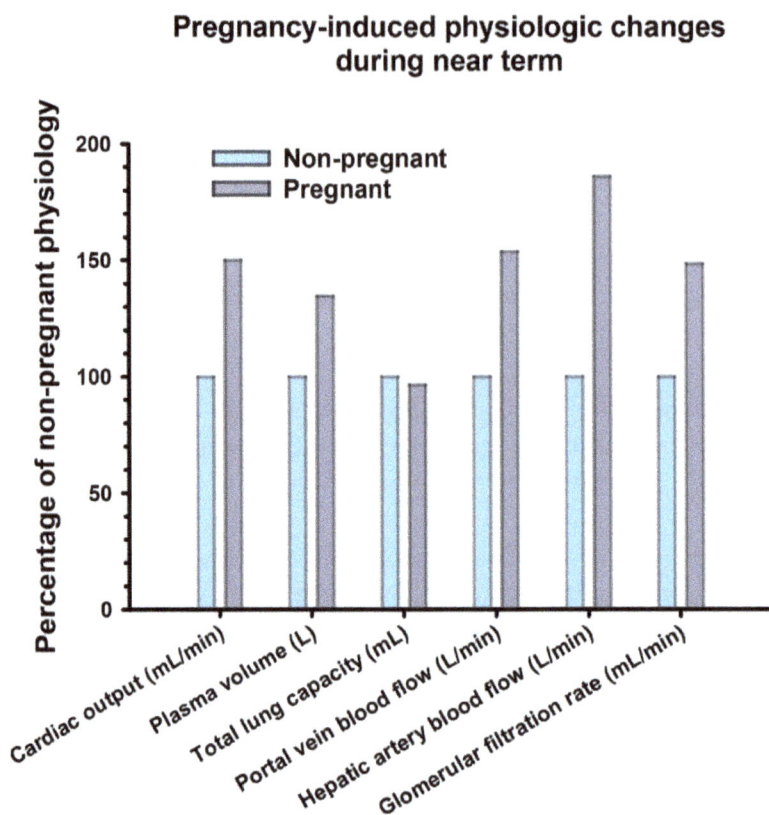

Figure 11-11. Pregnancy-induced physiologic changes during near term. Data are presented as % relative to non-pregnant women. *This figure was made based on information in Feghali M, et al. Semin Perinatol. 2015; 39(7): 512–519.*

The change in activities of drug metabolizing enzymes during pregnancy indicates that the plasma exposure of drugs which are substrates will be altered. As shown in Figure 11-12, midazolam, a CYP3A substrate, demonstrated a lower plasma exposure during pregnancy, which can be explained by increased intestinal and/or hepatic CYP3A and subsequent enhanced first-pass clearance. Amoxicillin is mainly renally eliminated, and its decreased plasma exposure during pregnancy (Figure 11-12, right figure) likely is the result of increased glomerular filtration rate and subsequent increase in renal clearance.

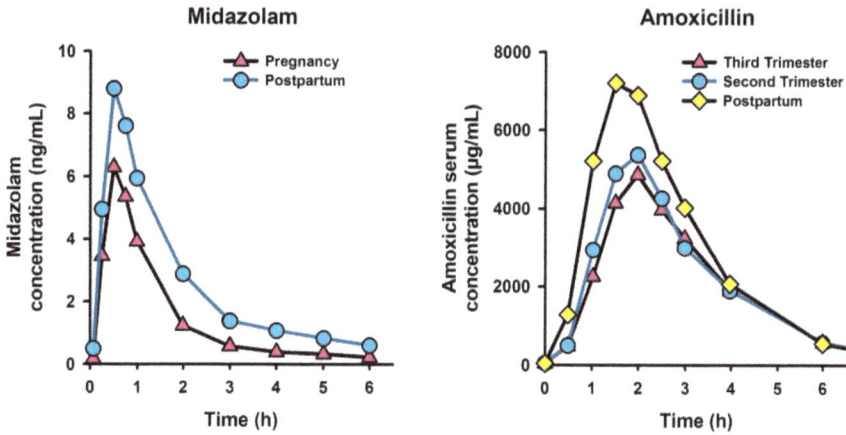

Figure 11-12. Pregnancy-induced changes in pharmacokinetics of midazolam (left) and amoxicillin (right). Mean concentration-time profiles are presented. *Midazolam figure was adapted from Herbet MF, et al. Clin Pharmacol Ther 2008;84(2):248-253. Amoxicillin figure was adapted from Andrew MA et al. Clin Pharmacol Ther 2007;81(4):547-556.*

Key References

Apovian CM, Bruno CD, Kyle TK, Chow CR and Greenblatt DJ (2023) Incomplete Data and Potential Risks of Drugs in People with Obesity. Curr Obes Rep 12:429-438.

Clinical Pharmacokinetics and Pharmacodynamics (2011). The 4th edition. Lippincott Willams & Wilkins, a Wolters Kluwer business.

Feghali M, Venkataramanan R and Caritis S (2015) Pharmacokinetics of drugs in pregnancy. Semin Perinatol 39:512-519.

Hanley MJ, Abernethy DR and Greenblatt DJ (2010) Effect of obesity on the pharmacokinetics of drugs in humans. Clin Pharmacokinet 49:71-87.

Lu H and Rosenbaum S (2014) Developmental pharmacokinetics in pediatric populations. J Pediatr Pharmacol Ther 19:262-276.

van Groen BD, Nicolai J, Kuik AC, Van Cruchten S, van Peer E, Smits A, Schmidt S, de Wildt SN, Allegaert K, De Schaepdrijver L, Annaert P and Badee J (2021) Ontogeny of Hepatic Transporters and Drug-Metabolizing Enzymes in Humans and in Nonclinical Species. Pharmacol Rev 73:597-678.

Winter's Basic Clinical Pharmacokinetics (2018). The 6th edition. Wolters Kluwer.

PART III

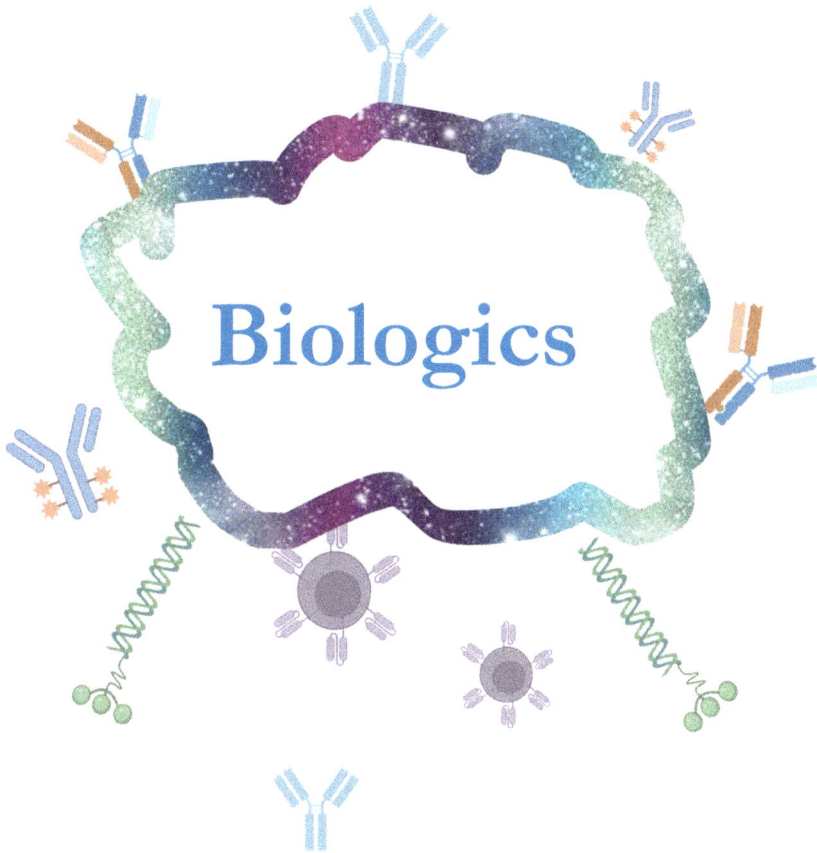

Biologics

Chapter 12.
Introduction to Biologic Medicines

Learning Objectives

After reading this chapter, the reader shall be able to:
1. Get familiar with the history of the development of biologic drugs.
2. Describe several general considerations of the biologics.
3. Describe the differences between small-molecule drugs and biologic products.

So far, I have walked you through Part I (Chapters 1-4) and Part II (Chapters 5-11) of this book, both of which only focus on small-molecule drugs. We all know that small molecule is no longer the only actor in the play – large molecule, including various types of biologic medicines, accounts for more than 30% of all new drugs launched during the last two decades. While most fundamental pharmacokinetics concepts learned in Part I of the book still apply to biologics, there are considerable differences between small-molecule drugs and large-molecule products in terms of mechanism of action, ADME, clinical pharmacology, drug-drug interaction, and safety. It is important to understand these differences and keep them in mind when dealing with the rational use of biologic medicines in clinical practice (if you are a healthcare professional) or the dose regimen selection and clinical trial design of large-molecule compounds in drug development (if you are a researcher in the pharmaceutical industry). The goal of Part III of this book (Chapters 12-16) is to serve as a "primer" on pharmacokinetics, pharmacodynamics, and clinical pharmacology of biologic medicines, especially antibodies (Chapter 13), antibody-drug conjugates (Chapter 14), oligonucleotide products (Chapter 15), and Chimeric antigen receptor (CAR) T-cell therapy (Chapter 16). Prior to discussing these individual drug modalities, I will first provide a basic introduction to biologics in this chapter (i.e., Chapter 12).

Biologics are defined as a large molecule derived from living organisms and used in the treatment, diagnosis, or prevention of disease. Biologics are also called *biotherapeutics* and *large-molecule drugs. In this book, these terms are interchangeable.* Biologics can be composed of sugars, proteins, nucleic acids, or complex combinations of these substances, or they could be living cells or tissues. Biologic medicines include therapeutic proteins, vaccines, blood, blood components, antibodies, cells, genes, tissues, to name some. Biologics has a rich history. I will share a few stories in section 12.1. Several basic considerations of large-molecule drugs, including a summary of the key differences between small-molecule drugs and large-molecule drugs, are covered in section 12.2.

12.1 History of Biologics

Among various types of biologics, blood represents one of the earliest biological products. The first blood transfusion from animal to human was performed in 17th century. Another type of biologic product that was introduced very early on is vaccine. The basis for vaccination began in 1796 by Edward Jenner (Figure 12-1), who used cowpox to inoculate against smallpox and is considered as the founder of modern vaccinology. The Centers of Disease Control and Prevention (CDC) has provided a nice description on Edward Jenner's first immunological experiment. I made a few minor revisions and provided the story below:

{Smallpox was a terrible disease. On average, 3 out of every 10 people who got it died. In 1796, the English doctor Edward Jenner noticed that milkmaids who had gotten cowpox were protected from smallpox. Jenner guessed that exposure to cowpox could be used to protect against smallpox. To test his theory, Dr. Jenner took material from a cowpox sore on milkmaid Sarah Nelmes' hand and inoculated it into the arm of James Phipps, the 9-year-old son of Jenner's gardener. Months later, Jenner exposed Phipps several times to variola virus, but Phipps never developed smallpox. More experiments followed, and, in 1801, Jenner published his treatise "On the Origin of the Vaccine Inoculation." In this work, he summarized his discoveries and expressed hope that "the annihilation of the smallpox, the most dreadful scourge of the human species, must be the final result of this practice.".

Almost two centuries after Jenner hoped that vaccination could annihilate smallpox, the 33 World Health Assembly declared the world free of this disease on May 8, 1980. Many people consider smallpox eradication to be the biggest achievement in international public health.} [https://www.cdc.gov/smallpox/]

It is estimated that smallpox led to 300 million deaths in the 20th century. Cowpox is similar to smallpox but is much less deadly. People infected by cowpox had milder symptoms. After cowpox inoculation, through battling with cowpox, the body learned to recognize smallpox and produced antibodies to eliminate it; this is fundamentally how vaccines function in general.

While vaccines and blood products are highly valuable, they are susceptible to contamination during manufacturing; this is a general issue with biologic medicines. In the early days, there was no regulatory control on biological products. A law on biologics control was finally passed in 1902, and it was triggered by Jim, an ordinary horse who had an extraordinary effect on public health. Following is the story from the FDA website:

{Jim's prominence stemmed from a tragedy in St. Louis in 1901. At that time, the standard treatment for children with diphtheria was an antitoxin serum made from the blood of horses. Jim had produced over 30 quarts of antitoxin in three years, but the horse was destroyed after contracting tetanus. The serum from Jim's

tainted blood was accidentally bottled and used to treat diphtheria patients, causing the death of 13 children. The serum had been manufactured in local establishments with no central or uniform controls in place to ensure potency and purity. Nor were there inspections or testing of the final product.

Around the time of the St. Louis deaths, a similar tragedy occurred in Camden, N.J. Nine children died from tetanus after receiving contaminated smallpox vaccine. Recognizing the critical need for regulatory safeguards, Congress passed the Biologics Control Act in 1902. Also known as the "Virus-Toxin Law," the act gave the government the first control over the processes used to make biological products, or biologics, and the responsibility to ensure their safety for the American public.} *[By Linda Bren; FDA Consumer magazine, Centennial Edition (Jan.-Feb. 2006)]*

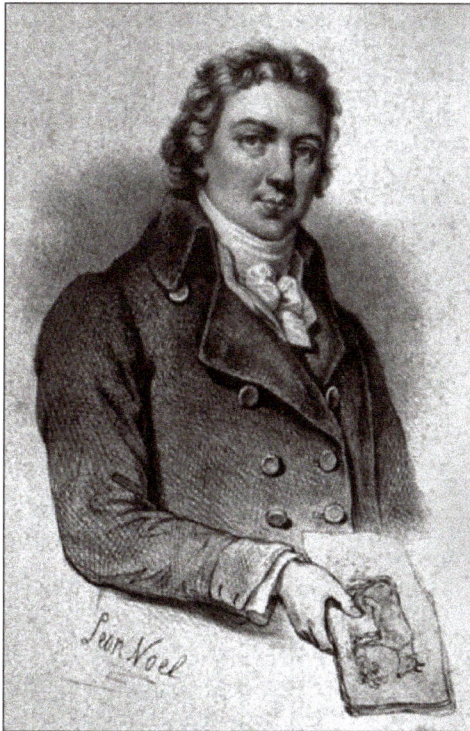

Figure 12-1. Edward Jenner, the founder of modern vaccinology. Photo courtesy of the National Library of medicine.

In addition to blood products and vaccines, the next biologic product available in the clinic was insulin. In 1910, researchers had figured out that diabetes resulted from the lack of insulin. The challenge was to find a way to extract insulin from the pancreas prior to its destruction. In 1921, Frederick Banting successfully established an experimental procedure which could destroy the trypsin-secreting cells but not the insulin. In 1922, the first ever injection of insulin was given to a 14-year-old boy who was dying from diabetes, and within 24 h, that boy's dangerously high blood glucose levels dropped to near normal levels. The news about insulin spread around the world like wildfire. Frederick Banting was awarded the 1923 Nobel Prize in Physiology or Medicine for his groundbreaking work.

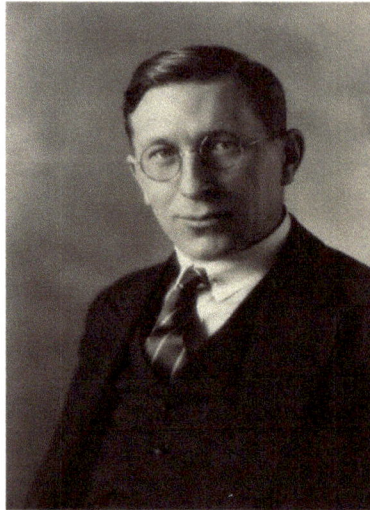

Figure 12-2. Frederick Banting. From Wikipedia

Cattles and pigs were the primary commercial sources of insulin for several decades before human insulin derived from recombinant DNA was made in 1982. Human insulin represents the first human protein therapeutic. Three years later, recombinant human erythropoietin (rHuEPO) was approved in 1985. In 1986, the first licensed antibody, namely Orthoclone OKT3® (muromonab-CD3) was available in the market, and its production was based on the Nobel-winning work of Kohler and Milstein on murine hybridoma technology. Since then, the development of biologic medicines has been accelerated thanks to further advances in molecular biology as well as giant technology leaps. To date, almost 300 biologic medicines, covering several different modalities, have been brought to the market. There are several common features among these biologic products; this is elaborated in the next section.

12.2 General Considerations of Biotherapeutics

Size: Small-molecule drugs typically consist of 20-100 atoms and their molecular weight (MW) is usually less than 1000 Dalton (Da). In contrast, biologics are considerably larger, often 100 to 1000 times their size. The upper panel of Figure 12-3 provides a size comparison using examples of aspirin, a small molecule composed of 21 atoms (MW=180 Da); filgrastim, a small biological drug composed of approximately 2700 atoms (MW=18,802 Da); and IgG antibody, a large biological drug consisting of more than 20,000 atoms (MW $\approx$ 150,000 Da).

Complexity: In addition to size, large molecule drugs exhibit greater structural complexity. Small molecule drugs are relatively simple chemical compounds that can be synthesized by chemical reactions. In contrast, biotherapeutics are extracted from genetically engineering living organisms or cells through complex and lengthy purification processes. The lower panel of Figure 12-3 uses objects (bicycle, car, and airplane) to reflect the size and complexity of the example drugs (aspirin, filgrastim, and antibody).

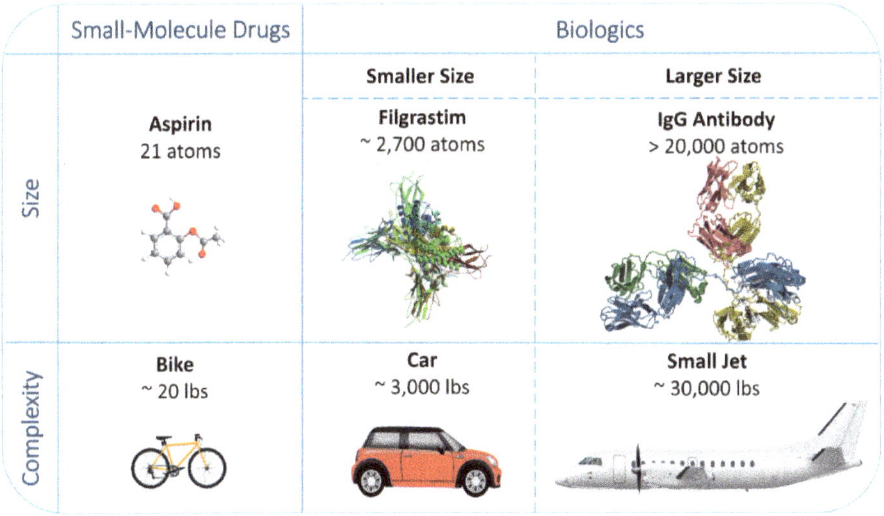

Figure 12-3. The differences in size and complexity between small-molecule and large-molecule drugs.

Immunogenicity: The immune system functions as a safeguard and protects our body from invaders. Due to their small size, small-molecule drugs usually enter the body without being noticed by the immune system. The situation is different for biologics. Because biologics have large sizes, they are often recognized by the immune system, marked as "foreigners", and then attacked by the antibodies produced by the body. This process is known as *immunogenicity*, which is also defined as the ability of a foreign substance to provoke an immune response in the body of a human or other animal. Immunogenicity against biotherapeutics is considered an undesirable physiological response. All biologics have the potential to trigger immunogenicity, and the incidence is often unpredictable. In practice, immunogenicity in the clinic is assessed by the detection of Anti-Drug Antibody (ADA).

There are different types of ADAs. Some ADAs have no harmful effect. Some ADAs bind and inactivate the biologic product administered, leading to disease progression. Some other ADAs can bind and inactivate both the administered biologics and endogenous protein, which may cause severe side effects. One such example is EPREX (Epoetin alfa made by Johnson & Jonson), a product that had been marketed for a decade without immunogenicity issues. Based on the request from the European Health Authorities, Johnson & Johnson made a change in the manufacturing procedure for EPREX, which caused severe side effects in a small number of patients. The ADA generated in these patients inactivated both EPREX and endogenous erythropoietin. As a result, these patients permanently lost their ability to make red blood cells and had to receive regular blood transfusions.

Manufacturing process: The manufacture of biologics is more difficult and more complicated than that in use to produce small-molecule drugs. Biologic medicines are extracted from genetically modified cell lines through complex and lengthy purification processes. Each of the numerous steps in the manufacturing process requires precise technique. It is important to use the same steps, same cell line, same equipment, and same conditions (e.g. temperature, pH, culture medium, raw materials, etc.) because even minor differences in production processes can generate variations in the resulting protein drug, leading to immunogenicity or reduced efficiency. The EPREX case example mentioned earlier clearly demonstrated that biotherapeutics are highly sensitive to their manufacturing and handing conditions.

In addition, compared to small molecule drugs, biologic products are easier to be contaminated during manufacturing; the horse Jim story reported above is an example of this issue. Because of the highly complex manufacturing process and the high susceptibility to contamination during manufacturing, quality control is extremely important for biologic medicines.

Biosimilar: In the small molecule arena, a generic drug is an *exact copy* of the innovator drug (Figure 12-4, upper). Small-molecule generics contain the identical chemical composition of the innovator products, although they may differ in excipient such as binders or fillers. Small-molecule generics are considered bioequivalent to their brand-name counterparts. Upon approval, small-molecule generics are automatically deemed interchangeable with the brand-name medication, which means that they can be substituted for the original products without consulting the prescribers.

The situation is different for biotherapeutics. As noted earlier, a minor change in the manufacturing process can lead to variations in the resulting biologic product. As commented in an article published in Nature - "Living cells may chemically modify the proteins they make by adding complex sugars and other compounds at certain positions. The exact conditions under which cells are grown can alter the pattern of these modifications, and thus the molecule's structure and behavior." (Ledford, 2015). As the manufacturing process of the innovator product is protected by patent, it is nearly impossible to replicate any product. Therefore, the biologics made by generic companies are only similar (NOT identical) to the innovator biologic products; that's why the products are called *biosimilars*. Different from small-molecule generics, biosimilars are *inexact copies* of the original biologic products (Figure 12-4, lower).

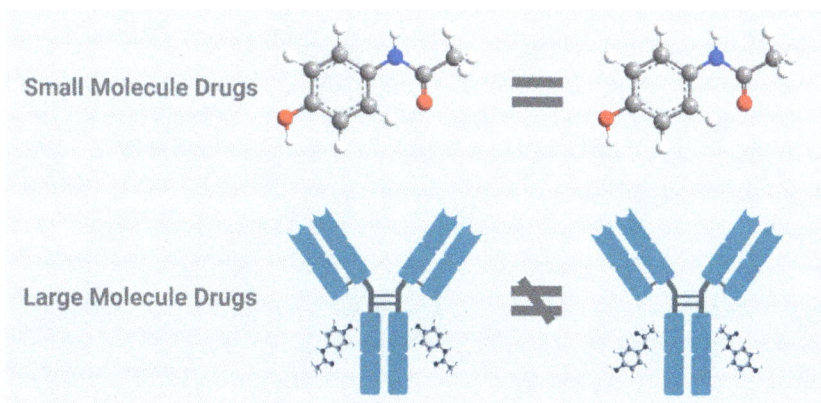

Figure 12-4. Illustration of the differences between small molecules and large molecules in terms of reproducibility and interchangeability.

Like snowflakes, biosimilars from different manufacturers differ from their originator biologic products and from each other; this fact is illustrated in Figure 12-5. Among the biosimilars approved so far, most of them are not interchangeable, which means that auto-substitution is not allowed. Up to now, only a few interchangeable biosimilars have been approved. As explained by the FDA- "An interchangeable biosimilar is a biosimilar that meets additional requirements outlined by the law that allows for the FDA to approve biosimilar and interchangeable biosimilar medications. An interchangeable biosimilar product may be substituted for the original product without consulting the prescriber, much like how generic drugs are routinely substituted for brand name drugs. This is commonly called pharmacy-level substitution and is subject to state pharmacy laws."

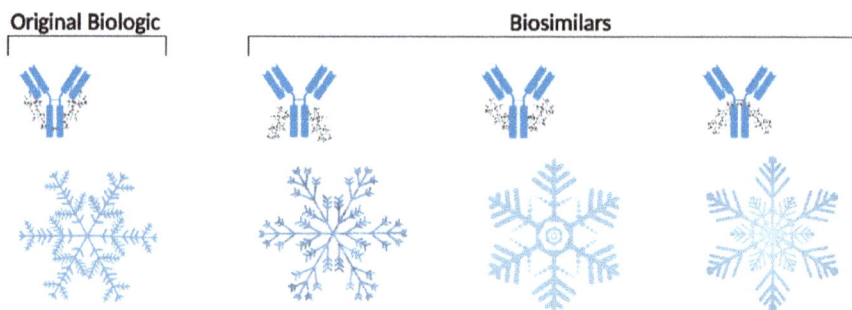

Similar to snowflakes, biosimilars from different manufacturers differ not only from their originator biologic medicines but also from each other.

Figure 12-5. Illustration of the differences between original biologics and biosimilars. Similar to snowflakes, biosimilars from different manufacturers differ from their originator biologic products and from each other.

**ADME**: As biotherapeutics are susceptible to rapid breakdown and digestion by gastrointestinal proteases/enzymes, they are not given orally. The common routes of administration are intravenous (I.V.) and subcutaneous (S.C.) injections. When biotherapeutics are given via S.C. administration, absorption is often a slow process because they travel in the lymphatic system, and lymphatic flow is known to be much slower than the blood flow. Regarding distribution, most biologic medicines have a limited volume of distribution due to their large size. In terms of metabolism, biologics are catabolized to endogenous amino acids (e.g., protein drugs) or nucleic acids (e.g., oligonucleotides products), which is fundamentally different from small molecules that are usually metabolized by drug metabolizing enzymes (e.g., CYP450s) present in the liver. For large biologics such as antibodies, there is minimal renal excretion because their size is bigger than the pores of glomerulus and therefore cannot be filtered by the kidney. For smaller biotherapeutics (e.g., peptides), extensive renal clearance can happen. Most small-molecule drugs demonstrate linear pharmacokinetics with short half-lives (e.g., in hours). In contrast, large-molecule drugs often have nonlinear pharmacokinetics with long half-lives (e.g., days or weeks for antibody drugs).

Summary of the characteristics of small molecules versus large molecules.

Table 12-1 compares the characteristics of small molecules and large molecules. Most of the information in the table has already been described in the above subsections and will not be elaborated on again. As mentioned at the beginning of this chapter, there are many different types of biotherapeutics, among which the largest and fastest growing one is antibody drugs; this will be the topic of the next chapter.

Table 12-1. Characteristics of Small Molecules Versus Large Molecules

	Small-molecule drugs	**Biologic Medicines**
Molecular Size	Small	Large
Method of Synthesis	Chemical reaction	Genetically engineering living organisms or cells
Structure	Usually fully known	Complex, frequently partially unknown
Sensitivity to physical environment (heat, light)	Low	Higher
Species	Interdependent	Specific
Susceptibility to contamination during manufacturing	Low	High
Manufacturing process	Relatively simple	Highly complex
Immunogenicity	Non antigenic	Usually antigenic
ADME		
Absorption	Faster	Slower
Distribution	Larger volume of distribution	Usually low/limited volume of distribution
Metabolism	Metabolized to inactive and active metabolites by the liver	Catabolized to endogenous amino acids (for protein drugs) or nucleic acids (for oligonucleotides products)
Excretion	Excreted as unchanged drug by the kidney (urine excretion) or the liver (biliary excretion)	Usually too big to be filtered by the glomerulus.
Pharmacokinetics profile	Frequently linear. The disposition is rarely target-mediated. Half-life is short(er)	Often non-linear. The disposition is often target-mediated. Half-life is usually longer
Safety	Toxicity (variable mechanisms)	Exaggerated pharmacology
Generic products	Bioequivalent; usually interchangeable	Biosimilar; usually not interchangeable

Key References

Kristina M. Lybecker. The biologics revolution in the production of Drugs. Fraserinstitute.org 2016.

Linda Bren (2006) The road to the biotech revolution - highlights of 100 years of biologics regulation. FDA Consumer magazine, Centennial Edition (Jan.-Feb. 2006).

CDC. History of Smallpox. https://www.cdc.gov/smallpox/

Ledford, Heidi (2015). First biosimilar drug set to enter US market. Nature 517 (January 15): 253-254.

Chapter 13.
Antibody Drugs

Learning Objectives

Learning Objectives

After reading this chapter, the reader shall be able to:

1. Be familiar with the history of development of therapeutic antibodies.

2. Describe the role of physiological antibodies.

3. List the different types of therapeutic antibodies.

4. Describe the various modes of actions of therapeutic antibodies.

5. Describe the ADME of antibody drugs and understand the difference in pharmacokinetics between therapeutic antibodies and small-molecule drugs.

6. Describe the mechanism of antibody-drug interactions.

7. List the common adverse effects of therapeutic antibodies. Understand of mechanism of immunogenicity and cytokine release syndrome.

Among different biological therapeutic modalities, antibodies represent the largest and fastest growing one, with more than 100 monoclonal antibody (mAb) drugs approved in the United States and/or European Union. The extent to which therapeutic antibodies have transformed healthcare can never be overstated. The development of antibody-based therapies has a long history. I will share several key events in section 13.1. Then I will provide a brief overview of the immune system and physiological antibodies (section 13.2) before I walk you through different types of therapeutic antibodies (section 13.3). Therapeutic antibodies exhibit their effects via many different modes of actions, which are elaborated in section 13.4. Antibody drugs have substantially different ADME properties compared with small-molecule drugs. The clinical pharmacology aspects of antibodies, including ADME, drug-drug interaction (DDI), and safety will be covered in section 13.5.

13.1 History

"Though many lay unburied, birds and beasts would not touch them, or died after tasting them... The bodies of dying men lay one upon the other... [But] those who had recovered from the disease... had now no fear for themselves; for the same man was never attacked twice-never at least fatally." - Thucydides, History of the Peloponnesian War, 431-428 B.C. [Quoted in Masopust et al. Eur. J. Immunol. 2007; 37:S103-110]

The above information described the outbreak of plague at Athens, and it was written by the great historian Thucydides almost 2500 years ago. For many centuries, keen observers of epidemic diseases, such as Thucydides for plague, noticed that individuals who survived the disease remained unharmed the next time the same disease passed their way. This observation laid the foundation for some of the earliest interventions against smallpox, such as taking material from the pustules of infected individuals and injecting it into healthy individuals so that the latter had "no fear" when the disease attacked them. The way Edward Jenner used cowpox to inoculate against smallpox was based on the same rationale (see Chapter 12 for more detailed information). It is impressive that all these early interventions/treatments were done with little understanding of how the human immune system worked.

In 1890s, Emil von Behring worked with Shibasaburo Kitasato on a number of important experiments, and the results showed that the serum from animals infected with tetanus or diphtheria could give immunity to other animals previously not exposed to these diseases (Figure 13-1). In collaboration with Paul Ehrlich, von Behring developed a diphtheria antitoxin for humans which was first used on Christmas Eve in 1891. In the next year, a significant decrease in mortality from diphtheria was observed, with the death rate dropped from 48% to 13% in Berlin children's hospitals. von Behring was considered as one of the founders of immunology and was the recipient of the first Nobel Prize in Physiology or Medicine awarded in 1901.

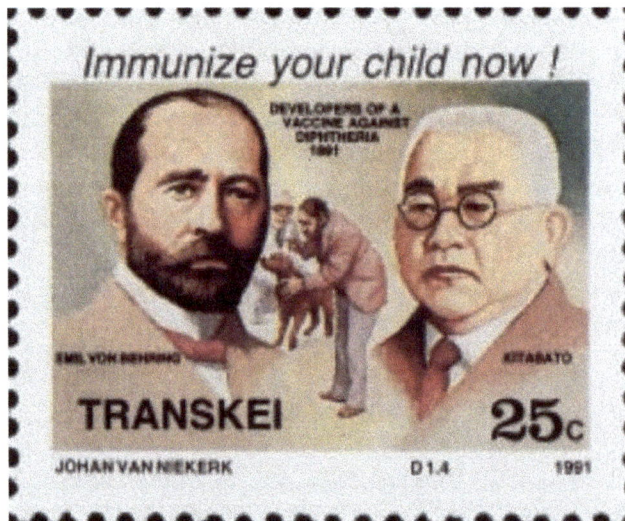

Figure 13-1. Emil von Behring and Shibasaburo Kitasato were honored philatelically on a stamp issued by Transkei in 1991. *Reprint with permission from BMJ Publishing Group Ltd.*

Following von Behring's work, Paul Ehrlich identified that the power of protection in serum came from antibodies. He raised the concept of "magic bullets" and hypothesized that antibodies could be used in a day as magic bullets for medicine. Since then, researchers began hunting for a means to isolate and purify desired antibodies. Purifying individual antibodies from the billions produced by the body was not an easy task. The earliest antibodies were produced by immunizing animals with an antigen and subsequently harvesting the antibody fraction from their serum. However, antibodies produced from such experiments were a mixture of antibodies produced from different B-lymphocytes, which are known as polyclonal antibodies. The drawback of polyclonal antibodies is the heterogeneity in specificity and affinity. Later, a method to create monoclonal antibodies was developed, where a single plasma cell clone was isolated to generate a homogenous antibody, then proliferated by repeated passage of spleen cells into irradiated syngeneic mice. However, this method had the limitations of low antibody yield and short cell lifespan, which precluded large-scale production.

The inability to produce large quantity of individual antibodies with known specificity was a key issue restricting the whole field for many years. This problem was solved by Cesar Milstein and George Köhler in 1975. In a 3-page report published at Nature in 1975, Milstein and Köhler described the hybridoma technique, where antibody producing cells were fused with tumor cells, resulting in immortalized cells that can produce unlimited monoclonal antibodies with predefined specificity. The hybridoma technique not only revolutionized biomedical research and diagnostics, but also opened new doors for treatment of diseases. Milstein and Köhler were the recipients of the Nobel Prize in Physiology or Medicine in 1984 for their groundbreaking work. Based on hybridoma technology, the first licensed monoclonal antibody, namely Orthoclone OKT3® (muromonab-CD3), was made available in the market. Since then, the therapeutic antibody drug market has experienced explosive growth. Currently, various types of monoclonal antibodies are available on the market (see section 13.3 for more detailed information).

13.2 Human Immune System and Physiological Antibodies

13.2.1 Brief overview of human immune system

The major function of the immune system is to defend the body by identifying and removing invaders, such as bacteria, viruses, and other pathogens. The immune system has two fundamental lines of defense: *innate immunity* and *adaptive immunity*. The innate immune system represents the first line of defense against invading pathogens, and its response is immediate, non-specific, relatively weak, and short-lasting. In contrast, the adaptive immune response takes days or weeks to become established, and it is powerful, more specific to pathogens and has a long-lasting effect.

The adaptive immune responses include two types: *the cellular immune response,* which is carried out by T lymphocytes (T cells), and *the humoral immune response,* which is mediated by B lymphocytes (B cells) and antibodies. T cells, once activated, can directly kill infected cells by apoptosis (e.g. cytotoxic T cells) or help other cells to fight the infected cells (e.g. helper T cells). For B cells, once activated, most of them turn into plasma cells, which actively secrete antibodies. A small percentage of the activated B cells become memory cells. Unlike plasma cells, memory B cells are not fighters. Instead, they remember the invader so that the immune system recognizes it and quickly mounts a defense when the same pathogen enters the body again.

The scene of plague outbreak documented by Thucydides, a mystery that had remained for many centuries, can be easily explained once we understand how the immune system works. Plague is caused by the bacterium *Yersinia pestis*, and there are different types of plagues. Although we won't know the exact type, apparently the one that occurred at Athens was a fatal and contagious form of plague. In that event, people who were exposed to *Yersinia pestis* for the first time only had the innate immune system fighting against the bacteria during the first several days. *Yersinia pestis* caused fatal damage to the body, and many people died (*"the bodies of dying men lay one upon the other"*) before their adaptive immune system could build a customized defense to fight the bacterium. Some people survived because their adaptive immune system kicked in (before they were killed) and eliminated *Yersinia pestis* using antibodies that were specifically against this pathogen. In these survivors' bodies, there were memory B cells hanging around for years; these memory cells remembered *Yersinia pestis* and had the ability to identify, fight, and destroy it when *Yersinia pestis* entered their body again. That is why *"[But] those who had recovered from the disease... had now no fear for themselves; for the same man was never attacked twice-never at least fatally."*.

The fighting occurs in a similar way between the human body and smallpox, an acute contagious disease caused by the variola virus, and many other pathogens. Vaccination is a smart strategy that leverages the adaptive immune system. Vaccines contain weakened or inactive parts of a particular pathogen that trigger an immune response, including the adaptive immune response, within the body. The memory lymphocytes generated can quickly mount a defense to avoid a full-blown infection whenever the targeted pathogen reenters the body.

Since memory cells can last for many years, you may wonder why many people still get COVID-19 after vaccination or why we are recommended to be vaccinated against influenza every year. This is because both SARS-CoV-2 (i.e., the virus causing COVID-19) and influenza viruses are RNA viruses which are characterized by high mutation rates. Remember that both B cells and T cells are very specific to the pathogen that they battle with. After many rounds of mutation, the RNA virus is no longer the same virus that the adaptive immune system recognized originally. So, it is not because our adaptive immune system failed to do its job, it is because the RNA virus is too fickle.

13.2.2 Classes of physiological antibodies

Under physiological conditions, B lymphocytes in the body fight against pathogens by generating antibodies, which are also called immunoglobulins (Ig). Based on their configuration and function, antibodies can be divided into 5 classes: IgA, IgD, IgE, IgG, and IgM. It's hard to memorize the names of these 5 immunoglobulins. Dr. Brianne Baker shared her immunology course on YouTube. To help students memorize the names of these immunoglobulins, she suggested using the initials of the following words "**MD**s **G**ive **E**veryone **A**pples", which is rephrased from the aphorism "An apple a day keeps the doctor away". I came up with a different method, which will likely work equally well for people in the pharmacokinetics field. Among these 5 classes, IgG is the most important one, and the therapeutic antibody field is currently dominated by IgG-based mAbs. So, let's remember IgG first. The rest four classes can be arranged to the sequence of Ig**A**, Ig**D**, Ig**M**, Ig**E** – ADME, which is an abbreviation that is used extensively in pharmacokinetics. Table 13-1 lists the features and properties of the 5 different classes of immunoglobulins.

Immunoglobulins A, D, M, and E

- IgA is the second most abundant natural antibody in the body, accounting for approximately 15% of all immunoglobulins. IgA antibodies are found in mucous membranes, especially in the respiratory and digestive tracts, and play a central role in defending mucosal surfaces against attack by infectious microorganisms. The normal range of the serum concentration of IgA in adults is 0.5-3.2 mg/mL. Elevated IgA levels may indicate an underlying infection and inflammation.

- IgD represents about 0.25% of the total serum immunoglobulins and has a half-life of approximately 3 days. IgD is found on B cells during certain stages of maturation. The serum concentration of IgD is low (<0.04 mg/mL). Increased or decreased levels of IgD appear to have no clinical value, as there is no clear correlation between changes in IgD levels and diseases.

- IgM represents the first antibody that the body makes in response to a new infection. IgM is the largest antibody – it can be constructed with five units (i.e., pentamers) or six units (i.e., hexamers). In general, IgM pentamers occur more often than hexamers. Due to its large size, IgM can not diffuse well and is mainly confined to blood and lymph fluids. Owing to its large size, IgM has excellent binding avidity. As a result, IgM can pick up trace amounts of infection to mark for recognition by phagocytes.

- IgE has the lowest quantity and accounts for only 0.002% of total immunoglobulins. The serum concentration of IgE usually is less than 0.0006 mg/mL. IgE is an important antibody - it is responsible for 90% of allergic reactions. IgE also plays an important role in fighting against parasites, especially helminths and some protozoa. Elevated IgE level occurs when the body overreacts to allergens, or when the body is fighting an infection from a parasite or some immune system conditions.

Table 13-1. Properties of the five different classes of immunoglobulins.

Class	Subclass	Molecular form and MW [kDa]	Structure	Serum Concentration (mg/mL)	Proportion of total Ig (%)	Serum half-life (days)
IgG	IgG1	Monomer : 150		9.5-12.5	75	21
	IgG2					21
	IgG3					7
	IgG4					21
IgA	IgA1	Monomer : 160		0.5-3.2	15	6
	IgA2	Secretory Dimer:385				
IgD	IgD	Monomer : 180		<0.04	0.25	3
IgM	IgM	Pentamer : 900 Hexamer: 1050		0.7-1.7	7	5
IgE	IgE	Monomer : 190		<0.0006	0.002	3

Immunoglobulin G

IgG is the predominant antibody in the body and accounts for 75% of all immunoglobulins. The serum concentration of IgG is around 9.5-12.5 mg/mL. IgG represents the most important class of immunoglobulins, and most antibody drugs are IgG-based therapy. It has a powerful ability to bind pathogens and toxins and plays a vital role in biological defense. When an individual is exposed to an unknown pathogen for the first time, it takes two to three weeks to generate IgG that is specific to the pathogen (primary response). If the same pathogen enters the body for a second time, IgG will be produced more rapidly and in a larger quantity to get rid of the pathogen (secondary response).

Compared to other classes, IgG antibodies have the lowest molecular mass and are found in all body fluids. It is also the only class of immunoglobulin that is capable of crossing the placental barrier to provide protection to the fetus. The primary immunoglobulin of the newborn is the maternal IgG, which is lost about 3 months after birth due to catabolism.

IgG has four subclasses, namely IgG1, IgG2, IgG3, and IgG4, with a proportion of 70:20:7:3. Compared to other classes, IgG has the longest half-life (21 days), except for IgG3 (7 days). The factor responsible for the extraordinarily long half-lives of IgG1, IgG2, and IgG4 is Fc receptor of neonates (FcRn). It was named FcRn because it was originally discovered during the investigation of antibody absorption in the gastrointestinal tract of neonates (i.e., maternal transfer of IgG to neonates). FcRn represents one of the primary determinants of IgG disposition in mammals. As shown in Figure 13-2, IgG was cleared much faster in FcRn deficient mice, resulting in much lower serum IgG concentrations.

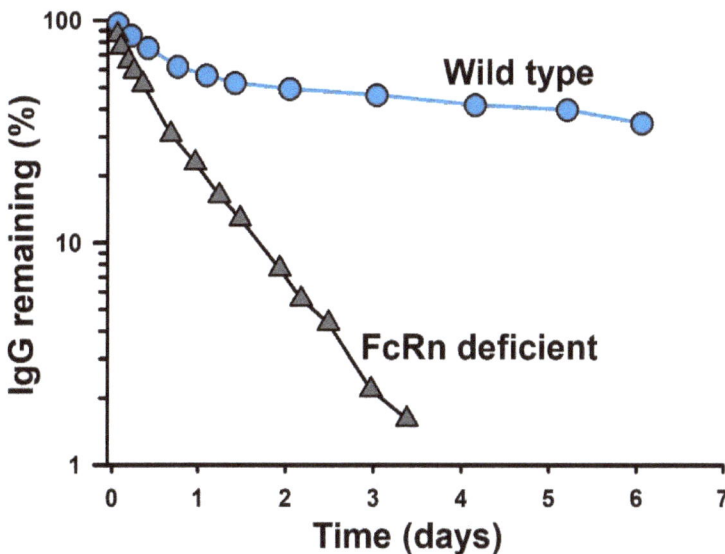

Figure 13-2. Concentration-time profile of IgG in wild-type mice and FcRn deficient mice. *This figure is adapted from Junghans and Anderson, Proc. Natl. Acad. Sci. 1996; 93:5512-5516.*

The proposed mechanism of FcRn protection is shown in Figure 13-3. FcRn is pH dependent and has high affinity at low pH (e.g. pH $\leq$6) and virtually no affinity at pH 7.4. IgG antibodies enter a cell by receptor-mediated endocytosis (i.e., pinocytosis). After pinocytotic vesicles fuse with acidic endosomes, pH drops, and FcRn can bind IgG. Excess unbound IgG antibodies enter the lysosome and are degraded. The intact IgG bound to FcRn is retained and transported to the cell membrane. Due to the increase in pH, IgG-FcRn complexes dissociate, and IgG antibodies are released to the cell surface by exocytosis. Because of the protection of FcRn, the residence time of intact IgG antibodies in the body is prolonged.

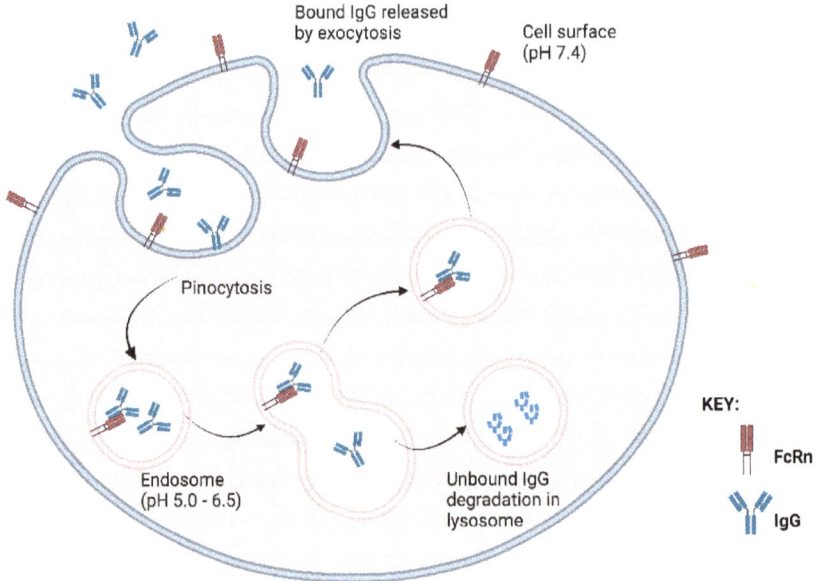

Figure 13-3. Protection of IgG from degradation by FcRn. IgG is ingested by receptor-mediated endocytosis (i.e.,pinocytosis). Pinocytotic vesicles fuse with acidic endosomes in which FcRn can bind IgG. Excess unbound IgG and other proteins enter the lysosome and are degraded thereafter. IgG bound to FcRn is retained and released by exocytosis. *This figure is adapted from Patel and Bussel. J Allergy Clin Immunol 2020;146:467-78.*

13.2.3 Structure of antibodies

Natural antibodies are commonly presented as monomers, which consist of two identical heavy and long chains (H-chains) and two identical light and short chains (L-chains). These chains are held together by disulfide bridges, forming a Y-shaped structure (Figure 13-4). There are five types of mammalian H-chains denoted by Greek letters: α, δ, μ, ε, and γ, which are found in IgA, IgD, IgM, IgE, and IgG antibodies, respectively. Different classes and subclasses of human immunoglobulins are distinguished by the type of heavy chain they contain, along with variations in the number and localization of disulfide bridges, as well as the glycosylation pattern.

As shown in Figure 13-4, The antibody includes a Fc region, which is referred to as "fragment crystallizable", and a Fab region, which is referred to as "fragment of antigen-binding". Pathogens and toxins that bind to antibodies are called *antigens*. Therefore, the Fab region represents the portion of antibody that interacts with the invaders. At the end of the Fab region, there is a variable domain (V), while the Fc region and the rest of the Fab region form constant domains (C). Within the variable domain, there are hypervariable sequences of amino acids known as complementarity-determining regions (CDR), which are responsible for the enormous diversity of antibodies. The specific portion of the antigen that is contacted by the antibody is called *epitope*. Antibodies recognize specific antigens through the interaction between CDR of the variable domain and the epitope of the antigen.

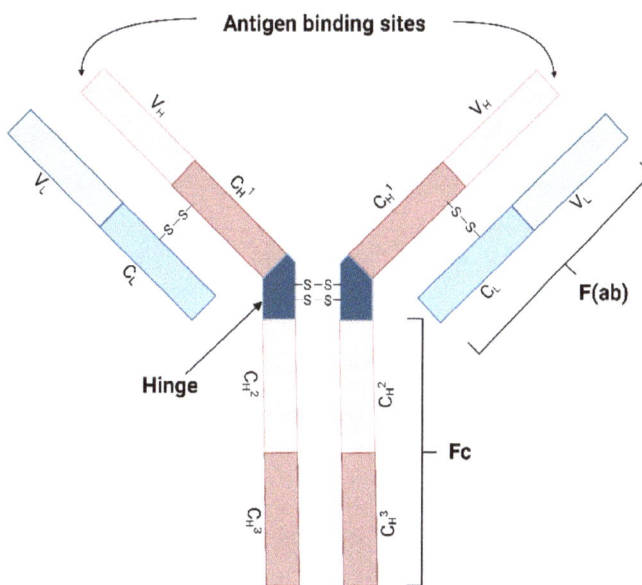

Figure 13-4. Antibody structure. The Y-shaped antibody is joined in the middle by a flexible hinge region. Antigen binding occurs at the variable domain (V), consisting of immunoglobulin heavy (H) and light chains (L). For illustration purpose, H-chains are colored in orange and L-chains are colored in blue. The base of the antibody includes constant domains (C). V_H – heavy chain variable domain, V_L- light chain variable domain, C_H – heavy chain constant domain, C_L – light chain constant domain.

13.3 Therapeutic Antibodies

Different from vaccines which stimulate the body to produce its own antibodies, therapeutic antibodies are directly administered to the body as drugs. Most antibody drugs currently on the market are therapeutic IgGs. Therapeutic antibodies can be broadly divided into two classes: polyclonal and monoclonal antibody drugs. mAbs are much more important in drug development due to their high specificity and other favorable properties compared to polyclonal antibodies. Many top-selling drugs in the pharmaceutical market are mAbs. In this section, I will only focus on mAbs.

As mentioned in section 13.1, the large-scale production of mAbs was made possible by the Nobel Prize-winning research of Kohler and Milstein on murine hybridoma technology. The procedure of the hybridoma method is shown in Figure 13-5.

The first step is to challenge an animal with a specific antigen, which subsequently triggers the immune reaction. As a result, B cells proliferate and secrete antibodies, which react with the antigen and accumulate in the spleen. Then B cells are isolated from the animal's spleen and fused with a malignant myeloma cell line to generate an immortalized cell line, a so called "hybridoma cell". The hybridoma cell inherits the ability of the B cell to produce a specific antibody and the capability of the myeloma cell to replicate indefinitely. After further testing, the hybridoma cell producing antibodies with predefined affinity is selected for further cloning to produce mAbs. As the selected hybridoma cells are from a single parent B cell, they are extremely specific because they recognize only a single epitope of an antigen. This remarkable specificity leads to low batch-to-batch variability and low cross-reactivity.

Murine mAbs: As the name suggests, these are antibodies of murine origin. The first licensed mAbs, muromonab-CD3, is a murine mAb. As shown in Figure 13-6, due to its non-human origin, murine mAbs have high incidence of immunogenicity which leads to the formation of the antibody against the administered therapeutic mAbs.

Chimeric mAbs: Based on recombinant gene technology, some of the limitations of murine mAbs are addressed by transferring the variable domain of a murine antibody to the constant domain of a human antibody, resulting in chimeric mAbs. According to Greek mythology, Chimera is a hybrid creature composed of different animal parts. The name "chimeric mAbs" nicely captures the feature of the mixed structure of mAbs. Although the murine part of mAbs is substantially reduced, immunogenicity still occurs, albeit with a lower incidence (Figure 13-6). Example chimeric mAbs include rituximab (approved in 1997).

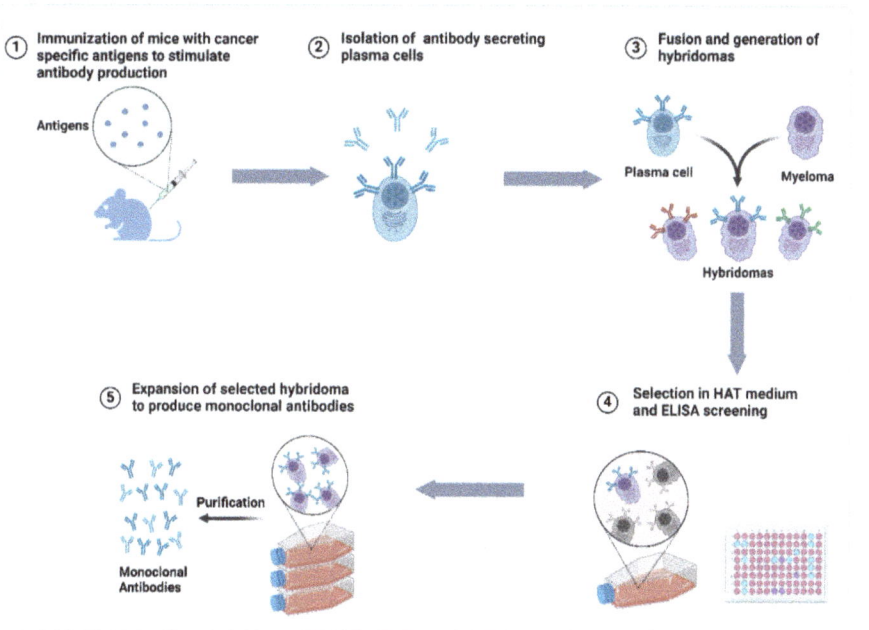

Figure 13-5. Hybridoma technique to produce monoclonal antibodies (mAbs).

Humanized mAbs: Further progress resulted in the generation of humanized mAbs, in which the only part originating from murine sources is the CDR portion of the variable domain. The incidence of immunogenicity was further reduced. Example humanized mAbs include trastuzumab (approved in 1998) and alemtuzumab (approved in 2001).

Human mAbs: With scientific and technological advancements, such as cDNA libraries of B cells and phage display technology, scientists were able to generate complete human mAbs. The first licensed human mAb was adalimumab (Humira) and it was approved in 2002.

In the past, antibody names used source infix like "-omab" for murine mAbs, "-ximab" for chimeric mAbs, "-zumab" for humanized mAbs, and "-umab" for human mAbs. The use of the source infix was discontinued in 2017 (announced by the WHO). Therefore, new antibodies approved after that do not follow the source infix.

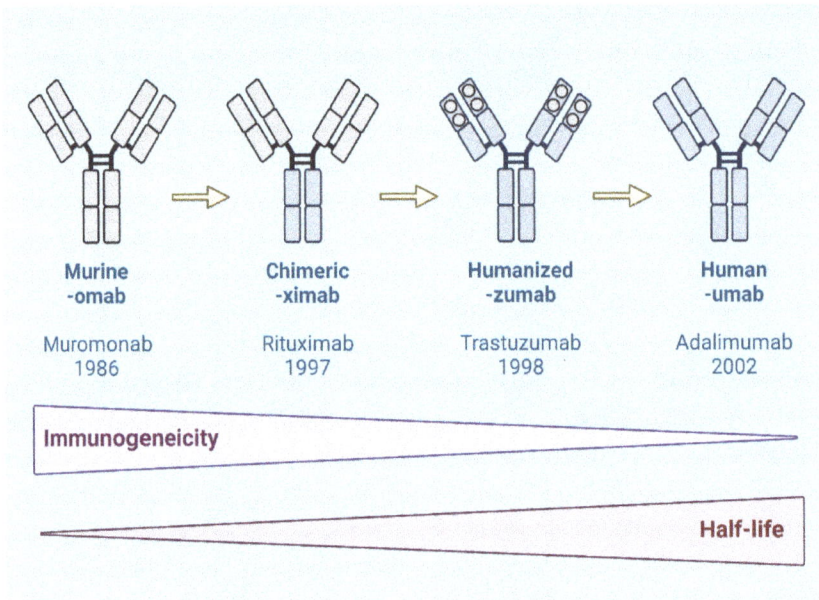

Figure 13-6. Evolution of therapeutic monoclonal antibodies (mAbs).

Bispecific mAbs

Bispecific mAbs (BsAbs) are the next generation of mAbs. In contrast to typical mAbs, which target one epitope, BsAbs have two distinct binding domains and accordingly can bind to two antigens or two epitopes of the same antigen simultaneously. The development of BsAbs was based on several technology advancements, including hybrid-hybridoma (quadroma) technology established in 1983, the single-chain variable fragment (scFv) invented in 1988 to minimize the refolding problems, as well as the knobs-into-holes technology developed in 1996 to ensure correct pairing (like puzzle pieces).

BsAbs can be separated into two categories: IgG-like and non-IgG-like. IgG-like BsAbs retain the traditional Y-shaped mAb structure, with the two Fab arms being merged from two different mAbs and binding two different epitopes (Figure 13-7, left). In contrast, non-IgG-like BsAbs do not have the Fc region, and there are different formats, such as chemically linked Fabs (Figure 13-7, middle) and connected scFvs (e.g. bi-specific T-cell engager (BiTE), Figure 13-7, right).

Each pathogen, toxin or cancer cell may have one or more antigens in its structure, with each antigen typically containing multiple epitopes. Different BsAbs may have different modes of actions based on the epitopes and antigens they are targeting. Below are some examples:

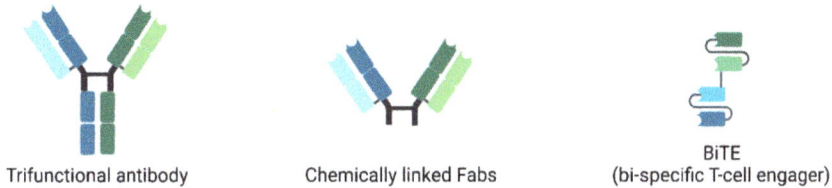

Figure 13-7. Three representative bispecific antibodies: trifunctional antibody (IgG-like), chemically linked Fabs (non-IgG-like) and bi-specific T-cell engager (non-IgG-like). Blue and Green parts distinguish parts from separate monoclonal antibodies.

- BsAbs may simultaneously target two antigens expressed on the same cancer cell, which may cause anti-tumor responses that are either independent or connected. This type of BsAbs may act like a "cocktail" of two mAbs. The advantage of using one BsAbs over two mAbs is that only one molecule needs to be manufactured. In addition, BsAbs targeting two antigens simultaneously may generate synergistic (or cooperative) responses, resulting in more significant treatment effects.

- BsAbs may simultaneously bind to an antigen expressed on the cancer cell and an antigen expressed on T cell. This represents the most common mode of action. Taking epcoritamab, a T-cell redirecting anti-cancer drug, as an example (Figure 13-8), one arm of epcoritamab binds CD20 on malignant B cells, and the other arm binds CD3 on T cells. As a result, cytotoxic T cells are recruited to the tumor site and activated to destroy the malignant B cells.

- BsAbs may simultaneously target two epitopes of the same antigen expressed on the pathogen. For example, SARS-CoV-2 viral spike protein is an antigen of SARS-CoV-2, the virus causing COVID-19. mAbs targeting the SARS-CoV-2 viral spike protein are not very effective due to the rapid emergence of SARS-CoV-2 variants that contain amino acid changes in the epitopes within the spike protein targeted by the mAbs. BsAbs are in a better position to address this challenge since they can simultaneously target two epitopes on the virus's spike protein, ensuring a broader spectrum of neutralization against emerging variants.

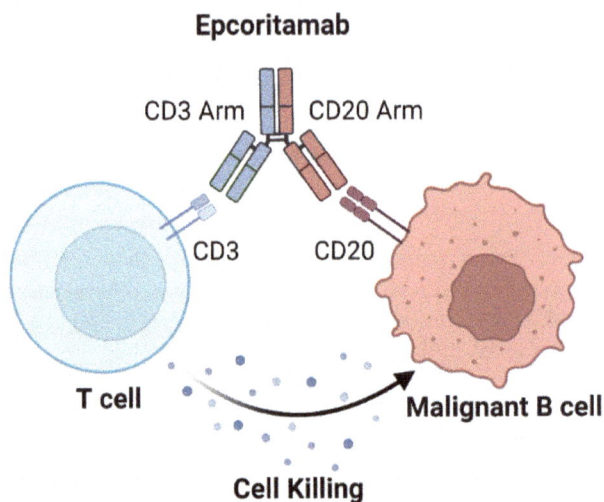

Figure 13-8. Mode of action of bispecific antibody Epcoritamab. One arm of epcoritamab binds CD20 on malignant B cells, and the other arm binds CD3 on T cells. As a result, cytotoxic T cells are recruited to the tumor site and activated to destroy the malignant B cells.

BsAbs have demonstrated great therapeutic potential and have become a hot spot in antibody drug research. So far, 10 BsAbs have been approved by the FDA (Table 13-2), among which 7 are T-cell redirecting anti-cancer drugs, and over 180 BsAbs are currently in clinical trials.

13.4 Mechanism of Action

Therapeutic antibody drugs demonstrate diverse mechanisms of action. I provide several representative ones in this section.

13.4.1 Antibody-dependent cellular cytotoxicity (ADCC)

The typical ADCC involves activation of natural killer (NK) cells by antibodies. The following is a brief description of the steps involved (Figure 13-9):

- The Fab region (i.e., the arm) of the mAb binds to the antigen on the surface of the target cell.
- The antigen-antibody interaction activates NK cells, which have Fc receptors on their surface. The Fc receptors on NK cells bind the Fc region (i.e., the leg) of the mAbs.
- The resulting complex triggers degranulation into a lytic synapse.

Table 13-2. Bispecific antibodies approved by the FDA (up to December 2023).

Trade Name	Active Ingredient	Targets	Year Approved	Approved Indication
Blincyto	Blinatumomab	CD3, CD19	2014	Philadelphia chromosome-negative relapsed or refractory B cell precursor acute lymphoblastic leukemia
Hemlibra	Emacizumab	Factor IXa, Factor X	2017	To prevent or reduce the frequency of bleeding episodes in hemophilia A with factor VIII inhibitors
Rybrevant	Amivantamab	EGFR, MET	2021	Locally advanced or metastatic non-small cell lung cancer with certain mutations
Vabysmo	Faricimab	VEGF, Ang-2	2022	Neovascular (wet) age-related macular degenerated and diabetic macular edema
Tecvayli	Teclistamab	CD3, BCMA	2022	Relapsed or refractory multiple myeloma
Lunsumio	Mosunetuzumab	CD3, CD20	2022	Relapsed or refractory follicular lymphoma
Epkinly	Epcoritamab	CD3, CD20	2023	Relapsed or refractory diffuse large B-cell lymphoma
Columvi	Glofitamab	CD3, CD20	2023	Relapsed or refractory diffuse large B-cell lymphoma or large B-cell lymphoma
Talvey	Talquetamab	CD3, GPRC5D	2023	Relapsed or refractory multiple myeloma
Elrexfio	Elranatamab	CD3, BCMA	2023	Relapsed or refractory multiple myeloma

Ang-2: angiopoietin-2; BCMA: B-cell maturation antigen; EGFR: Epidermal growth factor receptor; MET: mesenchymal epithelial transition; VEGF: vascular endothelial growth factor.

- Target cells die by apoptosis.

NK cells are part of the body's innate immune system. Therefore, for antibody drugs whose only (or main) mechanism of action is ADCC, the prerequisite of successful treatment is that the patient's innate immune system is intact.

13.4.2 Complement-dependent cytotoxicity (CDC)

Another common mechanism of action is CDC, in which target cells are lysed through activation and recruitment of the complement cascade to the targeted cell surface (Figure 13-9). The following is the brief description:

- The Fab region (i.e., the arm) of the mAb binds to the antigen on the surface of the target cell (e.g. bacterial or viral infected cell).
- The glycoprotein C1q, the initiating component of the classical complement pathway, is activated and bound to the Fc portion (i.e., the leg) of target-bound antibodies.
- The activation of C1q triggers the complement cascade, which involves the participation of C2, C3, C4, C5, C6, C7, C8, and C9. In the end, the membrane attack complex (MAC) pore is formed.
- The MAC pores allow water and salt ions into the targeted cell, leading to cell lysis and death.

Same as ADCC, CDC is an important part of the innate immune response. Therefore, for antibody drugs whose only (or main) mechanism of action is CDC, the prerequisite of successful treatment is that the patient's innate immune system is intact.

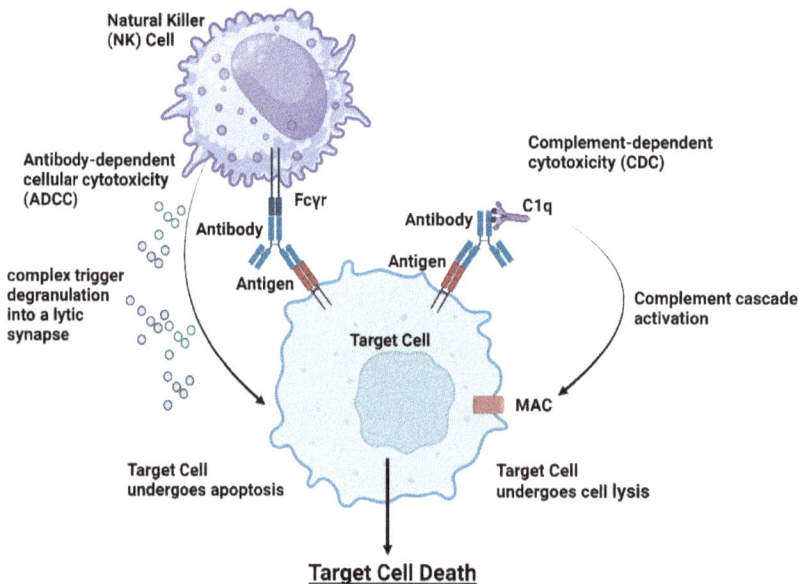

Figure 13-9. Two modes of action of mAbs – Antibody-dependent cellular cytotoxicity (ADCC) and Complement-dependent cytotoxicity (CDC). ADCC involves activation of natural killer (NK) cells, while CDC actives and recruits the complement cascade.

13.4.3 Blockage of interaction between antigen and pathophysiological ligand

In addition to ADCC and CDC, another mode of action is "blocking", where therapeutic antibodies act as either ligand antagonists or receptor antagonists as illustrated in Figure 13-10.

- *Ligand antagonist* Many pathogens, such as bacteria, fungi, and viruses, can produce toxins during infection. These toxins can be viewed as ligands, and they exhibit toxic effects by binding to receptors and triggering downstream reactions. Antibody drugs can bind to these toxins and block the interaction between toxins and their receptors. In this case, antibody drugs function as ligand antagonists, and they are often called neutralizing antibodies.

- *Receptor antagonist* In addition to interacting with the ligand, mAbs can also block the ligand-receptor interaction by binding the receptor expressed on the cell surface. In this case, antibody drugs function as receptor antagonists. Many anti-cancer therapeutic antibodies have this mode of action. For example, matuzumab binds the epidermal growth factor receptor (EGFR) and competitively blocks the binding of epidermal growth factor (EGF), the natural ligand of EGFR. As a result, the receptor-mediated downstream signaling is blocked, leading to impaired tumor cell proliferation.

13.4.4 Targeted delivery of toxin/radiation

In addition to "blocking", another mode of action of therapeutic antibodies is "targeting", as shown in Figure 13-10. Based on their remarkable specificity, mAbs can be utilized as drug delivery carriers. This is a smart strategy. Different from other modes of action where antibodies act as "soldiers", in this case, antibodies function as "vehicles" that transport the "soldiers", such as radiation, toxins, small-molecule cytotoxic drugs, to the target site. The targeted delivery of a defined dose of radiation by an antibody is used mainly in cancer therapy. An antibody carrying a small-molecule cytotoxic drug is called antibody-drug conjugate (ADC), which will be discussed in detail in Chapter 14.

13.4.5 Immuno-oncology related mode of action – Blocking checkpoint proteins to fight cancer

An area that is hot is using mAbs as checkpoint inhibitors. Figure 13-11 shows its mechanism of action. To prevent an immune response from being so strong that it destroys healthy cells, our immune system sets up a checkpoint process. The proteins involved in this process are called immune checkpoint proteins. Some of these proteins, such as programmed death-1 (PD-1), are expressed on the surface of T cells, and some others (e.g., programmed death ligand-1 (PD-L1)) function as

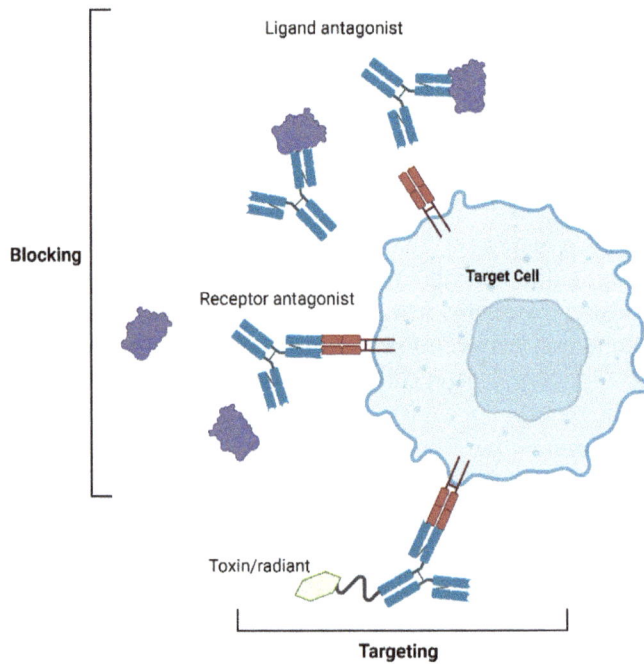

Figure 13-10. Two modes of action of mAbs – a) blocking, where antibodies act as either ligand antagonists or receptor antagonists, and b) targeting, where mAbs are utilized as drug delivery carriers.

partner proteins on other cells. When the checkpoint and partner proteins bind together, they send an "off" signal so that T cells won't attack the cells. Cancer cells are smart. They leverage this surveillance system by overexpressing immune checkpoint proteins, such as PD-L1.

With the fundamental understanding of how immune checkpoint system works, mAbs blocking checkpoint proteins have been developed to fight cancer. These mAbs are called immune checkpoint inhibitors. Some inhibitors block the immune checkpoint proteins on the T-cells. Example drugs include PD-1 inhibitors such as pembrolizumab, nivolumab and cemiplimab. Some inhibitors block the partner proteins expressed on the cancer cells. Example drugs include PD-L1 inhibitors such as atezolizumab, avelumab, and durvalumab.

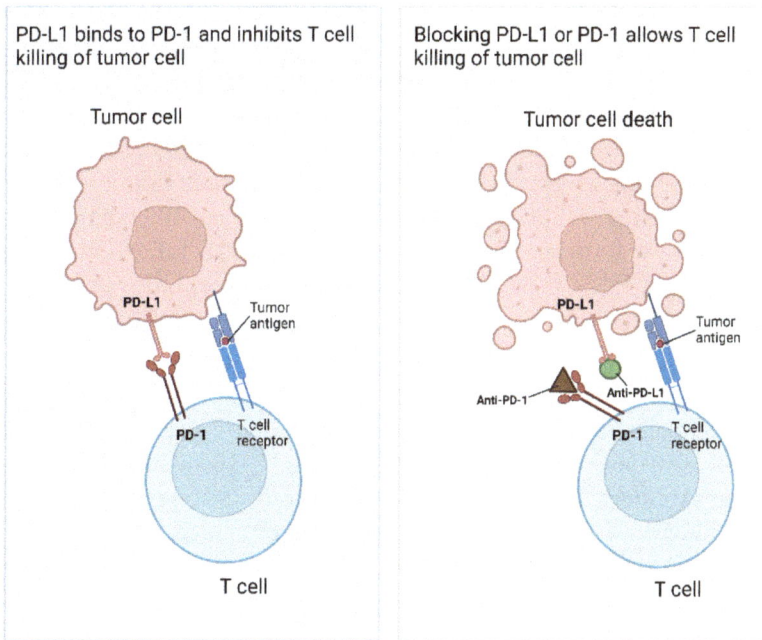

Figure 13-11. Additional modes of action of mAbs – Inhibition of checkpoint proteins, such as PD-1 on T cells and PD-L1 on the tumor cells.

13.4.6 Immuno-oncology related mode of action – Re-directing T cells to fight cancer

In addition to blocking checkpoint proteins to activate T cells for tumor killing, another promising immuno-oncology strategy is to redirect T cells to fight cancer. There are two different types of T-cell redirecting therapies. One is BsAbs, which simultaneously bind to an antigen expressed on the cancer cell and an antigen expressed on T cell (Figure 13-8). Through these interactions, cytotoxic T cells are recruited to the target site and activated to destroy the tumor cells. Another type of T-cell redirecting therapy is chimeric antigen receptor (CAR) T-cell therapy, which will be discussed in detail in the last chapter of this book (Chapter 16).

13.5 Clinical Pharmacology

13.5.1 ADME

Absorption: mAbs are commonly administered via intravenous (I.V.), subcutaneous (S.C.), and intramuscular (I.M.) routes. Oral administration of mAbs is generally considered not feasible at current stage due to the following barriers:

1) poor permeability due to their high molecular mass and high polarity; 2) poor stability because of the denaturation of mAbs in the acidic environment of the stomach; and 3) substantial degradation by proteases in the gastrointestinal tract. Regarding the S.C. and I.M. routes, mAbs are absorbed into the lymphatic system via convective flow of interstitial fluid. As the lymphatic vessels are porous, mAbs can easily pass through them. Because lymphatic flow is low, mAbs are absorbed over a long time period. The T_{max} of mAbs typically ranges from 1 to 8 days, which is much longer than the T_{max} of small-molecule drugs (usually within 2-6 hours for immediate-release forms). The bioavailability of mAbs following S.C. and I.M. injections ranges from 0.5-1. For example, a S.C. administration of 1 mg/kg efalizumab results in a bioavailability of 50% and a T_{max} of 2 days.

Distribution: Overall, the distribution of mAbs in the body is poor due to their large molecular mass and high hydrophilicity/polarity. The steady-state volume of distribution typically ranges from 5-10 L, indicating a limited distribution. Antibody fragments, such as Bi-specific T-cell engagers (BiTE), have a larger volume of distribution because of their small size. mAbs can be transported by different mechanisms, such as convection and endocytosis. Convection is considered the main mechanism responsible for the transport of mAbs from blood to the interstitial space of tissues, as well as from the interstitial space to the blood (via the lymphatic system). The cellular uptake of mAbs is accomplished by endocytosis, which can be either receptor-mediated or non-receptor-mediated. Receptor-mediated endocytosis is believed to be the predominant mechanism of cellular uptake of mAbs, and Fc-Rn, as mentioned in section 13.2.2, is often involved in this process. Non-receptor mediated endocytosis includes phagocytosis ("cell eating") and pinocytosis ("cell drinking"), which represent minor routes of cellular uptake of mAbs.

Metabolism and Excretion: For small-molecule drugs, the main elimination pathways include metabolism through drug metabolizing enzymes expressed in the liver and excretion via the kidney. The situation is different for mAbs. mAbs do not undergo metabolism medicated by drug metabolizing enzymes such as CYP450 isoforms. Additionally, mAbs do not undergo glomerular filtration either because their size (150 kDa) greatly exceeds the size limit of the glomerular filtration (20-30 kDa). However, small antibody fragments may undergo renal elimination due to their small size.

The elimination of mAbs involves the following pathways (Figure 13-12):

- *Endocytosis and subsequent proteolytic degradation*   As mentioned earlier, mAbs can be taken up by cells through endocytosis, which can be receptor mediated or non-receptor mediated. Receptor mediated endocytosis could happen by the interaction between the Fc portion of the mAbs and the Fcγ receptors on the cell surface. The non-receptor mediated endocytosis includes fluid phase phagocytosis and pinocytosis. Once inside the cells, FcRn often gets involved, and mAbs binding to FcRn escape proteolytic degradation and migrate to the cell surface, while the excessive mAbs that are not bound to FcRn are sorted to lysosomes for degradation. IgG fragment-based therapy does not get FcRn-mediated protection because they don't have the Fc portion. As a result, they often have extremely short half-lives. For example, abciximab does not have the Fc region and has a half-life of 30 minutes, which is much shorter than the half-lives of days to weeks seen in full length mAbs belonging to IgG1, IgG2, and IgG4.

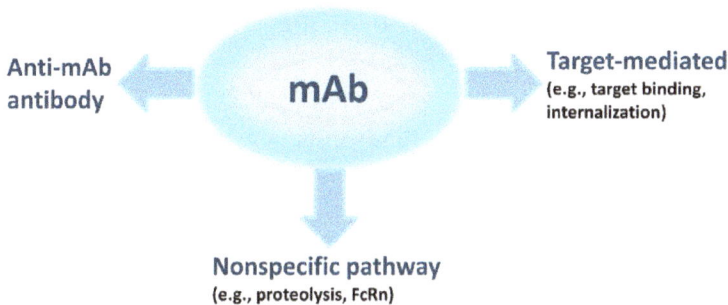

Figure 13-12. Diagram of elimination pathways for therapeutic mAbs. *This figure is adapted from Zhou and Mascelli. Annu. Rev. Pharmacol. Toxicol. 2011. 51:359–72.*

- *Target-mediated elimination*   The Fab portion of mAbs interacts with the antigen (i.e., the target), and the mAb-antigen complex formed elicits its pharmacological effect. If the antigen is a cell surface target (e.g. receptor, enzyme, transporter), the mAb-antigen complex undergoes internalization and subsequent lysosomal degradation; this phenomenon is known as target-mediated drug disposition (TMDD). At low concentrations, target-mediated elimination represents a major elimination pathway and the clearance of mAbs is high. With an increase in concentrations, target mediated elimination starts to saturate and the clearance of mAbs decreases. Figure 13-12 shows the target-mediated nonlinear pharmacokinetics of antibody drug TRX1. Due to the concentration-dependent biphasic clearance, mAbs concentration-time profiles often demonstrate S-shaped curves at high therapeutic doses if mAbs samples are collected over a prolonged time period (Figure 13-13).

- *Immunogenicity mediated elimination*   Most mAbs are immunogenic and the body may generate antibodies against therapeutic antibodies, which are commonly referred to as anti-drug antibodies (ADAs). Some ADAs bind to the Fc portion of mAbs, leading to accelerated clearance. Some ADAs may bind to the Fab region of mAbs and have impacts on efficacy, instead of pharmacokinetics, by inhibiting the binding to the target.

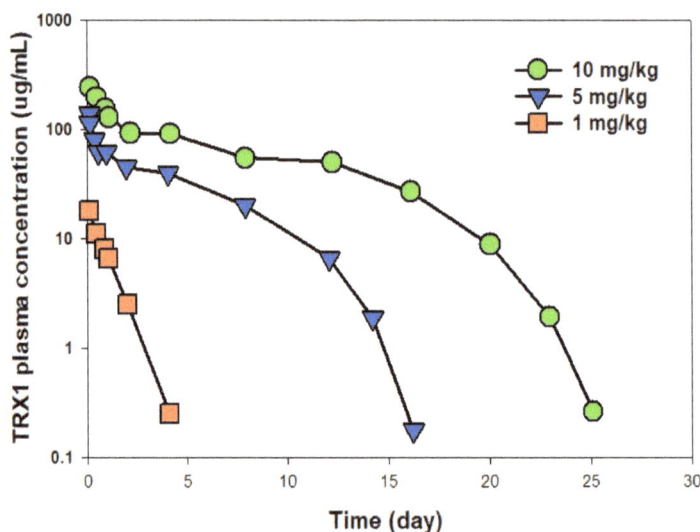

Figure 13-13. Nonlinear pharmacokinetics of TRX1 following doses of 1, 5, and 10 mg/kg. From: An G. Journal of Clinical Pharmacology 2020;60:149-163.

13.5.2 Drug-Drug Interactions

For small-molecule drugs, DDIs mediated by drug metabolizing enzymes and drug transporters are frequently observed. Antibody drugs are neither eliminated by drug metabolizing enzymes nor transported by drug transporters. Does that mean that DDI won't occur when a therapeutic antibody is co-administered with another drug? The answer is NO. Studies have shown that mAbs can interact with co-administered small-molecule drugs as perpetrators or victims. In addition, interactions between two mAbs could also occur.

- *DDI with mAbs being perpetrators* Proinflammatory cytokines, such as interleukin-6 (IL-6), are known to affect the expression of CYP enzymes. mAbs (e.g., blinatumomab) that cause increases in proinflammatory cytokine levels can downregulate CYP, leading to reduced hepatic clearance and increased plasma exposure of drugs that are substrates of CYP. Conversely, mAbs that reduce cytokine levels can relieve the CYP450 downregulation from an inflammatory environment. As a result, the expression of CYP is elevated, resulting in enhanced clearance and reduced exposure of drugs that are CYP substrates. For example, IL-6 concentration is elevated in rheumatoid arthritis (RA), which may cause reduced CYP activity. Tocilizumab binds to both membrane-bound and soluble IL-6 receptors, thus blocking IL-6 from activating the immune system. In a clinical study conducted in 12 patients with RA, the plasma exposure of simvastatin decreased by 57% when it was co-administered with tocilizumab.

- *DDI with mAbs being victims*   As noted earlier, ADAs are formed during immunogenicity, and they can cause increased elimination of the mAbs. Small-molecule drugs with immunosuppressive effects can reduce the incidence of immunogenicity and affect the pharmacokinetics of co-administered mAb by decreasing the ADA-mediated clearance. For example, methotrexate was reported to significantly decrease the elimination of infliximab, an anti-TNF-α mAb, and the decrease in clearance was found to directly correlate with the decreased immunogenicity incidence. Similar interactions were also observed when methotrexate was co-administered with a few other anti-TNF-α mAbs, such as adalimumab and golimumab.

- *DDI between two mAbs*   mAb-mAb interaction can occur when one mAb affects the interaction of another mAb with FcRn, by saturating, blocking, or interfering with the interaction between an mAb containing an Fc region of human IgG and FcRn. The affected mAb is expected to have increased clearance and decreased plasma exposure because it receives less FcRn-mediated protection.

13.5.3 Safety

Overall, therapeutic antibodies are considered a safe therapy. Instead of being metabolized by drug metabolizing enzymes, they are catabolized and degraded into amino acids, which are then recycled by the body for other biosynthetic processes. The following are the common adverse effects:

- *Immunogenicity*   This has already been discussed in Chapter 12 as a common feature among biologic products. In general, the less the non-human origin of the mAbs, the lower the incidence of immunogenicity.

- *Cytokine release syndrome*   Cytokine release syndrome (CRS) happens when the immune system responds to certain mAbs aggressively by rapidly releasing massive cytokines into the blood. The term "cytokine release syndrome" was first coined in the early 1990s when the anti-T-cell antibody muromonab-CD3 was introduced into the clinic. Later on, CRS was reported for several mAbs, such as TGN1412, rituximab, obinutuzumab, and alemtuzumab. CRS occurs more often in those T cell-engaging immunotherapies, such as BsAbs and CAR-T therapy. Symptoms of CRS include fever, fatigue, headache, nausea, vomiting, rash, rapid heartbeat, low blood pressure, and trouble breathing. The case of CRS observed with CD28 super-agonist TGN1412 was first published in the New England Journal of Medicine in 2006 and has been extensively cited since then; it provides valuable insights into the pathophysiology of this syndrome as the participants were healthy people. Following is the key summary that I copied from the article:

"Six healthy young male volunteers were enrolled in the first phase 1 clinical trial of TGN1412, a novel superagonist anti-CD28 monoclonal antibody that directly stimulates T cells. Within 90 minutes after receiving a single intravenous dose of the drug, all six volunteers had a systemic inflammatory response characterized by a rapid induction of proinflammatory cytokines and accompanied by headache, myalgias, nausea, diarrhea, erythema, vasodilatation, and hypotension. Within 12 to 16 hours after infusion, they became critically ill, with pulmonary infiltrates and lung injury, renal failure, and disseminated intravascular coagulation. Severe and unexpected depletion of lymphocytes and monocytes occurred within 24 hours after infusion. All six patients were transferred to an intensive care unit, where they received intensive cardiopulmonary support (including dialysis), high-dose methylprednisolone, and an anti–interleukin-2 receptor antagonist antibody. Prolonged cardiovascular shock and acute respiratory distress syndrome developed in two patients, who required intensive organ support for 8 and 16 days. Despite evidence of the multiple cytokine-release syndrome, all six patients survived." [quoted from Suntharalingam et al. N Engl J Med 2006;355:1018-28.]

The above case report is valuable as it documented the whole clinical course, which offered insights into the pathophysiology of CRS in the absence of contaminating pathogens, endotoxin, or underlying disease. Please note that severe CRS is rare if management is proactive. To reduce the incidence or severity of CRS during clinical trials, one strategy implemented in the development of BsAbs is to incrementally increase the dose administered to a patient before reaching the target dose level; this approach is known as "step-up dosing".

Key References

Pharmacokinetics and Pharmacodynamics of Biotech Drugs. (2006). 1st edition. John Wiley & Sons, Inc.

Masopust D, Vezys V, Wherry EJ and Ahmed R (2007) A brief history of CD8 T cells. Eur J Immunol 37 Suppl 1:S103-110.

Leavy O. The birth of monoclonal antibodies (2016). Nature Immunology 17: S13.

Bayer V (2019) An Overview of Monoclonal Antibodies. Semin Oncol Nurs 35:150927

Patel DD and Bussel JB (2020) Neonatal Fc receptor in human immunity: Function and role in therapeutic intervention. J Allergy Clin Immunol 146:467-478.

Zhou H and Mascelli MA (2011) Mechanisms of monoclonal antibody-drug interactions. Annu Rev Pharmacol Toxicol 51:359-372

Shimabukuro-Vornhagen A, Godel P, Subklewe M, Stemmler HJ, Schlosser HA, Schlaak M, Kochanek M, Boll B and von Bergwelt-Baildon MS (2018) Cytokine release syndrome. J Immunother Cancer 6:56.

Suntharalingam G, Perry MR, Ward S, Brett SJ, Castello-Cortes A, Brunner MD and Panoskaltsis N (2006) Cytokine storm in a phase 1 trial of the anti-CD28 monoclonal antibody TGN1412. N Engl J Med 355:1018-1028.

Chapter 14.
Antibody-Drug Conjugate

Learning Objectives

After reading this chapter, the reader shall be able to:

1. Describe the key elements of an ADC drug.
2. List the key considerations of the ADC design.
3. Describe the mechanism of action of ADCs.
4. Understand the barriers of the ADC development.
5. Describe the features of each generation of ADCs.
6. Familiar with the pharmacokinetics of ADCs and describe why its pharmacokinetics is more complicated than other modalities.

From the size perspective, the difference between small-molecule drugs and biologics is as dramatic as bicycles versus airplanes, or bunnies versus elephants. Size is not the only factor differentiating these two. As noted in Chapters 12 and 13, small molecule drugs and biologic products, including mAbs, are different in many other aspects, such as ADME, structure, method of synthesis, manufacturing process, adverse effects, and clinical pharmacology. Despite these differences, the development of small-molecule drugs and biologics is not mutually exclusive. Smart chemical designs can link these two fields to generate a new type of drug modality – antibody-drug conjugates (ADCs). Although the concept of ADC is not new, it took decades of effort to bring it to reality. I will share several key events in section 14.1. The structure of ADC and its design are more complicated than the antibody or small-molecule drug alone. I will go through the components of ADC and the key considerations of ADC design in section 14.2. The mechanism of action of ADCs is covered in section 14.3. From the early ADC products with suboptimal therapeutic windows to the newer generations of ADCs with great success in some highly treatment-refractory diseases, the development of ADCs has come a long way. The advances in the development of ADC will be briefly discussed in section 14.4. An ADC drug, after administration, may present in blood in multiple forms, including antibody-conjugated drug, unconjugated drug (i.e., naked drug), and unconjugated antibody (i.e., naked antibody). Which one(s) should be included for the pharmacokinetics evaluation of an ADC? What are the bioanalytical considerations for the measurement of ADC samples? Would the ADME of ADCs be different from therapeutic antibodies and small-molecule drugs? These questions will be addressed in section 14.5. Then this chapter ends with a brief discussion of current challenges and future direction of ADC development in section 14.6.

14.1 Introduction

Paul Ehrlich, a German physician and scientist, received the Nobel Prize for Physiology or Medicine in 1908 in recognition of his contribution to immunology. He coined the term "Antikörper" (German for "Antibody") and introduced the concept of "Zaberkugel" (German for "magic bullet"), as mentioned in Chapter 13. His impact, however, extended beyond immunology. He is also considered to be the founder of chemotherapy. In 1908, he discovered one of the first chemotherapeutic agents, salvarsan, which was used to treat syphilis until penicillin was introduced in 1945. He coined the term "chemotherapy" and in his vision, these "chemotherapies" were to be the new magic bullets, capable of killing pathogenic cells while sparing healthy tissues.

Unfortunately, the conventional small-molecule chemotherapeutic agents, such as anthracyclines (e.g., doxorubicin), topoisomerase inhibitors (e.g., topotecan), alkylating agents (e.g., cisplatin), and taxanes (e.g., paclitaxel) do not function as magic bullets because they damage all rapidly dividing cells, including not only cancer cells but also healthy cells (e.g., cells in bone marrow, GI tract, and hair follicles). Consequently, this indiscriminate action leads to myelosuppression, mucositis, vomiting, fatigue and many other adverse effects.

Considering the high specificity of antibodies, using them as carriers to transport small-molecule cytotoxic agents for targeted therapy represents an attractive strategy. In 1957, Mathe was the first to conjugate methotrexate with antileukemia 1210 antigen IgGs for the treatment of leukemia. In 1983, the first human clinical trial was conducted for the conjugates of vindesine-CEA. After decades of effort, the first ADC drug, mylotarg (gemtuzumab ozogamicin), was approved by the FDA in 2000, marking the beginning of ADC-based cancer targeted therapy. To date, there are 13 ADCs approved by the FDA for treating different hematological and solid tumor cancers (Table 14-1), with more than 100 ADCs under clinical development.

Table 14-1. ADC drugs approved by the FDA (up to December 2023)

ADC name; Approval	Brand name	Tumor target; Antibody type	Linker	Payload; DAR	Indication
Mylotarg; 2000; 2017*	Gemtuzumab ozogamicin	CD33; Humanized IgG4	Cleavable hydrazone linker	Calichea micin; 3-5	CD33 positive acute myeloid leukemia
Adcetris; 2011	Brentuximab vedotin	CD30; Chimeric IgG1	Cleavable maleimidocaproyl valine-citrulline linker	MMAE; 4	Hodgkin's lymphoma
Kadcyla; 2013	Trastuzumab emtansine	HER2; Humaized IgG1	Non-cleavable thioether linker	DM1; 3-4	HER2 positive breast cancer
Besponsa; 2017	Inotuzumab ozogamicin	CD22; Humanized IgG4	Cleavable hydrazone linker	Calichea micin; 6	B-cell acute lymphoblastic leukemia
Lumoxiti#; 2018	Moxetumom ab pasudotox	CD22; Recombinant murine IgG variable domain	Fusion protein (antibody and payload)	Pseudomo nas exotoxin	Hairy cell leukemia
Polivy; 2019	Polatuzumab vedotin	CD79b; Fully humanized IgG1k	Cleavable maleimidocaproyl valine-citrulline linker	MMAE; 3-4	Diffuse large B-cell lymphoma
Padcev; 2019	Enfortumab vedotin	Nectin4; Fully humanized IgG1k	Cleavable maleimidocaproyl valine-citrulline linker	MMAE; 3-4	Urothelial carcinoma
Enhertu; 2019	Trastuzumab deruxtecan	HER2; Fully humanized IgG1k	Cleavable maleimide tetrapeptide linker	Dxd; 8	HER2 positive breast cancer
Trodelvy; 2020	Sacituzumab govitecan	Trop-2; Humanized IgG1k	Cleavable carbonate linker	SN-38; 7-8	Triple-negative breast cancer
Blenrep; 2020	Belantamab mafodotin	BCMA, Humanized IgG1k	Non-cleavable maleimidocaproyl linker	MMAF; 4	Relapsed and refractory multiple myeloma
Zynlonta; 2021	Loncastuxim ab tesirine	CD19; Humanized IgG1k	Cleavable valine-alanine linker	SG3199, alkylating agent; 2-3	Relapsed or refractory DLBCL and high-grade B-cell lymphoma
Tivdak; 2021	Tisotumab vedotin	Tissue factor; Fully human IgG1κ	Cleavable mc-val-cit-PABC linker	MMAE; 4	Recurrent or metastatic cervical cancer
Elahere; 2022	Mirvetuxima b soravtansine-gynx	Folate receptor-alpha (FRα); Chimeric IgG1	Cleavable disulfide bond-based linker	DM4; 3-4	Epithelial ovarian, fallopian tube, or primary peritoneal cancer

DLBCL: diffuse large B-cell lymphoma.

*Mylotarg was first approved in 2000, withdrawn in 2010, and relaunched in 2017.
#Withdrawn from the US market in 2022.

14.2 Components and Key Considerations of ADC Design

As shown in Figure 14-1, an ADC drug is composed of an antibody, a small-molecule cytotoxic drug, and a chemical linker. The antibody acts as a navigator and carrier to bring the drug to the target site. The small-molecule cytotoxicity drug is often referred to as "payload" and functions as a "warhead" for destroying cancer cells. The chemical linker serves as a bridge between the antibody and the drug, controlling payload release inside tumor cells. Each component and their interactions play crucial roles in determining the overall physical and chemical properties of ADC drugs, as well as their pharmacokinetics, efficacy, and toxicity profiles.

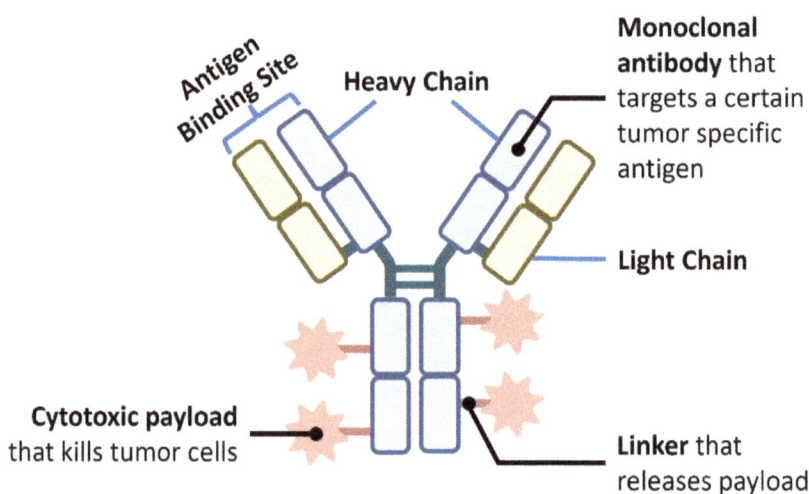

Figure 14-1. The structure and characteristic of an antibody-drug conjugate (ADC) drug. *Adapted from: Zuo P. AAPS J 2020;22:105.*

14.2.1. Antibody moiety

An ideal antibody moiety should have high specificity and affinity for binding to the target antigen, low immunogenicity, and a long plasma half-life. Humanized mAbs from the IgG class meet these prerequisites and naturally became the best choice in the current stage of ADC development. In the early days, mouse-derived antibodies were the only choice, and the ADCs generated had a high failure rate due to serious immunogenicity. With the emergence of recombinant technology, murine antibodies were first replaced with chimeric antibodies, then these were further replaced with humanized antibodies with significantly reduced immunogenicity. Among the 14 ADCs approved so far, none of them use murine antibody, only brentuximab vedotin uses chimeric antibodies, and the rest products all employ humanized antibodies.

The antibodies currently used for ADC drugs are predominantly IgG antibodies. As noted in Chapter 13, IgG has four subtypes: IgG1, IgG2, IgG3, and IgG4. Most ADCs are constructed with IgG1 because it is easy to prepare and has an intracellularly degradable hinge structure. In addition to IgG1, IgG4 has also been used in a number of approved ADCs. Regarding IgG2, it is not a popular option for ADCs due to its tendency to form dimers and aggregations in vivo, which can result in decreased ADC concentrations. In terms of IgG3, it is rarely employed in ADC because it does not get protection from the neonatal fragment crystallizable receptor (FcRn) and consequently has a much shorter half-life compared to the other three subtypes (7 days vs 21 days).

14.2.2 Cytotoxic payload

A payload is the warhead that exerts its tumor killing effect after being released from the ADC complex. An ideal payload should have the following features:

- **Ultra-high cytotoxicity**   After administration, only approximately 2% of ADCs eventually could reach the targeted tumor sites because of the low permeability of mAbs into tumor tissues, limited tumor antigen expression, as well as premature decomposition of ADCs in systemic circulation. Since only limited warheads can reach the site of action, they need to be very potent in order to fulfill their tumor killing duty. Current payloads usually have high cytotoxicity, with IC_{50} (i.e., half-maximal inhibitory concentration) of low nM (e.g., microtubule inhibitors) or even pM range (e.g., DNA damaging agents).

- **Appropriate payload characteristics**   Payloads need to be stable in physiological conditions, including the low pH environment of the lysosomes. Payloads need to have appropriate solubility to facilitate antibody coupling and contain function groups for conjugation with the antibody.

One type of cytotoxic payloads that is commonly used in ADCs is microtubule inhibitors, such as tubulin polymerization promoters (Figure 14-2), including auristatin derivatives monomethyl auristatin E (MMAE) and monomethyl auristatin F (MMAF), and tubulin polymerization inhibitors, including maytansinoid derivatives DM1 and DM4. As shown in Table 14-1, among the 14 approved ADCs, 5 of them use MMAE/MMAF as their payloads. In addition to microtubule inhibitors, DNA damaging agents, such as calicheamicin (for DNA double strand break), duocarmycin (for DNA alkylation), and DNA topoisomerase inhibitors (e.g., SN-38 and DXd for DNA intercalation), are also popular payload candidates due to their potent tumor killing effects (Figure 14-2).

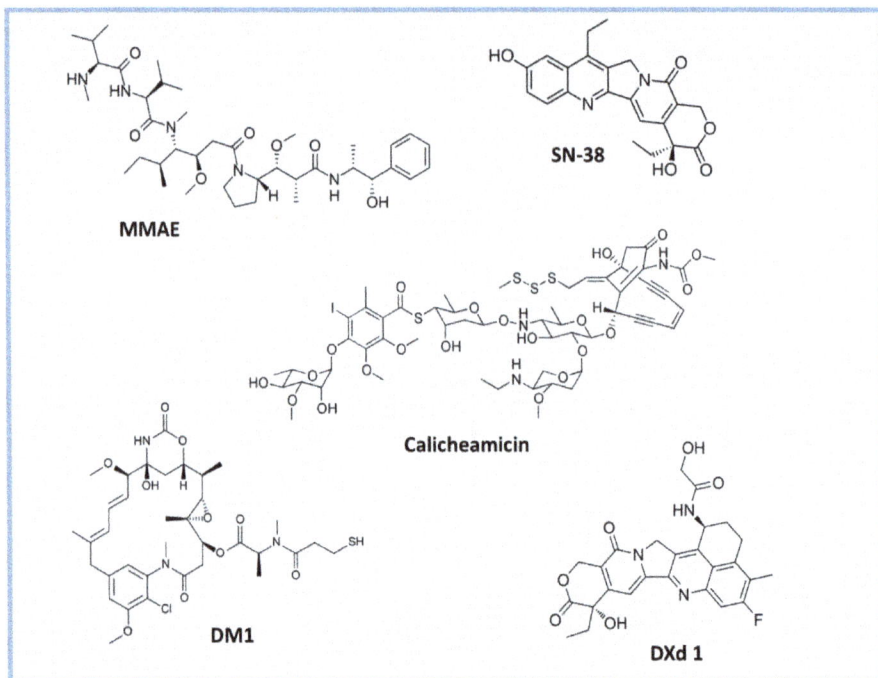

Figure 14-2. Structure of the representative payloads used in ADCs.

14.2.3. Linker

A linker connects the antibody with the payload and represents an important factor associated with ADC stability and payload release profile. An ideal linker should not induce ADC aggregation and is expected to have minimal premature payload release in systemic circulation and meanwhile active drug release at the target sites. Currently, there are two types of linkers employed in most ADC drugs: cleavable and non-cleavable linkers.

- *Cleavable linkers* Cleavable linkers achieve target payload release by leveraging the environmental differences between systemic circulation and tumor cells, such as pH difference (blood: pH 7.4 vs tumor cells: pH 4.8 in lysosomes and pH 5.5-6.2 in endosomes); difference in glutathione levels, where glutathione concentrations in blood is considerably lower than intracellular concentrations in cancer cells; or difference in lysosomal protease levels, where cancer cells have more lysosomal protease compared to blood. Based on the above mechanisms, different cleavable linkers have been developed, including hydrazone (pH sensitive linker), disulfide bond based linkers, and peptide based linkers. Hydrazone bond and disulfide bond linkers are chemical cleavable linkers, while peptide bond linkers are considered enzyme cleavable linkers.

- ***Non-cleavable linkers*** As the name indicates, this type of linkers are inert to in vivo chemical and enzymatic environments. For non-cleavable linkers, the entire ADC has to be degraded to release the "payload complex", which contains the payload, the linker, and the amino acid residue of the degraded antibody. The currently used non-cleavable linkers include thioether or maleimidocaproyl. Non-cleavable linkers consist of stable bonds that prevent proteolytic cleavage and therefore have greater plasma stability than their cleavable counterparts.

14.2.4. Other considerations – conjugation method

In addition to the selection of the antibody, the cytotoxic payload, and the linker, the conjugation approach to connect the small molecule moiety (i.e., linker plus payload) to the antibody is also important. In general, lysine and cysteine residues on the antibody are the most commonly used linker modification sites as these residues provide accessible reaction sites for conjugation. The conventional approach employes stochastic conjugation on pre-existing lysine or cysteine residuals and yields heterogeneous mixtures of multiple species, with a *drug-antibody ratio (DAR)* in the range of 0-8. As the lysine residues are distributed in both antibody light chain and heavy chain, conjugation occurring near the antigen recognition region may interfere with target binding. Cysteine based reaction represents a better method as there are fewer reaction sites, which reduces the heterogeneity of ADC. Products with DAR of 2, 4, 6, and 8 can be generated. So far cysteine-based reaction is the most commonly used conjugation method in approved ADC drugs.

The stochastic conjugation on lysine and cysteine residues has a number of disadvantages, such as premature payload release and corresponding off-target toxicity, and heterogeneous DAR. To address these issues, recently a number of site-specific conjugation methods have been developed. These methods either utilize engineered reactive cysteine residues (e.g., Thiomab technology) or introduce unnatural amino acids to achieve site-specific conjugation.

14.2.5. Other considerations – target antigen selection

The target antigen functions as the navigation direction for ADC drugs to identify tumor cells. The selection of target antigen is the first step of ADC design, and the importance of finding an appropriate target antigen is self-evident. Ideally, the target antigen should have the following features:

- Overexpressed in tumor cells, with minimal or low expression in normal tissues. In this case, off-target toxicity can be avoided. For example, HER2 represents a good option as its expression in certain types of tumors can be 100 times higher than in normal tissues. Among currently approved ADC drugs, three of them, namely ado-transtuzumab emtansine, fam-transtuzumab deruxtecan, and disitamab vedotin, target HER2.

- The target antigen should not be in secreted form. Antigen in the systemic circulation can cause ADC binding outside tumor sites, leading to reduced tumor targeting and increased adverse events. Therefore, a non-secreted antigen should be selected.
- The target antigen undergoes internalization upon ADC binding. In this case, the ADC-antigen complex can get in tumor cells, allowing active release of the payload.

For the approved ADC drugs, the target antigens are specific proteins overexpressed in tumor cells, such as HER2, CD22, CD30, CD33, BCMA, and CD79b. Recently, the target antigen selection has gradually expanded to targets in the tumor microenvironment.

14.3 Mechanism of Action

The main mechanism of action of an ADC is demonstrated in the right panel of Figure 14-3. Navigated by the target antigen, the antibody carries its cytotoxic payloads to the tumor site. The Fab portion of the antibody binds to the antigen, then the ADC-antigen complex undergoes endocytosis (i.e., internalization) to form early endosomes, which are subsequently matured into late endosomes and finally fused with lysosomes. Protected by FcRn, some ADC molecules in endosomes may be transported back to the cell surface instead of entering lysosomes. If the ADC is constructed with cleavable linkers, the payload can be released in early endosomes, late endosomes, and lysosomes. For an ADC with non-cleavable linkers, the payload usually is released in lysosomes after the antibody is degraded in that compartment. The payload, once released, can either cause damage to DNA or disrupt microtubules, leading to tumor cell apoptosis and cell death. If the cytotoxic payload is permeable, it may diffuse to the other tumor cells nearby and kill these neighbor antigen-negative tumor cells; this phenomenon is known as *bystander effect* (left panel of Figure 14-3).

In addition to payload-mediated tumor killing, the antibody may exert anticancer effects in a payload-independent manner. As elaborated in Chapter 13, the Fc portion of the antibody could bind to the Fc receptor of the effector cells (e.g., natural killer (NK) cells and macrophages), which triggers immune responses such as antibody-dependent cellular cytotoxicity (ADCC) and complement-dependent cytotoxicity (CDC). IgG1 is known to induce strong ADCC and CDC. Therefore, ADCs with IgG1 moiety often have these effector functions. In addition, the antibody component of ADCs could bind to the epitope antigen and block the downstream signaling pathway. Therefore, in addition to functioning as carriers, the antibody moiety of some ADC drugs could also act as fighters. For example, for trastuzumab emtansine (T-DM1), the antibody (i.e., trastuzumab) binds to the HER2 receptor and block the formation of heterodimer formation, resulting in the inhibition of the signal transduction pathways.

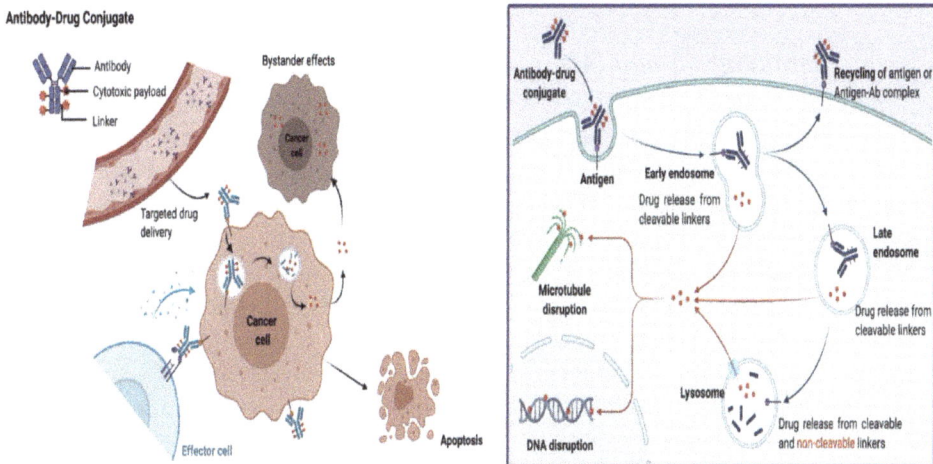

Figure 14-3. Mechanism of action of ADCs. *This figure is from Fu et al. Signal Transduction and Targeted Therapy 2022;7:93; used under Creative Commons CC-BY license.*

14.4 Advance in the Development of ADCs

Based on differences in drug composition and conjugated methods, ADC drug development has undergone three generations (Table 14-2).

- *First-generation ADCs*

In the early stage, the ADC candidates were composed of a conventional cytotoxic drug (e.g. doxorubicin), a murine antibody, and a non-cleavable linker. Due to the nature of the drug composition, these ADCs inevitably have the drawback of low potency and high immunogenicity. Later on, humanized mAbs and more potent cytotoxic agents were implemented in ADC design, which resulted in improved efficacy and safety profiles and thus market approval of the first-generation ADCs, including gemtuzumab ozogamicin and inotuzumab ozogamicin. These two drugs have many things in common. For example, both use IgG4 as the carrier, calicheamicin as the cytotoxic agent, and cleavable hydrazone as the linker. Although calicheamicin is very potent, its hydrophobicity can cause antibody aggregation, resulting in faster elimination and immunogenicity. The hydrazone linker can be cleaved in acidic conditions in other parts of the body, leading to uncontrollable release of cytotoxic payload and subsequent off-target toxicity. In addition, stochastic conjugation on pre-existing lysine or cysteine residuals was employed in the first-generation ADCs, which resulted in highly heterogeneous mixtures with variable DARs. Because of the issues mentioned above, the first-generation ADCs demonstrate suboptimal efficacy and safety profiles.

- **Second-generation ADCs**

With the effort of optimizing mAb isotypes, cytotoxic payloads and linkers, the second-generation ADCs, including brentuximab vedotin and trastuzumab emtansine, were subsequently launched. In contrast to IgG4 used in the first-generation products, the second-generation ADCs contain IgG1 isotype, which not only is more amendable for conjugation but also has higher tumor cell targeting ability. In addition to antibody moiety, better choices were also made on cytotoxic payload and linkers. For example, the payloads MMAE and DM used in the second-generation ADCs are more potent, have higher water solubility and increased conjugation efficiency. The linkers employed have higher plasma stability than those used in the first-generation ADCs. Although improvements in these key components resulted in better efficacy and safety of the second-generation ADCs, the system is not flawless. Off-target toxicity remains to be a concern. Aggregation and rapid clearance of ADCs are still observed in products with high DAR (e.g. ≥ 6).

- **Third-generation ADCs**

The experience gained from the first two generations has paved the way for the development of the third-generation ADCs. The representative products in this new generation include polatuzumab vedotin, endortumab vedotin, fam-trastuzumab deruxtecan, belantamab mafodotin, and other later approved ADCs. One major update is the implementation of the site-specific conjugation technology, which results in homogenous ADCs, less off-target toxicity, and better pharmacokinetic characteristics. In addition, there are moderate improvements in all three elements of ADCs (i.e., antibody, payload, and linkers). For example, fully humanized IgG1κ is utilized in the third-generation ADCs, further reducing immunogenicity. More options on payload are available (e.g., tubulysin, immunomodulators with novel mechanisms). Linkers with increased hydrophilicity are employed to reduce the aggregation of ADCs and the disturbance of immune system. Collectively, the third-generation ADCs have a better therapeutic index than early generations.

Table 14-2. The evolution of the ADC drug development. *This table is adapted from Fu Z et al. Signal Transduction and Targeted Therapy 2022;7:93.*

	First-generation ADC	Second-generation ADC	Third-generation ADC
Antibodies	Mouse-original or chimeric humanized antibodies	Humanized antibodies	Fully humanized antibodies or Fabs
Linkers	Unstable	Improved stability: cleavable and non-cleavable linkers	Stable in circulation; precise control drugs release into tumor sites
Payloads	Low potency, including calicheamicin, duocarmycin and doxorubicin	Potency, such as auristatins and mytansinoids	High potency, such as PBDs and tubulysin, and novel payloads like immunomodulators
Conjugation methods	Random lysines	Random lysines and reduced interchain cysteines	Site-specific conjugation
DAR	Uncontrollable (0-8)	4-8	2-4
Representative drugs	Gemtuzumab ozogamicin, inotuzumab ozogamicin	Brentuximab vedotin, adotrastuzumab emtansine	Polatuzumab vedotin, enfortumab vedotin, and fam-trastuzumab deruxtecan
Advantages	• Specific targeting •Increase therapeutic window to some extent	•Improved targeting ability • More potent payloads • Lower immunogenicity	• Higher efficacy though in cancer cells with low antigen • Improved DAR along with improved stability and PK/PD • More potent payloads • Less off-target toxicity
Disadvantages	• Heterogeneity • Lack of efficacy • Narrow therapeutic index •Off-target toxicity as premature drug loss • High immunogenicity	• Heterogeneity • Fast clearance for high DARs •Off-target toxicity as premature drug loss • Drug resistance	• Possible toxicity due to highly potent payloads • Catabolism may be different across species • Drug resistance

14.5 Pharmacokinetics

In general, the evaluation of the pharmacokinetics of ADCs is more complex than that of other therapeutic modalities because of the multiple elements contained in the structure, the heterogeneous species with varying number of drugs per antibody (i.e., a range of DAR) generated during the manufacturing process, as well as the dynamic DAR distribution caused by in vivo deconjugation and catabolism. As shown in Figure 14-4, after an ADC product is administered, multiple species are presented in the systemic circulation:

- *Conjugated antibody*, which includes any antibody that has at least one drug attached to them (DAR≥1).
- *Unconjugated antibody*, also known as naked antibody. As its name suggests, it only includes antibodies that have no drug attached to them.
- *Total antibody (Tab)*, which includes both conjugated and unconjugated antibody.
- *Antibody-conjugated drug*, which includes any cytotoxic payload that is attached to the antibody.
- *Unconjugated drug*, which only includes the payloads (i.e. the drug plus the linker) that are cleaved from ADC.

The heterogeneous and dynamic characteristics of an ADC bring a unique challenge to pharmacokinetic sample measurement because multiple bioanalytical assays are often required. The bioanalytical strategies for the development of ADCs, which have been the subject of intense discussion in the field, are beyond the scope of this book. The methods to measure different species usually include ELISA and LC/MS/MS methods. For most of the approved ADCs, the species (i.e., analytes) measured often include total antibody, conjugated antibody, and unconjugated drug. In some pharmacokinetic studies, the antibody-conjugated drug may also be quantified.

Figure 14-5 shows representative pharmacokinetic profiles following ADC administration. In this example, four analytes are evaluated, including two antibody related analytes, namely total antibody and conjugated antibody, as well as two small-molecule related analytes, namely antibody-conjugated drug and unconjugated drug. To avoid the bias introduced by the huge mass difference between a small-molecule and an antibody, molar concentration units were used across all analytes in the figure. As shown, antibody-conjugated drug has the highest molar concentrations, which is expected considering that the average DAR is usually more than 2. Compared to the total antibody, the conjugated antibody has a steeper terminal slope, indicating faster clearance in the systemic circulation. The accelerated clearance of the conjugated antibody can be caused by the linker and/or the small molecule drug attached to it. For example, when too many drugs

ADC Complexity

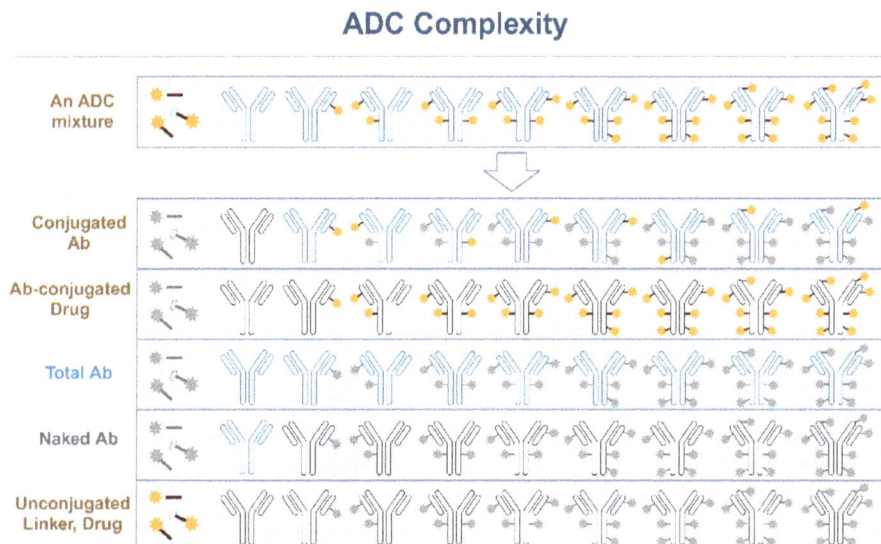

Figure 14-4. ADC complexity. After an ADC product is administered, multiple species are presented in the systemic circulation: conjugated antibody, which includes any antibody that has at least one drug attached to them (DAR ≥ 1); unconjugated antibody (i.e., naked antibody); total antibody (Tab), which includes both conjugated and unconjugated antibody; Antibody-conjugated drug, which includes any cytotoxic payload that is attached to the antibody; and unconjugated drug.

are attached to the antibody (e.g., DAR≥6), the ADC has increased hydrophobicity and tends to aggregate and then be cleared faster. In terms of the unconjugated drug, while it has no major impact on the disposition of the conjugated antibody, its plasma concentrations are often measured. This is because most of these cytotoxic agents have a narrow therapeutic index, and the pharmacokinetics of the unconjugated drug can be used to assess its safety.

The antibody moiety represents the backbone of an ADC and accounts for almost 99% of the total ADC molecular weight (mAb of 150 kDa vs (drug+ linker) of <2 kDa). As a result, the overall pharmacokinetics of an ADC is similar to the naked antibody. For example, ADCs also have relatively long half-lives due to FcRn-mediated protection and low volume of distribution because of their large size. ADCs also have the issue of immunogenicity, which may affect the clearance of ADCs. Another similarity is that ADC products also undergo target-mediated drug disposition (TMDD), a phenomenon that we have learned in Chapter 13 (see section 13.5.1 for detailed information). The TMDD of ADCs leads to nonlinear pharmacokinetics with higher clearance at low doses and a decrease in clearance at higher doses due to target saturation.

Despite the general similarities, there are a few subtle differences between ADCs and naked mAbs. For example, the half-life of an ADC is usually shorter than that of the naked antibody, which could be attributed to the linker and/or the drug as noted earlier. In addition, compared to the naked antibody, the ADC undergoes deconjugation, which represents an additional source of faster clearance.

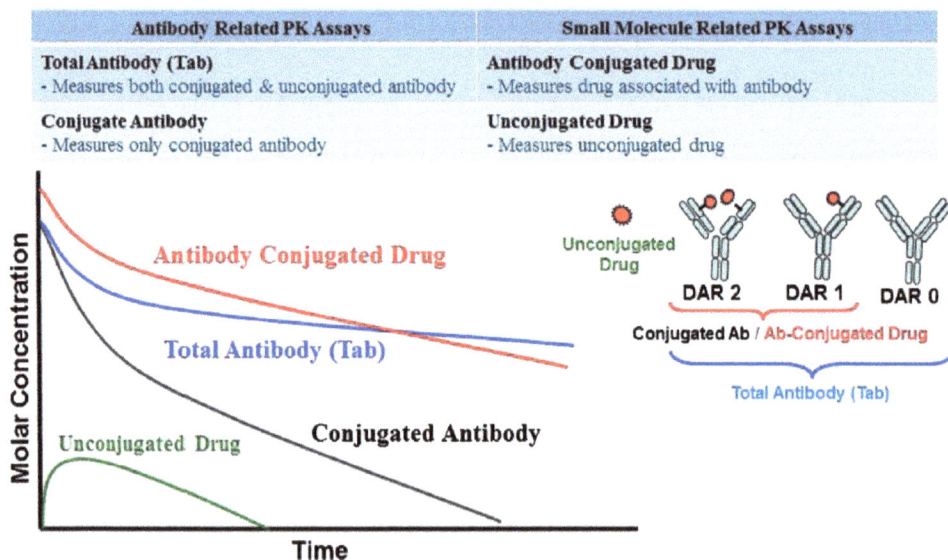

Figure 14-5. Example concentration-time profiles of different analytes following the administration of an ADC. Four analytes are measured, including two antibody related analytes, namely total antibody and conjugated antibody, as well as two small-molecule related analytes, namely antibody-conjugated drug and unconjugated drug. *From: Kamath AV and Lyer S. Pharm Res 2015;32:3470-3479; used under Creative Commons CC-BY license.*

14.6 Conclusions and Future Directions

ADC leverages the remarkable specificity of the antibody and the robust tumor killing ability of the cytotoxic agent, with the expectation of bringing synergy when putting these two types of modalities together. While the concept is attractive and straightforward, this is certainly not an easy task. The early stage of the ADC development faced numerous challenges, including poor plasma stability, premature payload release, highly variable DAR, high incidence of immunogenicity, off-target toxicity, minimal tumor penetration, and drug resistance. Decades of effort have been spent to overcome these obstacles by expanding antibody target ranges, utilizing humanized antibodies, developing super cytotoxic payloads, and advancing linker technologies and conjugation methods. Three generations of ADCs have been developed so far. In recent years, ADCs have received great attention because of the great success of the newer generations of ADCs for solid tumors, particularly breast cancer. The field is rapidly evolving, with more than 100 ADCs in different phases of clinical development. Lessons and experiences from over 20 years of clinical experience are critical in developing more effective and safe ADCs. There is still a large room in identifying new antigens, developing new antibodies and payloads, and designing new linkers with balanced stability and payload release for the next generation of ADCs. In addition, a number of novel ADC development strategies are currently under investigation, which include 1) connecting the payload to a bispecific antibody targeting different epitopes of the same antigen to facilitate receptor aggregation and target internalization; and 2) development of dual payload ADCs that incorporate two distinct cytotoxic agents in the product to reduce drug resistance. Although it has not been a smooth journey, the future of ADCs looks promising.

Key References

Fu Z, Li S, Han S, Shi C and Zhang Y (2022) Antibody drug conjugate: the "biological missile" for targeted cancer therapy. Signal Transduct Target Ther 7:93.

Jin Y, Schladetsch MA, Huang X, Balunas MJ and Wiemer AJ (2022) Stepping forward in antibody-drug conjugate development. Pharmacol Ther 229:107917.

Kamath AV and Iyer S (2015) Preclinical Pharmacokinetic Considerations for the Development of Antibody Drug Conjugates. Pharm Res 32:3470-3479.

Kaufmann SH (2008) Paul Ehrlich: founder of chemotherapy. Nat Rev Drug Discov 7:373.

Riccardi F, Dal Bo M, Macor P and Toffoli G (2023) A comprehensive overview on antibody-drug conjugates: from the conceptualization to cancer therapy. Front Pharmacol 14:1274088.

Zuo P (2020) Capturing the Magic Bullet: Pharmacokinetic Principles and Modeling of Antibody-Drug Conjugates. AAPS J 22:105.

Chapter 15.
Oligonucleotide Therapeutics

Learning Objectives

After reading this chapter, the reader shall be able to:

1. Get familiar with the history of the development of antisense oligonucleotides (ASOs) and small interfering RNAs (siRNAs).

2. Understand the mechanisms of action of ASOs and siRNAs.

3. Describe the ADME of ASOs and siRNAs.

4. List the advantages of oligonucleotides as therapeutic drugs.

5. Describe the potential safety concerns of ASOs and siRNAs.

6. Compare the differences among small-molecule drugs, ASOs, siRNAs, and antibody drugs.

Oligonucleotide therapeutics are an emerging therapeutic modality. Different from small-molecule drugs and antibodies, whose targets are mostly proteins, oligonucleotide therapeutics act on RNA and thus modify protein expression via gene modulation. As a novel class of drugs, oligonucleotide therapeutics are composed of a wide variety of short strings of synthetically modified RNA or RNA/DNA hybrids, such as antisense oligonucleotides (ASOs), small interfering RNAs (siRNAs), microRNAs (miRNAs), and aptamers. In this chapter, I only focus on ASOs and siRNAs, as these two are more established than others, and both have approved products on the market.

Oligonucleotide therapeutics have incredible potential in the treatment of genetic disorders and thus hold a particularly important position in rare disease area, as more than 70% of rare diseases were found to have a genetic origin. With small variations in the definition across different entities, a disease is considered rare when the incidence is less than 60 per 100,000 people (USA), 50 per 100,000 people (European Union), or 65 per 100,000 people (WHO). Although each rare disease has low prevalence, the aggregated number is large as there are approximately 8000 rare disorders. Rare diseases affect about 30 million people in the USA alone. Approximately 95% of all rare diseases do not yet have treatment, and among people who live with a rare disease, about two-thirds are children. Oligonucleotide therapeutics are of special interest for these rare diseases because of their potential ability to modify the pathogenic gene.

Same as other new modalities, the development of oligonucleotides as therapeutic drugs had faced numerous challenges in the early stage. The central problem is the poor drug profile of naked unmodified oligonucleotides, such as rapid degradation in blood and difficulty in entering cells on their own due to their size and charge. After several decades of efforts in overcoming these hurdles, this new modality has finally come to fruition, with 12 ASOs and 6 siRNA products being approved (as of April 2024) and numerous others in different phases of clinical development. Several approved ASO and siRNAs are very effective in treating a number of rare diseases, and these successes have given hope to the rare disease community.

As ASOs and siRNAs have different mechanisms of action and ADME profiles, I will discuss them separately in section 15.1 (for ASOs) and section 15.2 (for siRNAs). Compared to small-molecule drugs and antibody therapies, ASOs and siRNAs have their distinct advantages as therapeutic drugs; this is discussed in section 15.3. There are considerable differences in terms of structure, physicochemical properties, pharmacokinetics, pharmacodynamics, and clinical pharmacology related features among small-molecules, oligonucleotides (e.g., ASOs and siRNAs in this chapter) and therapeutic antibodies; I will summarize these differences in section 15.4.

15.1 Antisense Oligonucleotides (ASOs)

15.1.1 Introduction

ASOs are short *single-stranded* synthetic DNA/RNA molecules, typically comprised of 15-22 nucleotides. ASOs bind to RNA in a sequence specific manner via Watson-Crick base pairing. The first preclinical use of ASOs to modulate RNA function can be dated back to 1978. As noted earlier, the naked unmodified ASOs have poor drug profiles, and tremendous efforts have been made to enhance their clinical utility. It took 2 decades for the first ASO drug, fomivirsen, to be approved by the FDA in 1998, intended for use in HIV patients with cytomegalovirus (CMV) retinitis. Later on, CMV retinitis was no longer a medical problem for HIV patients owing to the development of highly efficacious HIV therapies. Accordingly, fomivirsen was withdrawn from the European market in 2002 and from the USA in 2006. Nevertheless, fomivirsen represents a milestone in the ASO field.

After the approval of fomivirsen, there was a slow pace of ASO development. It took 15 years to bring the second ASO drug to the market – mipomersen was approved by the FDA in 2013. Three years later, eteplirsen and nusinersen entered the market in 2016. Since then, the development of ASO therapeutics has been accelerating. So far, 12 ASOs have been approved by the FDA and/or EMA (Table 15-1), with numerous candidates under clinical development.

15.1.2 Mechanism of action

ASOs act on RNA and can reduce, restore, or modify protein expression through several mechanisms as detailed below:

   a) *Reduce protein expression via RNase H cleavage*

The physiological role of the enzyme RNase H is to recognize the DNA/RNA complex and degrade the redundant RNA primer after DNA replication has taken

Table 15-1. List of approved antisense oligonucleotides (ASOs).

Name	Modifi cation	Target	Mode of action	Therapeutic Indication	Approval	Route
Fomivirsen	PS	CMV IE2 mRNA	Expression inhibition	CMV retinitis	US 1998 EU 1999	IVT
Mipomersen	PS; 2'-O-MOE	ApoB-100 mRNA	Expression inhibition	HoFH	US 2013	SC
Eteplirsen	PMO	Dystrophin pre-mRNA	Splicing modulation	DMD	US 2016	IV
Nusinersen	PS; 2'-O-MOE	SMN2 pre-mRNA	Splicing modulation	Spinal muscular atrophy	US 2016 EU 2017	IT
Inotersen	PS; 2'-O-MOE	TTR mRNA	Expression inhibition	hATTR	US 2018 EU 2018	SC
Milasen*	PS; 2'-O-MOE	MFSD8	Splicing modulation	Batten's disease	US 2018	IT
Golodirsen	PMO	Dystrophin pre-mRNA	Splicing modulation	DMD	US 2019	IV
Volanesorsen	PS; 2'-OMe	ApoCIII mRNA	Expression inhibition	FCS	EU2019	IV
Viltolarsen	PMO	Dystrophin pre-mRNA	Splicing modulation	DMD	US 2020	IV
Casimersen	PMO	Dystrophin pre-mRNA	Splicing modulation	DMD	US 2021	IV
Eplontersen	GalNac - conjuga ted	TTR mRNA	Expression inhibition	ATTRv-PN	US 2023	SC
Tofersen	PS; 2'-MOE	SOD1 mRNA	Expression inhibition	ALS	US 2023	IT

* Milasen is a personalized drug which is developed for a single patient. ALS: Amyotrophic lateral sclerosis; ATTR: transthyretin amyloidosis; DMD: duchenne muscular dystrophy. FCS: familial chylomicronemia syndrome. IT: Intrathecal; IVT: Intravitreal.

place. ASO therapeutics can bind to their target RNA, which mimics the DNA/RNA complex recognized by RNase H, leading to mRNA degradation (Figure 15-1, left). For ASO drugs with this mechanism, they have unmodified DNA nucleotides in the middle (in order not to disturb the catalysis) and chemically modified nucleic acid analogs inserted at each end of the structure (to protect ASOs from degradation). Because of this DNA/RNA hybrid pattern, these ASOs are also called ASO "gapmers". Representative ASO drugs in this class include fomivirsen, mipomersen, inotersen, and volanesorsen.

b)   Reduce protein expression via steric hindrance

ASOs that do not recruit RNase H may still reduce protein expression through binding to their target RNA and causing translational arrest; this is known as steric hindrance. After pairing with its target mRNA, an ASO can block the translation process by hindering the contact of mRNA with the ribosomal 40s subunit or preventing the assembly on the 40S/60S subunits (Figure 15-1, middle). As ASOs do not activate RNase H-mediated cleavage, the structure of target mRNA is retained. None of the approved ASO drugs act through this mechanism.

c)   Restore protein expression via RNA splicing

Genes have coding segments (exons) interspaced by non-coding regions (introns). During DNA transcription process, pre-mRNA containing both exons and introns is produced first, then splicing factors are recruited to remove the introns, resulting in mature mRNA containing exons only. Some ASOs leverage the RNA splicing mechanism to modify protein production (Figure 15-1, right). There are two types of splice modulation- exon skipping and exon inclusion. In exon skipping, ASOs bind to the pre-mRNA and induce skipping of a mutated exon, thus producing a short but functional protein. Example ASO drugs functioning via this mechanism include eteplirsen, golodirsen, viltolarsen, and casimersen. In exon inclusion, ASOs bind to the pre-mRNA and prevent the splicing factors from accessing the transcript sites, leading to the inclusion of an exon (that is otherwise missed due to genetic disorder) and consequently the restoration of protein production. Example ASO drugs functioning via this mechanism include nusinersen.

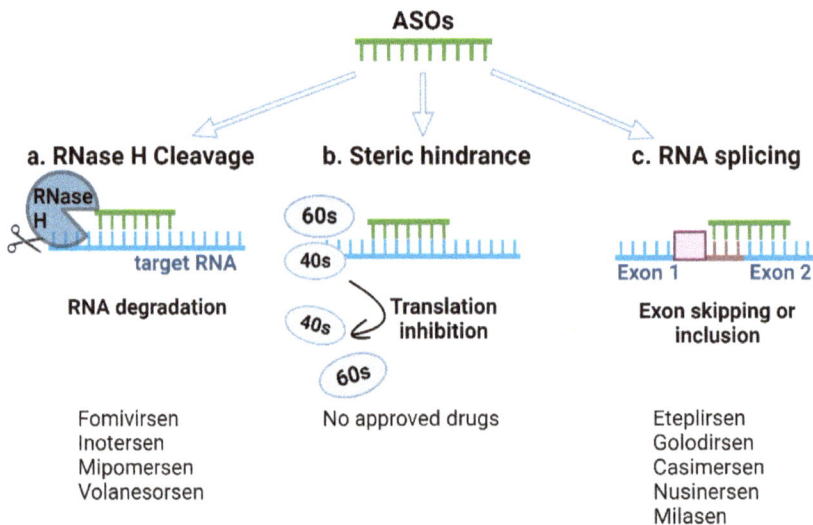

Figure 15-1. Mechanism of action of single strand antisense oligonucleotides. *This figure is adapted from Collotta et al. Frontiers in Pharmacology. 2023;14:1304342.*

15.1.3 Strategies used to enhance the clinical utility of ASOs

One major problem of ASOs is their rapid degradation mediated by endo- and exo-nucleases. To enhance their stability and pharmacokinetics characteristics, substantial efforts have been made to chemically modify the structure of ASOs. From the chemical modification perspective, the development of ASOs has undergone three generations.

- **First generation of modification**

The modification in this generation primarily focuses on the backbone chemistry of ASOs, with the phosphate (PO) backbone being replaced with a phosphorothioate (PS) backbone. Compared with the natural PO backbone, the PS backbone greatly increased the resistance of ASOs to nuclease-based degradation. In addition, ASOs with PS backbone have higher plasma protein binding, further reducing their renal clearance. However, this generation has drawbacks of off-target effects and other safety issues.

- **Second generation of modification**

The modifications in this generation focus on the sugar ring (ribose) instead of the phosphate backbone. Chemical modification of the hydroxyl in the 2' position of ribose sugars enhances their binding affinity and provides further resistance to nuclease-based degradation. The commonly used substitutions include 2'fluoro (2'F), 2'-O-methyl (2'-O-Me), and 2'-O-methoxyethyl (2'-O-MOE). Its worth pointing out that these modifications at the 2' position are not compatible with RNase H-mediated cleavage. This is why ASOs exerting their effects through RNase H require a gapmer pattern in their structure to make sure that the central region is unmodified and sugar-modified RNA-like nucleotides are only at each end. On the other hand, for ASOs acting via splicing, their structure can be fully modified with sugar substitution and PS bonds.

- **Third generation of modification**

Several major structural changes are considered as the third generation of modifications. Representative modifications include locked nucleic acids (LNAs) and alternative backbone structures such as phosphorodiamidate morpholino oligomer (PMO). LNAs increase binding affinity to the target RNA due to their preorganized structure. In PMOs, they are charge neutral and exert their antisense effect through steric hindrance or splice modulation.

As shown in Table 15-1, all approved ASOs are chemically modified. Popular modifications include 2'-O-Me/2'-O-MOE coupled with PS modification, as well as PMO.

While chemical modifications solve the problem of stability, they provide limited help in cellular uptake of ASOs. ASOs have a molecular weight of 6,000 to 10,000 Da. Although they can enter cells via endocytosis, this process may not be sufficient. Most of the approved ASOs are considered as "naked" ASOs, which means that they don't get any help with their delivery. With recent advances in conjugation technology, there is considerable interest in developing conjugated ASOs, particularly N-acetylgalactosamine (GalNAc)-ASO. GalNAc technology was originally developed for siRNA delivery, and now is expanded to ASO development. Detailed information on GalNAc conjugation will be provided in section 15.2. Among the approved ASOs, the only drug that is not "naked" is eplontersen, which is a GalNAc-ASO.

15.1.4 Treatment of ASO in rare diseases – case examples

The approved ASO drugs have been used to treat several rare diseases (Table 15-1), such as spinal muscular atrophy (SMA), Duchenne muscular dystrophy (DMD), transthyretin amyloidosis (TTR), CLN7 Batten disease, and amyotrophic lateral sclerosis (ALS). In this subsection, I will provide a few examples in SMA and DMD, both of which are neurodegenerative diseases.

- **Spinal muscular atrophy (SMA)**

SMA is an autosomal recessive disease caused by low expression of the survival motor neuron (SMN) protein. As the name suggests, this protein is essential for the development and survival of motor neurons. The SMN protein is encoded by the SMN1 gene. Patients with SMA no longer have a working copy of the SMN1 gene due to deletions or inactivating mutations. Humans have a second, almost identical gene called SMN2. However, it is a poor backup – due to a splice issue, exon 7 is excluded from most SMN2 transcripts, leading to the production of a truncated, unstable protein. Therefore, SMN2 only produces a small amount of functional SMN protein, and this amount is inversely correlated with the severity of SMA.

SMA has different types, with types 1-3 occurring in children and type 4 in adults. SMA is the number one genetic cause of infant mortality. For newborns and young children with SMA, their muscles get weak and shrink, and they gradually lose their ability to walk, crawl, or even hold their heads up.

Nusinersen (Spinraza) was approved to treat SMA. The mechanism of action of nusinersen is exon inclusion to restore the function of SMN2. Nusinersen binds to the SMN2 pre-mRNA and suppresses exon 7 splicing; the inclusion of exon 7 results in increased production of functional SMN protein.

Nusinersen is considered a game-changer for SMA patients. Nusinersen was approved by the FDA in December 2016, and many people called the FDA's announcement of nusinersen's approval "a Christmas surprise". Many children with SMA have benefited from nusinersen. One example is Emma Larson, whose story can be found on the internet and in magazines. Following is the story posted on the website of the Cold Spring Habor Laboratory (CSHL) (with minor revision for conciseness):

"Emma Larson was diagnosed with Type 2 SMA when she was one and half years old. When she reached her 2nd year birthday, she was already losing the ability to crawl, and to hold her head up without assistance. Within 2 months of receiving her first injections of nusinersen, Emma began to improve. "It was a miracle," Dianne (Emma's mom) recalls. One day Emma crawled all the way from

the living room to her mother's bedroom, catching her completely by surprise. "I was freaking out! I couldn't believe she had crawled all the way!" Dianne remembers. Today, Emma continues to receive injections and to improve. She is graduating from a walker to crutches, and getting ready to join her peers in preschool. "We are in tears over here, along with the rest of the community! Amazing! Still numb," Dianne said in an email the morning after the drug's FDA approval." [from the website of CSHL; this drug was conceived and developed by CSHL Professor Adrian Krainer and collaborators]

- ***Duchenne muscular dystrophy (DMD)***

DMD is a genetic disorder that leads to progressive muscle weakness and degeneration, and it is caused by mutations in the dystrophin gene, which is the longest gene in the human genome and encodes the dystrophin protein. Mutations in the dystrophin gene can disrupt the reading frame and produce an early stop codon, leading to premature termination of translation and ultimately the complete loss of the dystrophin protein. The majority of these mutations occur in exons 43-55. DMD occurs between the ages of 2-5 years with delayed walking, weakness, and loss of muscle function. Most children with DMD need a wheelchair by their teenage years.

Currently, there are 4 ASOs approved by the FDA to treat DMD, and all of them exert their antisense effect through exon skipping. For example, eteplirsen induces exon 51 skipping, casimersen targets exon 45, while both golodirsen and viltolarsen focus on exon 53. Through exon skipping, these ASO drugs correct the reading frame of the dystrophin mRNA. As a result, a short but functional dystrophin protein is produced, which can reduce the severity of DMD.

15.1.5 Pharmacokinetics

- ***ADME***

Due to their large molecular weight (6,000 to 10,000 Da) and charge, ASOs have low membrane permeability. Therefore, oral administration is generally not applicable for ASOs because of their low bioavailability. ASOs are commonly administered via IV and SC, with a few products given via nonconventional routes (e.g., intrathecal delivery to the central nervous system, intravitreal delivery to the eye). The bioavailability was found to be high following SC administration of ASOs. For example, both eterplirsen and mipomersen were fully absorbed via S.C. route, resulting in 100% bioavailability.

After entering systemic circulation, ASOs distribute to tissues extensively and rapidly, which is reflected by a marked drop in plasma concentration-time curve during the initial distribution phase. The distribution of ASOs from tissues back to plasma is a slow process, leading to an extended terminal phase of ASO plasma pharmacokinetics with a long half-life (days to weeks). The pattern of rapid decline in the distribution phase and slow terminal phase was clearly observed in the pharmacokinetic profiles of ISIS 104838 in both monkey and human (Figure 15-

2). ISIS 104838 is a gapmer ASO with PS and 2'-O-MOE modifications. with chemical modifications similar to approved gapmers ASOs, such as eterplirsen, mipomersen, and volanesorsen. The pharmacokinetics of ASOs are mainly driven by backbone chemistry and are sequence-independent within the same chemical class.

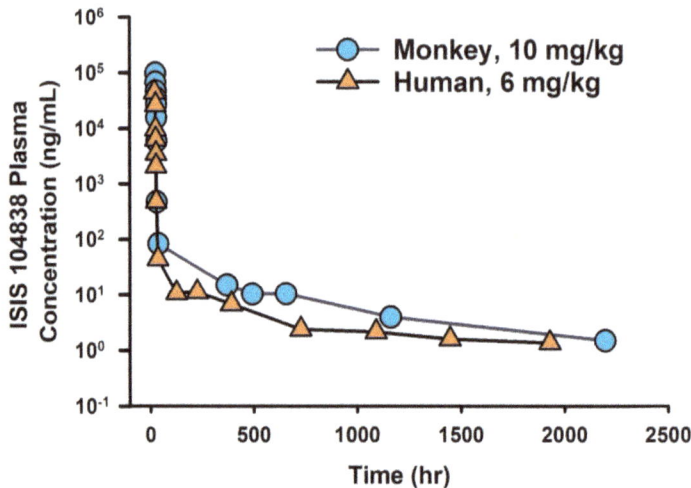

Figure 15-2. Pharmacokinetic profiles of ISIS 104838 in plasma after 1-h infusion in monkey and human. ISIS 104838 is a gapmer ASO with PS and 2'-O-MOE modifications. *This figure is adapted from Geary RS, et al. Drug Metabolism and Disposition 2003;31:1419–1428.*

In general, ASOs are readily distributed to tissues with fenestrated capillaries, such as the liver and kidney, but poorly distributed to tissues with tight continuous capillaries. The concentrations of ASOs in the liver can be several thousand-fold higher than in the plasma (Figure 15-3). Once reaching tissues, ASOs enter tissue cells by phagocytosis or endocytosis, followed by endosome escape and translocation into the nucleus, the final destination for ASOs to produce the desired biological response.

In terms of metabolism, ASOs are metabolized by both endonuclease and exonuclease, which cut the internal part and terminal site of ASOs, respectively, leading to shortened sequence metabolites that do not retain pharmacological activity. The approved ASO drugs have extensive modifications in their structure and thus have good resistance to nuclease degradation. ASOs with PMO modification are particularly stable in the presence of nucleases. For example, no metabolites were formed when eteplirsen was incubated with plasma and liver subcellular fractions.

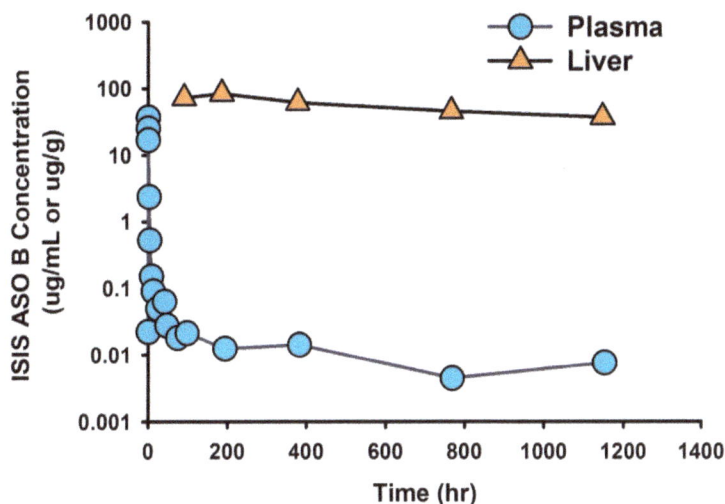

Figure 15-3. Pharmacokinetic profiles of an ASO in plasma and liver after 1-h infusion in monkey. This ASO contained PS and 2'-OMe modifications. *This figure is adapted from Geary RS, et al. Advanced Drug Delivery Reviews 2015;87: 46–51.*

Regarding excretion, the extent of renal excretion of ASOs depends on the type of chemical modifications. ASOs that contain a PS backbone are extensively bound to plasma proteins (≥85%). This high protein binding prevents substantial loss of drug to glomerular filtration. Accordingly, ASOs with PS modification only undergo limited renal excretion. For example, for 2′-MOE and PS-modified ASOs, their renal excretion only accounts for <3% of the total clearance in human. In contrast, ASOs that contain a PMO backbone are charge neutral and have low plasma protein binding. As a result, ASOs with PMO modifications are readily cleared via renal excretion and accordingly have plasma half-lives that are shorter than those containing a PS backbone.

- *Pharmacokinetics in special populations*

Recently, the pharmacokinetics of 2′-MOE and PS-modified ASOs were evaluated in subjects with renal or hepatic impairment. The results showed that moderate and mild renal impairment had no impact on the pharmacokinetics of the investigated ASOs, while severe renal impairment had a mild effect on pharmacokinetic exposure (up to 34%) relative to healthy volunteers. This result is consistent with the limited renal excretion for ASOs with 2′-MOE and PS modifications. Mild hepatic impairment had no effect on ASO disposition. As no subjects with moderate and severe hepatic impairment were enrolled in the study, it is unclear whether ASO pharmacokinetics will change under such conditions.

Since 2′-MOE and PS-modified ASOs share similar ADME characteristics, information learned from the tested ASOs may be applicable to other ASOs with same chemical modifications. However, this information should not be generalized to ASOs with different modifications, such as those containing a PMO backbone, because their ADME are quite different from those of 2′-MOE and PS-modified ASOs.

- ***Drug-drug interactions (DDIs)***

DDIs between ASOs and small-molecule drugs have been investigated in several in vitro and in vivo studies. The results showed that ASO drugs are neither substrates nor inhibitors/inducers of drug metabolizing enzymes and drug transporters. Therefore, when an ASO is co-administered with a small-molecule drug, the enzyme- or transporter-mediated DDI is low.

15.1.6 Safety

While ASO drugs are highly effective in treating several rare diseases, their potential toxicity should not be ignored. For example, mipomersen was approved in 2013 with a black box warning on the risk of liver enzyme elevation and hepatic steatosis, and it was withdrawn from the market in 2019 due to an unacceptable risk of hepatoxicity. As shown in Figure 15-4, many ASO drugs share common adverse effects, such as liver toxicity (e.g., mipomersen, inotersen), kidney toxicity (e.g., nusinersen, inotersen, golodirsen, viltolarsen, and casimersen), and hypersensitivity reactions (e.g., inotersen, eteplirsen, and golodirsen). One potential mechanism of ASO toxicity is RNase-H mediated off-target effects. It has been reported that 6-7 base pairs between the ASO and nontarget mRNA are sufficient to trigger RNase activity, resulting in the cleavage of wrong targets. The potential explanation for renal toxicity is the accumulation of the ASOs and their shortened sequence metabolites in the kidney.

15.2 Small Interfering RNAs (siRNAs)

15.2.1 Introduction

In 1998, Fire and Mello published a seminal paper on RNA interference (RNAi) in *Caenorhabditis elegans*. In this article, they demonstrated that double-stranded RNAs could regulate protein-coding genes through post-transcriptional gene suppression. Three years later, two research groups independently reported that synthetic 21-22 nucleotide double stranded RNAs can modulate protein expression in mammalian cells. These groundbreaking discoveries highlighted the

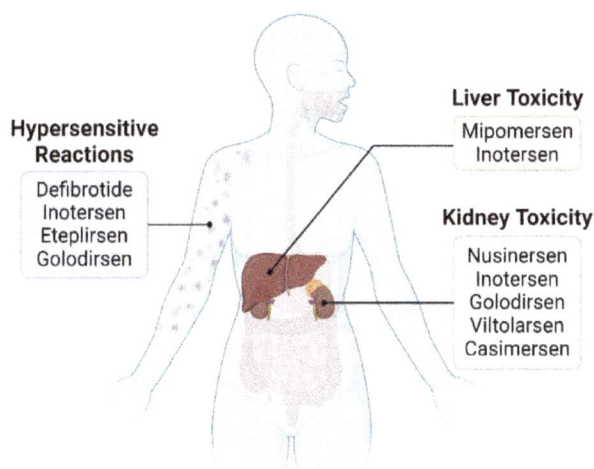

Figure 15-4. Toxicity of the FDA-approved ASO drugs.   *This figure is adapted from Alhamadani F, et al. Drug Metabolism and Disposition 2022;50:879-887.*

tremendous potential of these small interfering RNAs (siRNAs) to be used as a new therapeutic modality to treat previously "undruggable" diseases. Same as ASOs, naked unmodified siRNAs undergo rapid degradation in the blood. In addition, siRNAs are double stranded, which means that their molecular weight, on average, is twice that of the single stranded ASOs. Therefore, it is even harder for siRNAs to enter cells on their own due to their size and charge.

Same as ASOs, the journey of developing siRNA as a new therapeutic modality was not smooth. It took almost 2 decades for the first siRNA drug, patisiran, to be approved by the FDA in 2018. Patisiran is a lipid nanoparticle (LNP)-formulated siRNA and is indicated for the treatment of polyneuropathy caused by an illness called hereditary transthyretin-mediated amyloidosis (hATTR amyloidosis). In 2019, the second siRNA drug, givosiran, hit the market. Givosiran does not use LNP formulation; it is conjugated with GalNAc and represents the first GalNAc-siRNA conjugate. Soon after, three more GalNAc-siRNA conjugates were approved by the FDA; these drugs are lumasiran (2020 approval), inclisiran (2021 approval), and vutrisiran (2022 approval). The list of GalNAc-conjugated siRNAs approved or in different stages of clinical development is provided in Table 15-2.

Table 15-2. The list of GalNAc-conjugated siRNAs approved or in different stages of clinical development. *(adapted from An G. J Clin Pharmacol 2024;64(1):45-57.)*

Drug Candidate	Company	Clinical Phase	Target	Therapeutic Indication
Givosiran,	Alnylam	Registered	D-aminolevulinate synthase 1	Acute hepatic porphyria
Lumasiran	Alnylam	Registered	Glycolate oxidase 1	Hyperoxaluria type 1
Inclisiran	Alnylam/Novartis	Registered	PCSK9	Hypercholesterolemia
Vutrisiran	Alnylam	Registered	Transthyretin	TTR amyloidosis
Fitusiran	Alnylam/Sanofi	Phase 3	Antithrombin	Hemophilia/bleeding disorders
Nedosiran	Dicerna	Phase 3	Lactate Dehyrogenase	Primary hyperoxaluria
Olpasiran	Amgen	Phase 3	Lipoprotein A	Cardiovascular disease
Cemdisiran	Alnylam	Phase 2	Complement C5	Complement-mediated diseases
AB-729	Arbutus	Phase 2	Viral protein	Hepatitis B infection
JNJ-3989	Arrowhead/JNJ	Phase 2	HNV viral proteins	Hepatitis B infection
ALN-AAT02	Alnylam	Phase 1/2	AAT	AAT deficiency-associated liver disease
ALN-HBV02	Alnylam	Phase 1/2	HBV viral protein	Chronic HBV infection
ALN-HSD	Alnylam/Regereron	Phase 1/2	HSD17B13	Non-alcoholic steatohepatitis (NASH)
SLN-124	Silence	Phase 1/2	TMPRSS6	Thalassemia
DCR-HBVs	Dicerna/Roche	Phase 1	HNV viral protein	Hepatitis B infection
DCR-A1AT	Dicerna	Phase 1	SERPINA1	Alpha 1 anti-trypsin deficiency liver disease
Zilebesiran	Alnylam	Phase 1	Angiotensinogen	Hypertension

15.2.2 Mechanism of action

siRNAs are double-stranded RNAs. They are composed of 19-21 base pairs in length with two nucleotide overhangs at the 3' ends of each strand. Different from ASOs which have several mechanisms of action (e.g., RNase activation, steric hindrance, and splicing modulation), siRNAs only have one mechanism - inhibition of target gene expression through triggering the RNAi pathway. RNAi is an intrinsic mechanism of post-transcriptional gene silencing, occuring in the cytosol of cells. The siRNA enters cells through endocytosis to form endosomes; a small fraction exits the endosome and enters the cytosol, a process known as endosomal escape. Once in the cytoplasm, siRNA is incorporated into RNA-induced silencing complex (RISC) and subsequently unwound into the sense and antisense strands. The sense strand, also known as the passenger strand, is cleaved and discarded. The antisense strand, also called the guide strand, remains and serves as a guide to bind the target mRNA, resulting in degradation and silencing of the target gene. The schematic of s.c. delivery of GalNAc-conjugated siRNA is shown in Figure 15-5.

15.2.3 Strategies used to enhance the clinical utility of siRNAs

Similar to ASOs, naked unmodified siRNAs have poor drug profiles. The key challenge of siRNA development is to ensure that systemically administered siRNAs reach their site of action in sufficient amount. This is not a small task, as there are multiple hurdles on the road before siRNA molecules reach the targeted destination - the cytosol of relevant cells in a target tissue. These hurdles include 1) rapid degradation by a host of ubiquitous exonucleases and endonucleases within the plasma; 2) difficulty in entering cells on their own due to their large size (around 14,000 Da) and charge (around 40 negatively charged phosphates); and 3) difficulty in escaping the endosome after entering the cell via internalization. It has taken nearly two decades to overcome these hurdles. The following are two broad strategies that have been successfully implemented to enhance the "druggability" of siRNAs.

- *Chemical modification*

One strategy is modify the sugar-phosphate backbone of siRNAs. For example, replacing a natural PO backbone with a PS backbone enhances siRNA resistance to nuclease-mediated cleavage and increases the hydrophobicity of the backbone, leading to increased plasma protein binding and extended circulation time; these improvements result in a more favorable pharmacokinetic profile of siRNAs. To avoid the interference from PS in the central part of the strand with RISC recognition and activation, partial PS modification at the end of the strands is usually used.

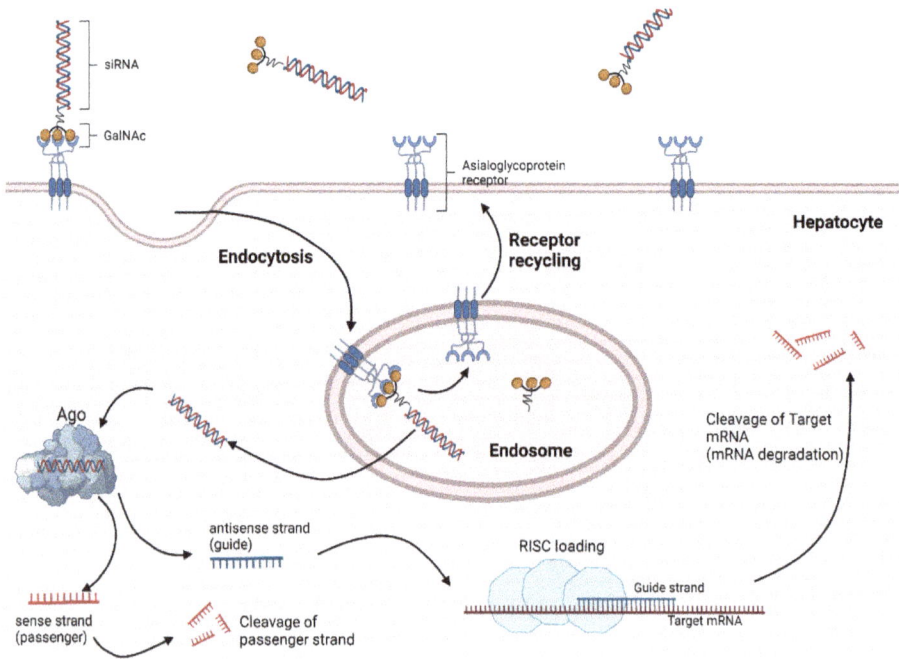

Figure 15-5. Mechanism of action of GalNAc-conjugated siRNAs. GalNAc-conjugated siRNA molecules, once reach systemic circulation, can be efficiently taken into the liver through ASGPR-mediated endocytosis and accumulated in endosomes. Due to a pH drop during endosomal maturation, GalNAc is dissociated from ASGPR. Then GalNAc and the linkers are degraded to free up siRNAs, while ASGPR recycles back to the cell surface. For the free siRNA molecules, most of them remain trapped in the endosome, with only a small fraction (<1%) being released into cytoplasm. Once in the cytoplasm, siRNA is incorporated into RISC. During siRNA-RISC assembly, the siRNA duplex is unwound into the sense and antisense strands, where the former (passenger/sense strand) is cleaved and discarded whereas the latter (guide/antisense strand) remains and serves as a guide to bind the target mRNA in a complementary fashion, leading to the degradation and silencing of the target gene. ASGPR, Asialoglycoprotein receptor; GalNAc, N-acetylgalactosamine; RISC, RNA-induced silencing complex. *This figure is from An G. J Clin Pharmacol 2024;64(1):45-57.*

Another strategy is modify the sugar 2'OH group since it is not involved in the catalytic activity of RISC and meanwhile is prone to endoribonuclease degradation. The 2'OH group is commonly replaced with a 2'-fluoro (2'-F) or 2'-O-methyl (2'-OMe), which greatly increases the stability of siRNA toward nucleases. In addition, these 2' modifications are well tolerated by the RNAi machinery and dramatically decrease immunogenic reactions. Nowadays, most of the siRNAs in clinical trials utilize fully 2' modified siRNAs containing multiple 2'-F and 2'-OMe modifications in the structure.

Over the years, several generations of siRNA chemistry design have been developed. These include 1) standard template chemistry (STC), which replaced all 2'OHs with an alternating 2'-F and 2'-OMe pattern; 2) enhanced stability chemistry (ESC), which increased 2'-OMe content, decreased 2'-F content, and added two PS on the 5' end of each strand; 3) advanced ESC, which further reduced 2'-F to 9-10 positions with the remaining being 2'-OMe, and 4) ESC+, which incorporated a glycerol nucleic acid (GNA) to reduce off-target seed interaction.

- Delivery systems – GalNAc conjugation technology

While chemical modifications greatly increase siRNA stability and reduce immunogenic reactions, this strategy alone is not enough as siRNAs have the inherent cell permeability issue. One early delivery strategy to address this issue was to encapsule siRNAs into nanocarriers, such as LNPs. As noted earlier, the first approved siRNA drug, patisiran, is formulated by LNP. However, LNPs are not ideal carriers. They can cause excipient-induced inflammation. In addition, large doses of encapsulated siRNA with frequent administration are often needed with LNP formulation.

Another delivery strategy is to conjugate a ligand directly to naked siRNAs to facilitate cell uptake. The most popular ligand is GalNAc, a sugar derivative of galactose that binds to asialoglycoprotein (ASGPR) with high affinity and specificity. As ASGPR is highly abundant on the surface of hepatocytes (about 500,000 copies per hepatocyte) with rapid recycling and turnover, using GalNac as the ligand ensures sufficient cell uptake of siRNAs. Indeed, it has been reported that a single administration of GalNAc-siRNA can yield high siRNA uptake. Compared to LNP-formulated siRNAs, GalNAc-siRNA conjugates have the following advantages: 1) more favorable safety profiles, 2) easier synthesis, 3) longer PD duration, 4) less frequent administration, and 5) allow for more convenient administration route (I.V. for LNP-formulated siRNAs vs S.C. for GalNAc-siRNA conjugates). GalNAc conjugation technology is by far the most successful and widely used approach for systemic delivery of siRNAs for liver-based diseases.

15.2.4 Pharmacokinetics

As most siRNA products approved or under various phases of clinical development are GalNAc-siRNA conjugates, in this section, I only focus on GalNAc-siRNA drugs.

- ***ADME***

GalNAc-conjugated siRNAs are quickly absorbed following S.C. administration, with T_{max} approximately 3-4 h in humans. Within the range of tested doses, GalNAc-conjugated siRNAs demonstrated linear pharmacokinetics, which has been consistently observed in rats, monkeys, and humans. The plasma protein binding of GalNAc-conjugated siRNAs is around 80% to 90% at clinically relevant concentration levels and decreases at toxicological dose levels (>100 mg/kg). The high plasma protein binding was found to have minimal impact on ASGPR-mediated uptake of GalNAc-conjugated siRNAs. Upon absorption into systemic circulation, GalNAc-conjugated siRNAs are quickly and predominately taken up by the liver, resulting in a much higher liver concentration than that in the plasma. Compared to the extensive distribution to the liver, there is a much smaller faction (up to 25-fold lower) distributed to the kidney.

After the GalNAc-siRNA enters the cell, the GalNAc moiety is cleaved by β-N-acetylglucosaminidase during endo/lysosomal trafficking. Like ASOs, the deconjugated siRNA undergoes metabolism through exonucleases and endonucleases. Exonucleases cut the end of siRNA strands, resulting in the release of mononucleotides, whereas endonucleases cut nucleotides from the middle of the chain, leading to strands of varying lengths. Due to extensive chemical modifications, GalNAc-conjugated siRNAs are stable in systemic circulation with limited metabolism in plasma (<10%); this has been consistently observed across conjugates and species. Preclinical mass balance data showed that only a small fraction (<25%) of siRNAs were excreted in their unchanged parent form, which has been observed for different GalNAc-siRNA conjugates designed for different targets. Preclinical data indicated that the majority of the GalNAc-conjugated siRNAs were metabolized slowly in the liver and excreted as shortmer metabolites into urine and bile. These preclinical data are in good agreement with the clinical data obtained from approved GalNAc-siRNA drugs, where the siRNA molecules excreted as intact forms in human accounted for less than 30% of the administered doses.

- ***Pharmacokinetics in special populations***

The pharmacokinetics of GalNAc-siRNAs in special populations have been evaluated for several approved products. Overall, no meaningful impact of renal impairment on the pharmacokinetics of GalNAc-siRNAs was observed in humans. For example, no clinically relevant difference in givosiran exposure was observed in patients with mild, moderate, or severe renal impairment compared to patients with normal renal function. A similar conclusion was also reached for lumasiran and vutrisiran. For inclisiran, although there was an increase in inclisiran exposure in patients with severe renal impairment (2.5-fold), the pharmacodynamic markers were comparable to those with normal renal function, indicating the lack of clinical impact. For all approved GalNAc-conjugated siRNAs, dose adjustment is not needed in patients with renal impairment. Regarding the impact of hepatic impairment on GalNAc-siRNA pharmacokinetics, the clinical experience and available literature data are much more limited due to the difficulty in recruiting participants, especially patients with severe hepatic impairment. Based on the data collected in patients with mild/moderate hepatic impairment, no dose adjustment is needed for givosiran, vutrisiran, lumasiran, and inclisiran.

- ***Drug-drug interactions***

Since GalNAc-conjugated siRNAs are metabolized by exonucleases and endonucleases, they are unlikely to be substrates of drug-metabolizing enzymes that are commonly involved in small-molecule metabolism (e.g. CYP enzymes). Indeed, in vitro DDI data showed that none of the tested GalNAc siRNAs are substrates of any CYP isoform evaluated. Therefore, there is low potential of enzyme-mediated siRNA-drug interaction with the siRNA being the victim drug. In addition, none of the tested GalNAc siRNAs are inducers or time-dependent inhibitors of any CYP450 isoform evaluated, indicating a low possibility of enzyme-mediated siRNA-drug interaction with the siRNA being the perpetrator. Additionally, none of the evaluated GalNAc-conjugated siRNAs are substrates of transporters; one has an inhibitory effect on P-gp, but is not clinically relevant.

So far, the only siRNA drug that has clinically meaningful DDI is givosiran, which indirectly modulates CYP enzymes through a different mechanism. Givosiran inhibits ALAS and can potentially lower hepatic heme content, which may subsequently reduce the activity of CYP enzymes. A recent clinical DDI study showed that givosiran increased the plasma exposure of caffeine (CYP1A2 substrate), dextromethorphan (CYP2D6 substrate), omeprazole (CYP2C19 substrate), midazolam (CYP3A4 substrate), and losartan (CYP2C9 substrate) by 3-fold, 2.4-fold, 1.6-fold, 1.4-fold; and 1.1-fold, respectively. In a separate report, two patients experienced a strong anticoagulant effect of vitamin K antagonists (CYP2C9 substrates) after the first dose of givosiran, indicating that givosiran likely inhibits CYP2C9 more substantially than originally reported.

15.2.5 Unique pharmacokinetics-pharmacodynamic relationships

The pharmacokinetics/pharmacodynamics relationship of GalNAc-conjugated siRNAs is very different from small-molecules and protein drugs. The key feature is that plasma pharmacokinetics of GalNAc-siRNAs and their PD effects are completely disconnected (Figure 15-6). As noted earlier, GalNAc-siRNAs in the circulation are rapidly taken into hepatocytes via ASGPR-mediated uptake. As a result, the plasma exposure of GalNAc-conjugated siRNAs is generally transient, with a short plasma half-life in humans ($t_{1/2}$ around 10 h). In sharp contrast, GalNAc-siRNAs have a delayed onset of action and prolonged duration of pharmacodynamic response, with the effect remaining for months in humans. For example, givosiran has transient plasma pharmacokinetics, but a sustained and dose-dependent pharmacodynamic response lasting for months after a single SC dose in human. Similar transient plasma pharmacokinetics and prolonged pharmacodynamic effect were also observed in human for all other approved GalNAc-conjugated siRNAs, namely lumasiran, inclisiran, and vutrisiran, as well as many other products that are under clinical development (e.g olpasiran, cemdisiran, and fitusiran). Due to the prolonged PD duration, givosiran and lumariran are administered to patients once monthly, vutrisiran is given once every 3 months. For inclisiran, it is given 3 months after the first dose, then every 6 months.

Results from animal studies demonstrated that the direct pharmacodynamic driver of GalNAc-conjugated siRNAs is not siRNA concentrations in plasma or in the liver, but the cytoplasmic concentrations of siRNA bound to RISC. Brown and colleagues conducted a mechanism study and found that siRNA accumulation and stability in acidic intracellular compartments are critical for long-term activity. GalNAc-siRNA conjugates were delivered through ASGPR-mediated endocytosis and accumulated in acidic intracellular compartments (e.g. endosomes). Then siRNAs were slowly released into the cytosol from these compartments followed by subsequent RISC loading. The slow releases over time from these intracellular compartments was believed to be the key reason for delayed onset of activity and prolonged PD duration. Interestingly, the pharmacodynamic duration of LNP-formulated siRNAs was much shorter than GalNAc-conjugated siRNAs, likely due to a one-time, bolus-like release of siRNA into the cytosol instead of the slow release over time as seen in conjugate delivery.

15.2.6 Safety

- **Immunogenicity**

The issue of immunogenicity of naked and unmodified siRNAs has been successfully addressed by extensive chemical modifications, especially the replacement of the sugar 2'OH group with 2'-F or 2'-OMe. All currently approved GalNAc-conjugated siRNAs are fully 2' modified siRNAs and their immunogenicity incidence is low (<2.5% for those approved GalNAc-siRNA drugs).

- **Off-target RNAi silencing**

The siRNA guide strand seed region contains only seven bases. Therefore, off-target RNAi silencing can occur if there is an unintended seed region match between siRNA guide strand and non-targeted mRNAs. This potential issue can be alleviated by careful sequence selection. During preclinical development phase, a subset of GalNAc-siRNAs was found to cause hepatotoxicity at supratherapeutic doses in rats due to off-target RNAi silencing. To address this potential safety concern, the ESC+ design was developed where these off-target effects can be mitigated by modulating seed-pairing using a thermally destabilizing chemical modification. None of the approved GalNAc-conjugated siRNAs has the issue of off-target-driven hepatotoxicity.

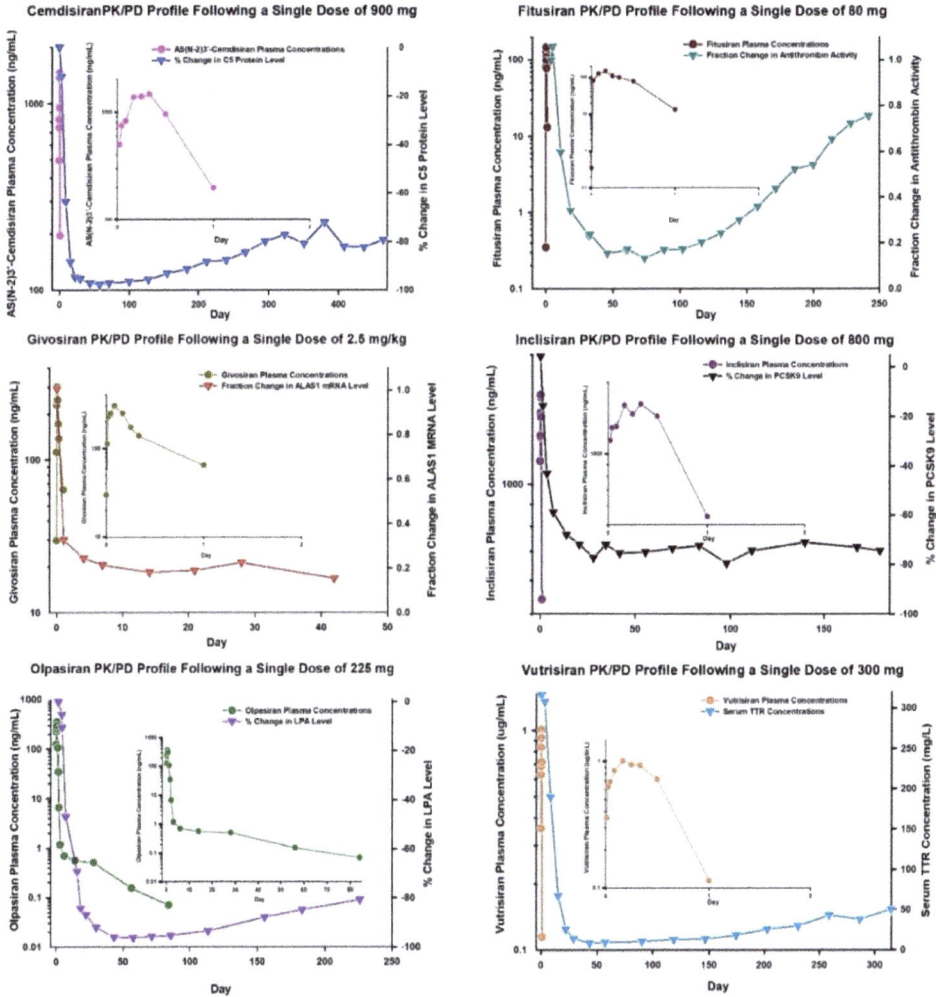

Figure 15-6. Human plasma PK (circles) and PD (triangles) of representative GalNAc-conjugated siRNA products, including cemdisiran (upper left panel), fitusiran (upper right panel), givosiran (middle left panel), inclisiran (middle right panel), olpasiran (lower left panel), and vutrisiran (lower right panel). .*This figure is from An G. J Clin Pharmacol 2024;64(1):45-57.*

15.3 Advantages of Oligonucleotides as Therapeutic Drugs

As a new therapeutic modality, oligonucleotide therapeutics, including both ASOs and siRNAs, have the following advantages over traditional small-molecules and protein-based therapeutics:

- *Battle intracellular and "undruggable" targets*

    Many disease targets located intracellularly are difficult to work with owing to significant structural disorder, large protein–protein interaction interfaces, and/or the lack of deep protein pockets. For those targets, small molecules and protein drugs won't work well because the former requires a specific or well-defined binding pocket, while the latter can only bind to extracellular targets. Oligonucleotide therapeutics generate knockdown at the mRNA level, instead of the protein level. Accordingly, they are not dependent on identifying a binding pocket of the target protein. Therefore, oligonucleotide therapeutics are in a unique position to battle those "undruggable" targets.

- *Simple drug design with lower production cost and a more rapid drug development cycle*

    Once a target mRNA sequence is defined, designing a complementary oligonucleotide molecule is a straightforward process. Because of the complete Watson-Crick base pairing with mRNA, the oligonucleotide product can be highly specific and highly efficacious. As there is no need for a cellular expression system and complex protein purification, the production cost of siRNA is considerably lower than that of protein drugs. In addition, the development process of oligonucleotide therapeutics could be more rapid than that of small molecules. It is well known that the lead compound identification and optimization process of small molecules is time consuming and challenging due to the requirement of sufficient specificity and affinity of drug candidates to the protein target of interest. The development of oligonucleotide therapeutics does not involve such a lengthy process, which is a clear advantage.

- *Extremely versatile with unrestricted choice of targets*

    As oligonucleotide therapeutics can be designed against virtually any gene, once a product is developed, "sister" products with slightly different sequences can rapidly come up to keep pace with the mutations in diseases driven by genetic changes or to battle a different disease with a similar genetic disorder; this is a property that neither small-molecule drugs nor protein products can perform.

For the three advantages of oligonucleotide therapeutics that I listed above, milasen, an ASO drug, serves as a perfect example. A 6-year-old girl was hospitalized after the rapid development of vision loss, frequent falls, dysarthria, and dysphagia. She was diagnosed with Batten's disease, a fatal genetic disorder affecting the retina and the central nervous system. At the time, there was no treatment option for this rare disease. Researchers at Boston Children's Hospital developed a patient-customized treatment for this little girl. After the muted MFSD8 gene was identified via whole-genome sequencing, they designed an antisense oligonucleotide to correct mis-splicing and restore MFSD8 expression. They named it "milasen", which is a 22-nucleotide ASO with the same backbone and sugar chemistry as nusinersen. The patient's condition continued to deteriorate. Due to the urgent nature of the situation, Milasen was rapidly developed in a race against time. From the beginning (e.g., target identification and ASO sequence design) to the FDA approval under Expanded Access Investigational New Drug Application, it only took a year; this is remarkable. The rapid development of milasen was possible, largely due to three factors: 1) ASO can be customized in a sequence-specific fashion; 2) the precedent set by nusinersen allowed for the direct use of same backbone, sugar, and base chemistry. Milasen is essentially a "sister" drug of nusinersen; 3) a relatively simple manufacturing process. If you are interested in learning more detailed information about milasen and the study, I recommend reading the original article (Kim J, et al. N Eng J Med 2019;381:1644-1652.)

15.4 Comparison of Oligonucleotide Therapeutics with Small-molecule drugs and Antibodies

Table 15-3 lists the differences of pharmacokinetics/pharmacodynamics related features among small-molecules, oligonucleotide therapeutics, as well as therapeutic antibodies. As it shows, oligonucleotide therapeutics differ from small-molecules and protein-based drugs in terms of size, mechanism of action, physicochemical and pharmacological properties, ADME, pharmacokinetics/pharmacodynamics relationship, as well as clinical pharmacology features. The ADME and clinical pharmacology features of oligonucleotide products are sequence-independent, which means that these properties can be similar and highly predictable as long as the oligonucleotide drugs have same/similar chemical modification in their structures.

Table 15-3. The differences of pharmacokinetics/pharmacodynamics related features among small-molecules, ASO, GalNAc-siRNA conjugates as well as therapeutic antibodies.

	Small molecules	Oligonucleotide therapeutics		Therapeutic antibodies
		ASO	**GalNAc-siRNA**	
Size	<1000 Da	6,000 to 10,000 Da	~ 16,000 Da	>150,000 Da
Route of delivery	Typically oral; other routes (e.g. IV, IM, SC, inhalation) possible	S.C., I.V., IT	S.C.	Mostly I.V. and S.C.
Plasma Protein binding	Often high plasma protein binding for lipophilic drugs and low binding for hydrophilic drugs	ASOs with PS backbone has high protein binding (>85%); ASOs with PMO backbone has low protein binding	High plasma protein binding (80-90%)	Low plasma protein binding
Binding to tissues	Often high volume of distribution (especially for lipophilic drugs)	Extensive liver distribution	Extensive liver distribution	Usually low volume of distribution, within systemic circulation and extravascular fluid
Metabolism	Metabolized by drug metabolizing enzymes (e.g. CYP450 enzymes)	Metabolized by exonucleases and endonucleases. No drug metabolizing enzyme involved.	Metabolized by exonucleases and endonucleases. No drug metabolizing enzyme involved.	Proteolytic degradation; catabolism by specific (receptor) and non-specific clearance mechanisms. No drug metabolizing enzyme involved.
Renal clearance	Often represents an important elimination pathway	ASOs with PS backbone undergo limited renal excretion. ASOs with PMO backbone are readily cleared by the kidney.	Full-length siRNAs can be cleared by the kidneys. However, not a major elimination route (<25%)	No renal clearance of intact antibody.
Plasma half-life	Relatively short half-life (hours)	Long half-life (days to weeks).	Short half-life (<10 hours)	Long half-life (weeks)
PK linearity	Usually linear PK over therapeutic dose range; Nonlinear PK can happen for some drugs	Linear PK	Linear PK	Often nonlinear at low doses due to target-mediated drug disposition (TMDD); linear PK at high doses

PK/PD relationship	PK usually is independent on PD;	PK is independent on PD;	PK is independent on PD;	PK is often dependent on PD (i.e TMDD);
	PD usually is dependent on PK		Large disconnect between plasma PK and PD;	PD usually is dependent on PK
			PD is dependent on siRNA loaded on RISC, instead of plasma PK	
Drug-drug interaction (DDI)	Commonly seen	Low potential	Low potential	Low potential.

PK: Pharmacokinetics; PD: Pharmacodynamics.

Key References

Alhamadani F, Zhang K, Parikh R, Wu H, Rasmussen TP, Bahal R, Zhong XB and Manautou JE (2022) Adverse Drug Reactions and Toxicity of the Food and Drug Administration-Approved Antisense Oligonucleotide Drugs. *Drug Metab Dispos* **50**:879-887.

An G (2024) Pharmacokinetics and Pharmacodynamics of GalNAc-Conjugated siRNAs. *J Clin Pharmacol* **64**:45-57.

Brown CR, Gupta S, Qin J, Racie T, He G, Lentini S, Malone R, Yu M, Matsuda S, Shulga-Morskaya S, Nair AV, Theile CS, Schmidt K, Shahraz A, Goel V, Parmar RG, Zlatev I, Schlegel MK, Nair JK, Jayaraman M, Manoharan M, Brown D, Maier MA and Jadhav V (2020) Investigating the pharmacodynamic durability of GalNAc-siRNA conjugates. *Nucleic Acids Res* **48**:11827-11844.

Collotta D, Bertocchi I, Chiapello E and Collino M (2023) Antisense oligonucleotides: a novel Frontier in pharmacological strategy. *Front Pharmacol* **14**:1304342.

Debacker AJ, Voutila J, Catley M, Blakey D and Habib N (2020) Delivery of Oligonucleotides to the Liver with GalNAc: From Research to Registered Therapeutic Drug. *Mol Ther* **28**:1759-1771.

Geary RS, Norris D, Yu R and Bennett CF (2015) Pharmacokinetics, biodistribution and cell uptake of antisense oligonucleotides. *Adv Drug Deliv Rev* **87**:46-51.

Geary RS, Yu RZ, Watanabe T, Henry SP, Hardee GE, Chappell A, Matson J, Sasmor H, Cummins L and Levin AA (2003) Pharmacokinetics of a tumor necrosis factor-alpha phosphorothioate 2'-O-(2-methoxyethyl) modified antisense oligonucleotide: comparison across species. *Drug Metab Dispos* **31**:1419-1428.

Humphreys SC, Thayer MB, Campbell J, Chen WLK, Adams D, Lade JM and Rock BM (2020) Emerging siRNA Design Principles and Consequences for Biotransformation and Disposition in Drug Development. *J Med Chem* **63**:6407-6422.

Jiang R, Hooshfar S, Rebecca Eno M, Yun C, Sonego Zimmermann E and Shinkyo R (2023) Factors Influencing ADME Properties of Therapeutic Antisense Oligonucleotides: Physicochemical Characteristics and Beyond. *Curr Drug Metab* **24**:536-552.

Kim J, Hu C, Moufawad El Achkar C, Black LE, Douville J, Larson A, Pendergast MK, Goldkind SF, Lee EA, Kuniholm A, Soucy A, Vaze J, Belur NR, Fredriksen K, Stojkovska I, Tsytsykova A, Armant M, DiDonato RL, Choi J, Cornelissen L, Pereira LM, Augustine EF, Genetti CA, Dies K, Barton B, Williams L, Goodlett BD, Riley BL, Pasternak A, Berry ER, Pflock KA, Chu S, Reed C, Tyndall K, Agrawal PB, Beggs AH, Grant PE, Urion DK, Snyder RO, Waisbren SE, Poduri A, Park PJ, Patterson A, Biffi A, Mazzulli JR, Bodamer O, Berde CB and Yu TW (2019) Patient-Customized Oligonucleotide Therapy for a Rare Genetic Disease. *N Engl J Med* **381**:1644-1652.

Lundin KE, Gissberg O and Smith CI (2015) Oligonucleotide Therapies: The Past and the Present. *Hum Gene Ther* **26**:475-485.

McDougall R, Ramsden D, Agarwal S, Agarwal S, Aluri K, Arciprete M, Brown C, Castellanos-Rizaldos E, Charisse K, Chong S, Cichocki J, Fitzgerald K, Goel V, Gu Y, Guenther D, Habtemariam B, Jadhav V, Janas M, Jayaraman M, Kurz J, Li J, Liu J, Liu X, Liou S, Maclauchlin C, Maier M, Manoharan M, Nair JK, Robbie G, Schmidt K, Smith P, Theile C, Vaishnaw A, Waldron S, Xu Y, Zhang X, Zlatev I and Wu JT (2022) The Nonclinical Disposition and Pharmacokinetic/Pharmacodynamic Properties of N-Acetylgalactosamine-Conjugated Small Interfering RNA Are Highly Predictable and Build Confidence in Translation to Human. *Drug Metab Dispos* **50**:781-797.

Setten RL, Rossi JJ and Han SP (2019) The current state and future directions of RNAi-based therapeutics. *Nat Rev Drug Discov* **18**:421-446.

Shadid M, Badawi M and Abulrob A (2021) Antisense oligonucleotides: absorption, distribution, metabolism, and excretion. *Expert Opin Drug Metab Toxicol* **17**:1281-1292.

Takakusa H, Iwazaki N, Nishikawa M, Yoshida T, Obika S and Inoue T (2023) Drug Metabolism and Pharmacokinetics of Antisense Oligonucleotide Therapeutics: Typical Profiles, Evaluation Approaches, and Points to Consider Compared with Small Molecule Drugs. *Nucleic Acid Ther* **33**:83-94.

Wang Y, Diep JK, Yu RZ, Hurh E, Karwatowska-Prokopczuk E, Schneider E, Henry S, Bhanot S and Geary RS (2023) Assessment of the Effect of Organ Impairment on the Pharmacokinetics of 2'-MOE and Phosphorothioate Modified Antisense Oligonucleotides. *J Clin Pharmacol* **63**:21-28.

Chapter 16.
Chimeric Antigen Receptor T-cell (CAR-T) Therapy

Learning Objectives

After reading this chapter, the reader shall be able to:

1. Understand the mechanism of action of CAR-T therapy
2. Familiar with the manufacture procedure of CAR-T therapy
3. List the FDA-approved CAR-T products
4. Describe the adverse effect of CAR-T products
5. Understand the mechanisms underlying relapses of CAR-T therapy
6. Describe the pharmacokinetics of CAR-T products
7. List the difference between kinetics of a small-molecule drug and CAR-T therapy

---

This is the last chapter of the book. For those of you who have reached this far, thank you for staying with me. For this chapter, I would like to start with a story published in Dec 2023 in the New Yorker Magazine on Christian Wiman, who is among the most distinguished Christian writers of his generation. When he was 39 years old, Wiman was diagnosed with Waldenström's macroglobulinemia, a rare form of lymphoma. He has been fighting against it for 19 years.

"Whenever Wiman's cancer threatened to kill him, a new intervention saved his life. After years of chemotherapy and cancer drugs like rituximab, he got an autologous bone-marrow transplant, which worked for a few years before he got sick again. A new drug, ibrutinib, came along, which gave him a few more years. Another, venetoclax, gave him a few more months after that. Last spring, Wiman became so sick that he could barely get out of bed. He was accepted into an experimental trial and became one of the first people with Waldenström's to undergo chimeric-antigen-receptor T-cell therapy, or CAR-T. The treatment involves intravenous drips of the patient's own T cells, re-engineered in a laboratory to bind with specific antigens on the surface of the patient's cancer cells. "I don't think anyone thought it would work," Wiman's friend the novelist Naeem Murr said. The drip, Murr said, "looks like nothing, a thimble of clear nothing. But it worked, he went into complete remission. It was miraculous."" [with minor revision to keep the content concise]

https://www.newyorker.com/magazine/2023/12/11/a-poets-faith

I share this story because it serves as a good example showing that CAR-T therapy may represent the last resort of relapse and/or refractory blood cancers (such as the one that Wiman has). In addition, from this story you can get a good perspective regarding how people outside of the healthcare field (e.g. Wiman and his friends) think about CAR-T therapy. Wiman's friend Murr said that *"It was miraculous"*. Wiman and his wife commented that *"We've moved beyond the edge of knowledge"*. For this "miracle" drug which *"looks like a thimble of clear nothing"*, how is it made and how does it work? These questions are addressed in sections 16.1 and 16.2, respectively.

16.1 Manufacturing of CAR-T

CAR-T cells are derived from patients' own T cells, which means that they are *autologous*. The advantage of autologous cell therapy is that it can avoid the problem of allogeneic rejection. CAR-T cell manufacturing usually involves in the following steps (Figure 16-1):

Leukapheresis: Leukapheresis is a procedure for removing white blood cells from the blood. During the procedure, blood is collected and goes through a leukapheresis machine, which is a cell separator. White blood cells are then extracted by the machine, while the remaining blood, including the plasma and red blood cells, is returned to the same patient. After white blood cells are collected, they are cryopreserved and shipped to the manufacturing facility.

T-cell activation and transduction: Next step is T-cell activation, which is accomplished by stimulating CD3 and CD28. The stimulation of CD3 (signal 1) triggers T-cell activation while CD28 activation can provide the necessary co-stimulation (signal 2). After T cells are activated, the CAR gene is inserted into the T cell genome. So far, all FDA-approved CAR-T cell products use lentiviral or retroviral transduction to achieve CAR transgene integration.

Ex vivo CAR-T cell expansion: Once T cells are successfully modified to express the CAR transgene, the next step is cell expansion to grow a sufficient number of CAR-T cells in order to meet the required dose for administration. Different methods, such as plates/T-flasks, static culture bags, and rocking motion bioreactors, can be used to grow cells, among which rocking motion bioreactors is the most popular one.

Product release testing: Before the CAR-T cells are shipped back to the clinic, rigorous testing is performed to ensure that they meet defined product characteristics relating to safety, purity, potency, identity, and stability.

Lymphodepleting chemotherapy: Before CAR-T cell transfusion, the patient may receive chemotherapy for pretreatment to wipe out any bad white blood cells that are still circulating around and make room for the new T cells. This chemotherapy pretreatment is known as lymphodepleting conditioning regimen.

CAR-T cell infusion: The CAR-T product is shipped back to the clinic and infused into the patient.

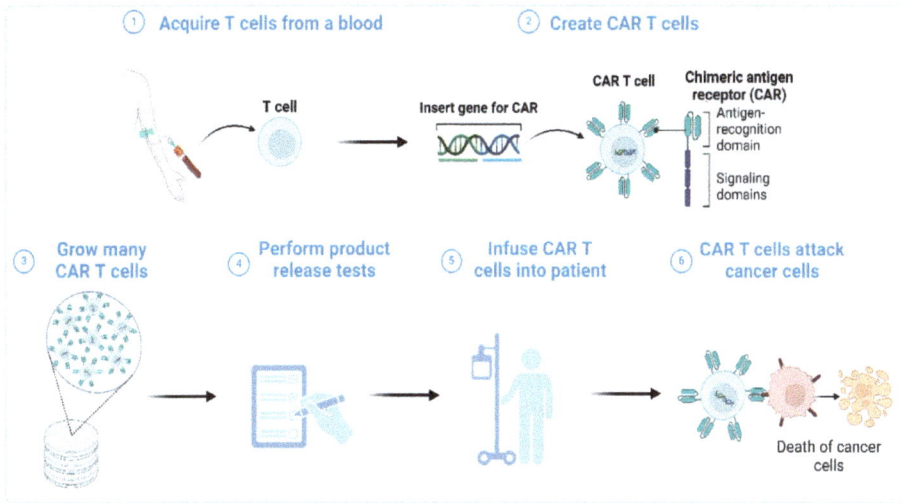

Figure 16-1. CAR-T cell manufacturing process.

16.2 Mechanism of Action

As shown in Figure 16-2, the structure of CARs is typically composed of four domains/regions, namely, extracellular antigen recognition domain, hinge region, transmembrane domain, and intracellular T cell signaling domain. The extracellular domain contains the single-chain variable fragment (scFv), which recognizes specific tumor-associated antigens (TAAs). The intracellular domain includes co-stimulatory and signaling regions. After CAR-T cells are administered in the body, they are navigated to the tumor cells through the interaction between the scFv of the CAR and TAA expressed on the surface of the tumor cells. The binding between the scFv and TAA activates the intracellular co-stimulatory and signaling pathways, resulting in CAR-T-cell mediated tumor killing via cytokine secretion of granzyme and perforins.

The development of CARs has undergone five generations, as shown in Figure 16-3. The first generation of CARs is efficient at antigen recognition but has low proliferation abilities due to the lack of the co-stimulatory component. This limitation has been addressed in the second-generation CAR, in which a co-stimulatory region containing CD28 or 4-1BB is integrated to enhance cell proliferation and cytotoxicity. The third-generation CAR was built on top of the second generation and contains two co-stimulatory regions. Regarding the fourth generation, the CAR-T cells redirected for universal cytokine killings (TRUCKs) contain IL12 expression system, with the goal of enhancing the ability to attach

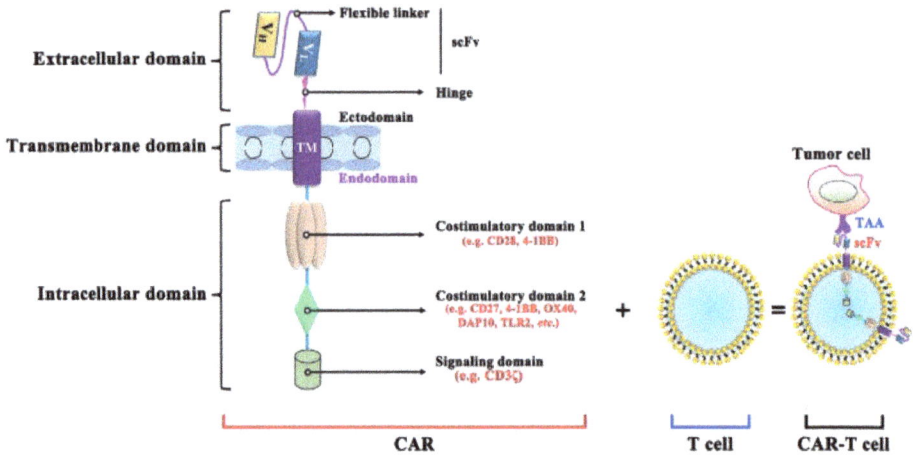

Figure 16-2. CAR-T cell structure and mechanism of action. *This figure is from Chen L, et al. Front. Immunol. 2022; 13: 871661; used under Creative Commons CC-BY license.*

tumor cells. The fifth generation is constructed based on the second generation, and the only difference is that a truncated cytoplasmic IL-2 receptor β-chain (IL-2R β) domain is incorporated in the fifth generation. Although CARs evolve rapidly with five generations being developed, it is unclear which generation provides the best clinical efficacy since currently there are no head-to-head studies to compare the result.

16.3 FDA Approved CAR-T Products

So far, six CAR-T products have been approved by the FDA. The following is a brief description of each product:

- Kymriah (Tisagenlecleucel)

Kymriah represents the first approved CAR-T therapy by the FDA in August 2017. The target antigen is CD19, which is the most frequently used target due to its high expression in most B-cell malignancies. The indications of Kymriah include 1) Patients (below 25 years of age) with B-cell precursor acute lymphoblastic leukemia (B-ALL) that is refractory or in second or later relapse; 2)

Adult patients with relapsed or refractory (r/r) large B-cell lymphoma after two or more lines of systemic therapy, including diffuse large B-cell lymphoma

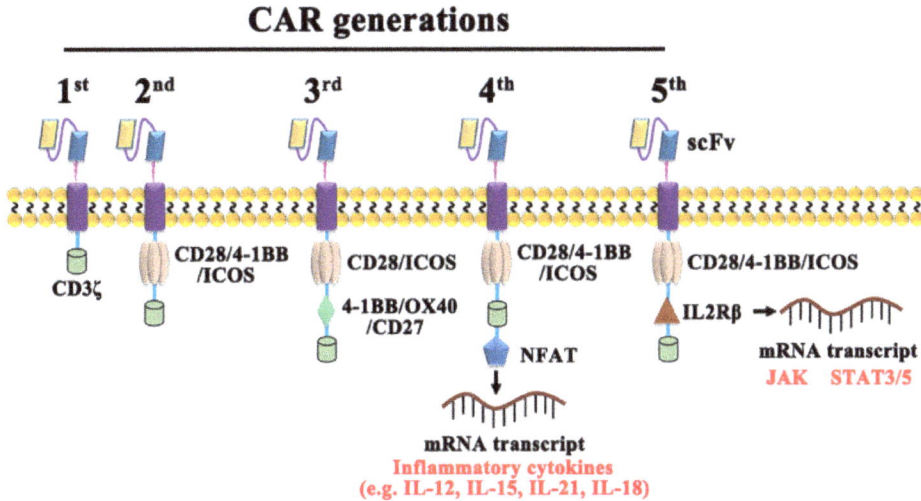

Figure 16-3. The development of CARs, which has undergone five generations. *This figure is from Chen L, et al. Front. Immunol. 2022; 13: 871661; used under Creative Commons CC-BY license.*

(DLBCL) not otherwise specified, high grade B-cell lymphoma, and DLBCL arising from follicular lymphoma; and 3) Adult patients with relapsed or refractory follicular lymphoma (FL) after two or more lines of systemic therapy. The key clinical trials of Kymriah development include JULIET, ELIANA, and ELARA. Among these trials, Kymriah has achieved high objective response rates (ORR, 52-86%) and impressive complete responses (CR, 40-69%) in different blood cancer populations (Table 16-1).

- Yescarta (Axicabtagene ciloleucel)

Yescarta is the second CAR-T therapy available on the market, and it was approved by the FDA in October 2017. Same as Kymriah, the target antigen of Yescarta is also CD19. The intended indications include 1) Adult patients with large B-cell lymphoma (LBCL) that is refractory to first-line chemoimmunotherapy or that relapses within 12 months of first-line chemoimmunotherapy; 2) Adult patients with relapsed or refractory LBCL after two or more lines of systemic therapy, including DLBCL, primary mediastinal LBCL, high grade B-cell lymphoma, and DLBCL arising from follicular lymphoma; and 3) Adult patients with relapsed or refractory FL after two or more lines of systemic therapy. The key clinical trials of Yescarta development include ZUMA-1 and ZUMA-5. Among these trials, Yescarta has achieved high ORR (82-92%) and CR (54-74%) in different blood cancer populations (Table 16-1).

- Tecartus (Brexucabtagene Autoleucel)

Tecartus represents the third CAR-T drug, with intended indications in adult patients with relapsed or refractory mantle cell lymphoma (MCL) as well as adult patients with relapsed or refractory B-ALL. The target antigen of Tecartus is CD19. The key clinical trials include ZUMA-2 and ZUMA-3. Same as Kymriah and Yescarta, Tecartus also achieved high ORR (71-93%) and CR (56-67%) in different blood cancer populations (Table 16-1).

- Breyanzi (Lisocabtagene Maraleucel)

Breyanzi was approved by the FDA in February 2021, with intended use in adult patients with LBCL, high grade B-cell lymphoma, primary mediastinal LBCL, and FL grade 3B. Same as previous CAR-T drugs, the target antigen of Breyanzi is also CD19. The key clinical trials include TRANSCEND and TRANSFORM, in which Breyanzi achieved high ORR (73-86%) and CR (53-66%) in different blood cancer populations (Table 16-1).

- Abecma (Idecabtagene Vicleucel)

Abecma was approved by the FDA in March 2021 for the treatment of adult patients with relapsed or refractory multiple myeloma (MM) after four or more prior lines of therapy, including an immunomodulatory agent, a proteasome inhibitor, and an anti-CD38 monoclonal antibody. The target antigen is BCMA. The key clinical trial performed during Abecma development is KARMMA, in which 128 relapsed or refractory MM patients received the treatment, with an ORR of 73% and a CR of 33%.

- Carvykti (Ciltacabtagene Autoleucel)

Carvykti was approved by the FDA in February 2022. Same as Abecma, the target antigen of Carvykti is also BCMA, and the intended indication is also adult patients with relapsed or refractory MM. The key clinical trial is CARTITUDE, in which 113 relapsed or refractory MM patients received the treatment, with high ORR (93%) and CR (67%).

Table 16-1. FDA-approved CAR-T products and the associated efficacy and toxicity profiles from key clinical trials.

Product, Approval	Trial	Indication	ORR	CR	CRS any/grade ≥3 (%)	ICANS any/grade ≥3 (%)
Kymriah (tisagenlecleu cel), 2017	JULIET (N=93)	DLBC TFL	52	40	58/22	21/12
	ELIANA (N=75)		81	60	77/46	40/13
	ELARA (N=97)	FL	86	69	49/0	37/3
Yescarta (axicabtagene ciloleucel), 2017	ZUMA-1 (N=111)	DLBCL TFL PMBCL	82	54	93/13	64/28
	ZUMA-5 (N=104)	FL MZL	92	74	82/7	59/19
Tecartus (brexucabtage ne autoleucal), 2020	ZUMA-2 (N=60)	MCL	93	67	91/15	63/31
	ZUMA-3 (N=71)	B-ALL	71	56	89/24	60/25
Breyanzi (lisocabtagene maraleucel), 2021	TRANSCEN D (N=256)	LBCL MCL	73	53	42/2	30/10
	TRANSFOR M (N=92)	LBCL	86	66	49/1	12/4
Abecma (idecabtagene vicleucel), 2021	KARMMA (N=128)	MM	73	33	84/5	18/3
Carvykti (ciltacabtagen e autoleucel), 2022	CARTITUD E-1 (N=113)	MM	97	67	95/5	21/10

Abbreviations: DLBCL, diffuse large B-cell lymphoma; TFL, transformed follicular lymphoma; PMBCL, primary mediastinal B-cell lymphoma; FL: follicular lymphoma; MZL: marginal zone lymphoma; LBCL: large B-cell lymphoma; MCL, mantle cell lymphoma; B-ALL, B-cell precursor acute lymphoblastic leukemia; MM, multiple myeloma; ORR, objective response rate; CR, complete response; CRS, cytokine release syndrome; ICANS, immune effector cell-associated neurotoxicity syndrome.

For the CAR-T products listed above, they are used as the last resort of relapse and/or refractory blood cancers, and all of them have demonstrated high ORR and CR. I would like to share the story of Emily Whitehead, who probably holds a spot not only in CAR-T field but also in the cancer history books, considering that she was the first pediatric patient receiving Kymriah, the first CAR-T product, when the drug was still in the development phase.

"At only six-years-old, Emily Whitehead was facing a life-threatening recurrence of acute lymphoblastic leukemia. Emily's cancer resisted over 16 months of chemotherapy treatments when her parents were told that her cancer had relapsed and that she would not survive. Determined to save their child's life, her parents enrolled her in a clinical trial of a new immunotherapy treatment, called CAR-T cell therapy, which had never been tested in a child before. The treatment worked, and Emily's cancer went into complete remission immediately. In June 2012, at age 7, Emily was discharged from the hospital. Nearly 1,000 people gathered in Emily's town to welcome her home and celebrate her triumph over leukemia. Emily Whitehead's story made national headlines. Emily held her father's hand as he spoke at the FDA approval hearing for the Kymriah, which was approved in August 2017. It has been over 10 years since her treatment, Emily remains cancer-free." [*I made minor revision to keep the content concise. The whole story can be found from https://www.cancerresearch.org/stories/patients/emily-whitehead*]

Emily's story clearly indicated the impact of CAR-T therapy, which indeed has been revolutionary with remarkably effective response. However, it's worth pointing out that the impressive efficacy of CAR-T therapy does not come without a cost. As shown in Table 1, high incidences of toxicities were observed during the treatment; this is the topic of section 16.4.

16.4 Safety Considerations

For Emily Whitehead's story that I shared in the previous section, that is not the whole story. Before Emily achieved complete remission, she experienced a severe side effect of the CAR-T therapy. The following is the story from two posts on the website of Children Hospital of Philadelphia.

"As momentous as the promise of T-cell therapy was, the actual delivery was very simple. The family stayed nearby, and Emily came in for the injection of her reprogrammed T cells as an outpatient. An hour after the infusion, she was free to leave, with instructions to stay nearby and come back if she started to show signs of a reaction. Emily did have a reaction. It began as a fever about six hours after the infusion, and she was admitted to the oncology floor. Within two days, her blood pressure became unstable, and she was moved to the Pediatric Intensive Care Unit (PICU).

The medical team worked quickly to determine what had caused her sudden illness. They learned that the level of a certain protein had become very elevated as a result of the T cells growing in her body. This same protein is involved in rheumatoid arthritis, and there is a drug for that disease that turns off production of that particular protein. The team administered the drug to Emily, with dramatic results: her condition improved faster than anyone could have hoped for. Almost overnight, her breathing improved, her fever dropped, and her blood pressure was back to normal. In the weeks that followed, Emily recovered completely from the illness, called **cytokine release syndrome***, which resulted from the therapy. " [I made minor revision to keep the content concise.* https://www.chop.edu/stories/t-cell-therapy-relapsed-leukemia-emily-s-story   and https://www.chop.edu/stories/relapsed-leukemia-emilys-story *]*

16.4.1 Cytokine release syndrome (CRS)

The adverse effect that Emily Whitehead experienced is cytokine release syndrome (CRS), also known as "cytokine storm", which is an on-target and the most common type of toxicity of CAR-T therapy. The severity of CRS can range from mild to life-threatening, and the symptoms of CRS may include fever, hypotension, hypoxia, capillary leak, and end-organ dysfunction. CRS usually occurs within the first several days after CAR-T infusion. The pathophysiology underlying CRS is the activation of T cells upon CAR-antigen interaction, which subsequently leads to the proliferation and release of several cytokines. A marked elevation in cytokines, especially interleukin-6 (IL-6), is the hallmark of CRS. The fact that IL-6 is a key mediator of CRS forms the basis of using tocilizumab, an IL-6 receptor monoclonal antibody, to improve the symptoms associated with CRS. Nowadays, tocilizumab represents the main treatment option of CRS management.

16.4.2 Immune effector cell-associated neurotoxicity syndrome (ICANS)

In addition to CRS, another common adverse effect of CAR-T therapy is immune effector cell-associated neurotoxicity syndrome (ICANS). The symptoms of ICANS include headache, dizziness, delirium, confusion, seizures, dysphasia, hallucinations, and impaired cognitive skills, which usually occur within the first several weeks of CAR-T infusion. ICANS can occur with or without CRS, indicating that there are some underlying pathophysiological differences between these two conditions. For patients with ICANS, the management of toxicities relies on supportive care such as corticosteroids. Anti-epileptics may also be prescribed as needed. The symptoms are often resolved within a few days after treatment.

16.4.3 Other adverse effects

Infections associated with CAR-T therapy are also relatively common adverse effects. In addition, tumor lysis syndrome (TLS) can occur during CAR-T therapy because of the rapid necrosis of tumor cells, especially in large volume and high metabolism blood cancers. Lastly, cytopenia, including neutropenia, thrombocytopenia, and anemia, could also occur during CAR-T therapy, which can be managed through supportive care and anti-infective treatment.

16.5 Issue of Relapse and Potential Strategies

While CAR-T therapy has generated substantial excitement among the cancer community, we need to be aware that it does have limitations. For example, durable remission is not guaranteed, as reflected by relapse occurring in more than half of patients who received CAR-T therapy. The following are the two main groups of relapses:

- Antigen-negative relapse

Initially, single antigen targeting CAR-T therapy can deliver high response rates. However, cancer cells are smart. Over time, the cancer cells undergo gene mutation and may display either partial or complete loss of target antigen expression, a phenomenon known as *antigen escape*. Without the target antigen, CAR-T cells lose their ability to attack. As a result, relapse occurs. For example, the CD19-negative relapse accounts for up to 20% of the relapsed CAR-T treated patients.

The potential strategy to overcome the issue of antigen-negative relapse is to design novel CAR containing two scFVs to target two different antigens expressed on the tumor. This concept has been tested pre-clinically and is currently in the clinical phase of research.

- Antigen-positive relapse

Relapse can occur even when tumor cells still express antigens on their surface. This type of relapse is associated with poor CAR-T cell expansion and persistence, which is often caused by *T cell exhaustion*. Therefore, the development of strategies to counteract T cell exhaustion is essential in overcoming antigen-positive relapse. It is believed that T cell exhaustion is triggered by co-inhibitory pathways, such as increased expression of inhibitory immune checkpoint receptors (e.g., PD-1, CTLA-4, TIM-3, and LAG-3).

The potential strategies to overcome the issue of antigen-positive relapse are illustrated in Figure 16-4 using PD-1 blockage as an example. One strategy is to combine CAR-T therapy with a checkpoint inhibitor, such as pembrolizumab for PD-1 blockage. Another strategy is to engineer novel CAR-T cells which can autosecrete immune checkpoint molecules (e.g., anti-PD-1/PD-L1). Another potential strategy is genetic perturbation of CAR-T cell autoimmune checkpoint genes, such as knockout of CAR-T cell-encoding PD-1 gene using CRISPR-Cas9, thus enhancing the clearance of PD-L1 positive tumor cells in vivo.

16.6 Pharmacokinetics

So far, we have learned how CAR-T is made, how it works, its remarkable efficacy, as well as its limitations, including issues of toxicity and relapse. The last topic that I would like to bring up is pharmacokinetics of CAR-T therapy, which is fundamentally different from all other drug modalities because CAR-T is a

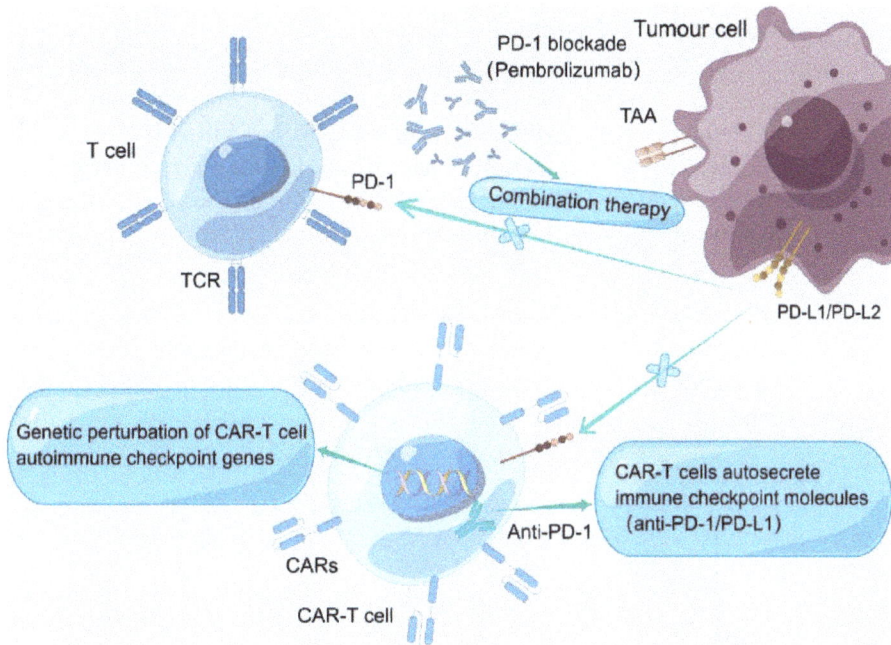

Figure 16-4. Immune checkpoint blocking strategies in overcoming antigen-positive relapse during CAR-T therapy, including 1) combination therapy with anti-PD-1 drug (e.g. pembrolizumab); 2) CAR-T cells self-secrete immune checkpoint molecules; and 3) Genetic perturbation of CAR-T cell autoimmune checkpoint genes. *This figure is from Lu J and Jing G. Molecular Cancer 2022; 21:194; used under Creative Commons CC-BY license.*

"living drug". Following a single dose, the cellular kinetics of CAR-T can be divided into four phases, as shown in Figure 16-5:

- *Lag/distribution*   After CAR-T cells are administered, the cells are rapidly distributed into tissues. The CAR transgene level in the blood, measured in a unit of copies/ug DNA, is either stable or transiently decreased during the lag/distribution phase. The distribution of CAR-T cells is the result of the complex interplay between T-cell trafficking, migration from the blood to the bone marrow and other secondary lymphoid tissues. This phase usually lasts 1-3 days.

- *Expansion*   In the next several days, CAR-T cells undergo rapid expansion, which can result in an increase of several logs beyond the infused cell dose. This expansion is caused by the binding of CAR-T cells to their target antigens, which subsequently activates intracellular co-stimulatory and signaling pathways, resulting in CAR-T-cell mediated tumor killing and CAR-T cell proliferation. The expansion phase can last 1-2 weeks.

- *Contraction*   After the CAR-T product reaches the maximum level in the blood, it decays with a biphasic pattern. The initial steeper decline is known as the contraction phase, which is thought to correspond to programmed cell death of activated CAR-T cells. The contraction phase can last several weeks to a few months.

- *Persistence*   The second shallower decline is known as the persistence phase, which is associated with the long-lived memory CAR-T cells. The duration of the persistence phase varies and can last for several years.

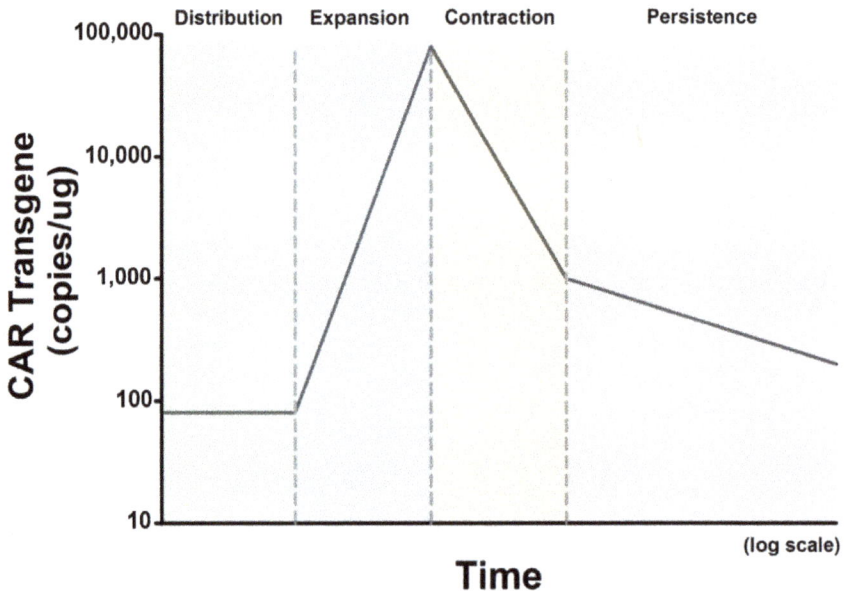

Figure 16-5. Graphical representation of the cellular kinetics of CAR-T therapy. CAR-T is a "living drug" and can be divided into four phases: a) distribution phase, which usually lasts 1-3 days; b) expansion phase, which can last 1-2 weeks; c) contraction phase, which can last several weeks to a few months, and d) persistence phase, with duration of several years.

Unlike traditional drugs, there is either no or weak relationship between CAR-T dose and blood exposure (e.g., AUC, C_{max}). This dose-exposure disconnection can be explained by the fact that the extent of the expansion of CAR-T cells is independent of dose and driven by factors such as antigen abundance, tumor burden, target cell type, native immune system, etc. The exposure of CAR-T product can be linked to its efficacy and toxicity. For example, high in vivo CAR-T expansion indicates that these cells are active in the body, and accordingly, patients have a higher chance to be responders. Indeed, higher CAR-T cell expansion was observed in responders than non-responders for Kymriah in B-ALL and CLL, Yescarta in LBCL, Tecartus in MCL, and Breyanzi LBCL. Higher in vivo CAR-T cell expansion was also associated with a higher incidence of CRS, which is not surprising since CRS is an on-target adverse effect.

Key References

Awasthi R, Maier HJ, Zhang J and Lim S (2023) Kymriah(R) (tisagenlecleucel) - An overview of the clinical development journey of the first approved CAR-T therapy. Hum Vaccin Immunother 19:2210046.

Ayala Ceja M, Khericha M, Harris CM, Puig-Saus C and Chen YY (2024) CAR-T cell manufacturing: Major process parameters and next-generation strategies. J Exp Med 221.

Chen L, Chen F, Niu H, Li J, Pu Y, Yang C, Wang Y, Huang R, Li K, Lei Y and Huang Y (2022) Chimeric Antigen Receptor (CAR)-T Cell Immunotherapy Against Thoracic Malignancies: Challenges and Opportunities. Front Immunol 13:871661.

Chohan KL, Siegler EL and Kenderian SS (2023) CAR-T Cell Therapy: the Efficacy and Toxicity Balance. Curr Hematol Malig Rep 18:9-18.

Gumber D and Wang LD (2022) Improving CAR-T immunotherapy: Overcoming the challenges of T cell exhaustion. EBioMedicine 77:103941.

Lu J and Jiang G (2022) The journey of CAR-T therapy in hematological malignancies. Mol Cancer 21:194.

Ogasawara K, Dodds M, Mack T, Lymp J, Dell'Aringa J and Smith J (2021) Population Cellular Kinetics of Lisocabtagene Maraleucel, an Autologous CD19-Directed Chimeric Antigen Receptor T-Cell Product, in Patients with Relapsed/Refractory Large B-Cell Lymphoma. Clin Pharmacokinet 60:1621-1633.

Qi T, McGrath K, Ranganathan R, Dotti G and Cao Y (2022) Cellular kinetics: A clinical and computational review of CAR-T cell pharmacology. Adv Drug Deliv Rev 188:114421.

Stein AM, Grupp SA, Levine JE, Laetsch TW, Pulsipher MA, Boyer MW, August KJ, Levine BL, Tomassian L, Shah S, Leung M, Huang PH, Awasthi R, Mueller KT, Wood PA and June CH (2019) Tisagenlecleucel Model-Based Cellular Kinetic Analysis of Chimeric Antigen Receptor-T Cells. CPT Pharmacometrics Syst Pharmacol 8:285-295.

Sterner RC and Sterner RM (2021) CAR-T cell therapy: current limitations and potential strategies. Blood Cancer J 11:69.

Uscanga-Palomeque AC, Chavez-Escamilla AK, Alvizo-Baez CA, Saavedra-Alonso S, Terrazas-Armendariz LD, Tamez-Guerra RS, Rodriguez-Padilla C and Alcocer-Gonzalez JM (2023) CAR-T Cell Therapy: From the Shop to Cancer Therapy. Int J Mol Sci 24.

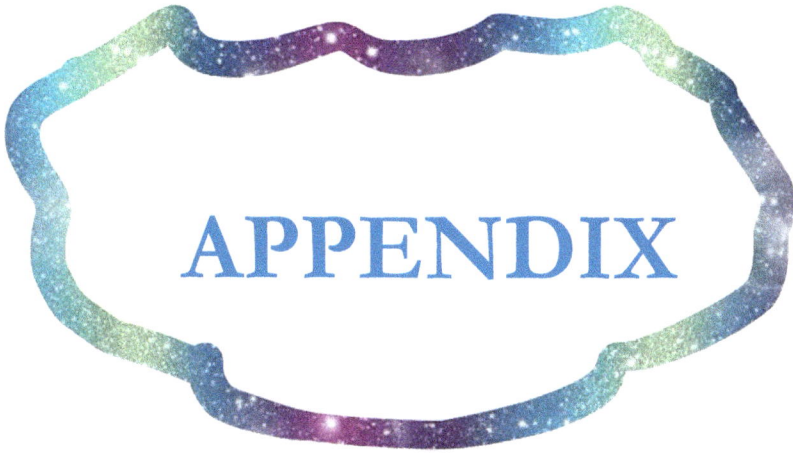

APPENDIX

Answer Key to Study Problems

Chapter 1

1. B
2. B
3. B
4. B
5. B
6. A
7. B
8. A
9. B
10. A

Chapter 2

1. B
2. A
3. F=0.75 (i.e., 75%)
4. A, C
5. B
6. A, B, D, E
7. A
8. B
9. A
10. B

Chapter 3

1. B
2. B
3. B
4. 33 L
5. B
6. B
7. A
8. 22 L
9. C, D
10. A

Chapter 4

1. F, T, T, F, F
2. B
3. A

4. A
5. B
6. A, B, C
7. B
8. A
9. B
10. C

Chapter 5

$$k_e = -slope = -\frac{\ln C_2 - \ln C_1}{t_2 - t_1} = -\frac{\ln 2.5 - \ln 8}{9 - 1} = 0.145 \, h^{-1}$$

$$t_{1/2} = \frac{0.693}{k_e} = \frac{0.693}{0.145} = 4.77 \, h$$

$$8 = C_0 \cdot e^{-0.145 \cdot 1} \quad \rightarrow C_0 = 9.25 \, mg/L$$

$$V_d = \frac{Dose}{C_0} = \frac{100}{9.25} = 10.8 \, L$$

$$CL = V_d \cdot k_e = 10.8 \times 0.145 = 1.57 \, L/h$$

$$AUC_{inf} = \frac{Dose}{CL} = \frac{100}{1.57} = 63.6 \, mg \cdot h/L$$

Since this drug is mainly eliminated via the liver, we can assume it total clearance = hepatic clearance. Therefore, CL_H=1.57 L/h.

$$E = \frac{CL_H}{Q_H} = \frac{1.57}{87} = 0.018$$

Drug B is a low extraction drug. Its clearance is dependent on CL_{int} and fu. When Drug B is co-administered with a CYP3A inducer (i.e., CL_{int} increases), its CL increases, and AUC will decrease.

Since Drug B is a low extraction drug, its oral bioavailability is close to 1, which means that it is not dependent on CL_{int}. When it is given a CYP3A inhibitor, its F will remain the same.

Chapter 6

1.   Please pay attention to units before you work on parameter calculations. The unit of CL is 100 mL/min. If we want the unit of time in h and volume in L, we need to convert CL to L/h: CL = 100 mL/min = 100/1000*60 = 6 L/h

$$F' = \frac{C_{max,ss}}{C_{min,ss}} = \frac{4}{2} = 2$$, this is the maximum allowable fluctuation.

$$k_e = \frac{CL}{V_d} = \frac{6}{400} = 0.015 \; h^{-1}$$

$$\tau = \frac{lnF'}{k_e} = \frac{ln2}{0.015} = 46.2 \; h$$, this is the maximum allowable dosing interval.

$$C_{ave,ss} = \frac{C_{max,ss} - C_{min,ss}}{lnC_{max,ss} - lnC_{min,ss}} = \frac{4-2}{ln4 - ln2} = 2.89 \; mg/L$$

If we decide to give the drug every 24 h, the dose will be:

$$Dose = C_{ave,ss} \cdot CL \cdot \tau = 2.89 \left(\frac{mg}{L}\right) \cdot 6 \left(\frac{L}{h}\right) \cdot 24 \; (h) = 416 \; mg$$

2.   Since there are two data points, ke can be calculated directly:

$$k_e = -slope = -\frac{lnC_2 - lnC_1}{t_2 - t_1} = -\frac{ln10 - ln20}{4} = 0.173 \; h^{-1}$$

Based on the equation $C_{max,ss} = \frac{Dose}{V_d} \cdot \frac{1}{(1 - e^{-k_e \cdot \tau})}$ and the $C_{max,ss}$ of 20 mg/L, we can calculate V_d:

$$20 = \frac{200}{V_d} \frac{1}{(1 - e^{-0.173 \cdot 8})} \quad \rightarrow V_d = 13.3 \; L$$

$$C_{ave,ss} = \frac{Dose}{CL \cdot \tau} = \frac{200}{0.173 \cdot 13.3 \cdot 8} = 10.9 \; mg/L$$

$$t_{1/2} = \frac{0.693}{k_e} = \frac{0.693}{0.173} = 4 \; h$$

It will take 20 h (i.e., 5 half-lives) to reach steady state.

Loading dose $= C_{max,ss} \cdot V_d = 20 \cdot 13.3 = 266\ mg$

Therefore, if you don't want to wait that long, you can give a loading dose of 266 mg.

Chapter 7

$$k_o = C_{ss} \cdot CL = C_{ss} \cdot k_e \cdot V_d = 25 \cdot \frac{0.693}{8} \cdot 1 \cdot 80 = 173\ mg/_h$$

It will take 40 h (i.e., 5 half-lives) to reach steady state. If we don't want that long, we can give a loading dose, which is an I.V. bolus dose at the beginning:

Loading dose = $1.44 \cdot$ ko $\cdot t_{1/2} = 1.44 \cdot 173 \cdot 8 = 1993$ mg, which is around 2 g.

If the total infusion time is 8 h, it means that the drug has not reached steady state before the infusion is stopped. The concentration of drug Y at 4 h, 8h, and 11 h are:

$$C_{4h} = \frac{k_o}{k_e \cdot V_d}(1 - e^{-k_e \cdot t}) = \frac{173}{6.93}(1 - e^{-0.0866 \cdot 4}) = 7.31\ mg/_L$$

$$C_{8h} = \frac{k_o}{k_e \cdot V_d}(1 - e^{-k_e \cdot T}) = \frac{173}{6.93}(1 - e^{-0.0866 \cdot 8}) = 12.5\ mg/_L,\ \text{please note, C8h}$$

is the maximum concentration since the infusion time is 8 h.

$$C_{11h} = C_{max} \cdot e^{-k_e \cdot t'} = 12.5 \cdot e^{-0.0866 \cdot 3} = 9.62\ mg/_L$$

If the total infusion time is 50 h, the drug reaches steady state before infusion stops.

$$C_{53h} = C_{ss} \cdot e^{-k_e \cdot t'} = 25 \cdot e^{-0.0866 \cdot 3} = 19.3\ mg/_L$$

www.ingramcontent.com/pod-product-compliance
Lightning Source LLC
Chambersburg PA
CBHW052337210326
41597CB00031B/5282